Nursing Fundamentals

DeMYSTiFieD

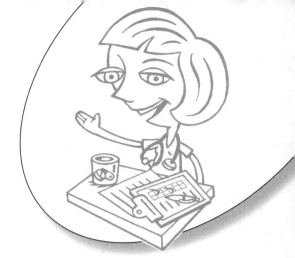

Nursing Fundamentals

DeMYSTiFieD

Second Edition

Bennita W. Vaughans, MSN, RN
Adjunct Faculty Member
Auburn University Montgomery
Montgomery, Alabama
Formerly Nursing Instructor and Allied Health Program Coordinator
H. Councill Trenholm State Technical College
Montgomery, Alabama

Jim Keogh, DNP, RN-BC

New York   Chicago   San Francisco   Athens   London   Madrid
Mexico City   Milan   New Delhi   Singapore   Sydney   Toronto

Nursing Fundamentals Demystified, Second Edition

Copyright © 2019 by McGraw-Hill Education. All rights reserved. Printed in the United States of America. Except as permitted under the United States Copyright Act of 1976, no part of this publication may be reproduced or distributed in any form or by any means, or stored in a data base or retrieval system, without the prior written permission of the publisher.

1 2 3 4 5 6 7 8 9   LCR   23 22 21 20 19 18

ISBN 978-1-259-86226-7
MHID 1-259-86226-7

This book was set in Minion Pro by Cenveo® Publisher Services.
The editors were Susan Barnes and Kim J. Davis.
The production supervisor was Richard Ruzycka.
Production management was provided by Radhika Jolly, Cenveo Publisher Services.

This book is printed on acid-free paper.

Library of Congress Cataloging-in-Publication Data

Names: Vaughans, Bennita W., author. | Keogh, James Edward, 1948- author.
Title: Nursing fundamentals demystified / Bennita Vaughans, MSN, RN, Adjunct
    Faculty Member, Auburn University Montgomery, Montgomery, Alabama,
    Formerly Nursing Instructor and Allied Health Program Coordinator, H.
    Councill Trenholm State Technical College, Montgomery, Alabama, Jim Keogh,
    DNP, RN-BC.
Description: Second edition. | New York: McGraw-Hill Education, [2019] |
    Includes bibliographical references and index.
Identifiers: LCCN 2018009739 (print) | LCCN 2018013288 (ebook) | ISBN
    9781259862274 (Ebook) | ISBN 1259862275 (Ebook) | ISBN 9781259862267
    (paperback)
Subjects: LCSH: Nursing. | BISAC: MEDICAL / Nursing / Psychiatric.
Classification: LCC RT41 (ebook) | LCC RT41 .V38 2019 (print) | DDC
    610.73—dc23
LC record available at https://lccn.loc.gov/2018009739

McGraw-Hill Education books are available at special quantity discounts to use as premiums and sales promotions or for use in corporate training programs. To contact a representative, please visit the Contact Us pages at www.mhprofessional.com.

To God for His everlasting love and the gifts He has given me. To my husband, Charles, and my children, Kedrick and Kendra, for their unyielding support, especially my daughter Kendra who is my number one cheerleader and artistic assistant. In memory of my parents, Benjamin and Juanita Witherspoon, who gave me life and love and made it possible for me to even have this experience. Also, in memory of my mother-in-law and father in law Gertie and Charles Vaughans who were both the most loving and supportive surrogate parents anyone could ever ask for. To my sisters, Brenda and Priscilla Witherspoon, for their belief in me and the countless encouragement they provided. Last but not least, to my students, who continuously inspire me.

B. W. V.

This book is dedicated to Anne, Sandy, Joanne, Amber-Leigh Christine, Shawn, Eric, and Amy, without whose help and support this book could not have been written.

J. K.

About the Authors

Bennita W. Vaughans, MSN, RN, currently serves as an adjunct faculty member at Auburn University at Montgomery. She is employed as a Nurse Case Manager at a local hospital. Ms. Vaughans has been a nurse for 30 plus years and a nurse/allied health educator for over 20 years. She received her bachelor of science degree in nursing from the University of Alabama Capstone College of Nursing and her master's degree in nursing from Troy University. Ms. Vaughans has experience in the area of quality and safety. She previously served as a Patient Safety Manager and Performance Improvement coordinator. Additionally, she previously served as a level chairperson and assistant dean at Tuskegee University. She has taught various courses at the baccalaureate, associate, and technical levels of nursing. She has also served as an instructor and coordinator in an allied health program. She has coauthored multiple nursing textbooks and has written several publications.

Jim Keogh, DNP, RN-BC, is an assistant professor at New York University and is on the faculty of St. Peter's University in Jersey City, New Jersey. He is board-certified in psychiatric-mental health nursing and is the author of more than 87 books, including 20 nursing titles published by McGraw-Hill.

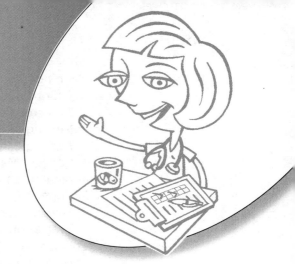

Contents

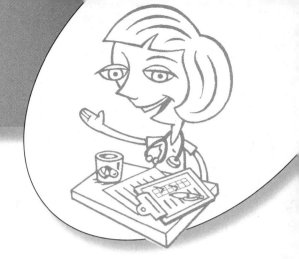

Contributors

Peggy Hall, MSN, CRNP
Women Veteran Program Coordinator
Central Alabama Veterans Health Care System
Montgomery, Alabama

Joyce Y. Johnson, PhD, RN, CCRN
Dean and Professor, Department of Nursing
College of Sciences and Health Professions
Albany State University
Albany, Georgia

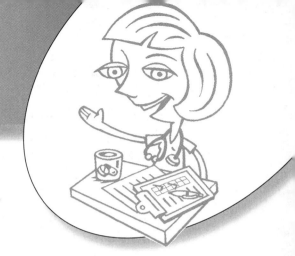

Preface

Nursing students usually have their first formal introduction to nursing concepts in Fundamentals of Nursing courses. As the course name implies, the intent of the course is to provide students with foundational information that will be used throughout the remainder of the nursing curriculum. Assimilating the information presented in the course can be quite an overwhelming task. Students are challenged not only to learn a new body of knowledge but also to begin to analyze, synthesize, and apply this information in clinical situations.

The intent of *Nursing Fundamentals Demystified* is to facilitate students' understanding of this new and uncharted territory of information. This book is not intended to replace core "fundamentals of nursing" textbooks; instead, it emphasizes the most critical concepts. This book can be used as a supplemental resource for both novice students and nurses who need a quick and simple reference resource.

Key features included in this edition of *Nursing Fundamentals Demystified* include the following:

- A list of Learning Objectives at the start of each chapter with supporting content location identifiers in the text to assist the reader to easily find answers for the objectives
- Key terms with accompanying definitions embedded within the body of the text to facilitate immediate understanding
- Tables and boxed information that summarize critical concepts and serve as easy study tools

- Nursing Alerts, which spotlight key quality and safety for nurses using the QSEN framework.
- Spotlights on Evidence-Based Practice when applicable.
- Nursing Care Plans in selected chapters, which assist readers in identifying key assessment data, nursing diagnoses, and interventions
- Selected Procedure Tips to assist readers with clinical application of content
- "Routine Checkup" questions at various checkpoints throughout each chapter, which enable readers to evaluate their individual learning
- NCLEX-style questions at the end of each chapter, which readers can use to evaluate their overall understanding of the content presented

The book is divided into three parts. *Part I: Introduction to the Nursing Profession* includes two chapters. Chapter 1 provides a discussion of key precepts that define the nursing profession, including nursing history, theoretical foundations, legal and ethical perspectives, cultural perspectives, practices settings, and the future of nursing. Chapter 2 is devoted to an in-depth discussion of the nursing process. Each phase of the nursing process is discussed in detail. The role that critical thinking plays in the implementation of the nursing process is also explored. Updated information pertaining to the nursing process has been integrated into the second edition of this textbook.

Part II: Fundamental Principles of Nursing Care is divided into five chapters. The section opens with Chapter 3: Communication and Documentation. Basic communication principles and methods of documentation and reporting are presented. Vital sign assessment and health assessment are presented in Chapters 4 and 5, respectively. Part II closes with a discussion of principles of medication administration and safety.

The remaining chapters of the textbook are devoted to topics that relate to meeting basic human needs, as the title of the part implies: *Part III: Meeting Basic Human Needs*. A new chapter on mental health needs has been added to this edition. Each chapter in this section starts with an overview and includes a description of the underlying physiology of the need, influencing factors, effects of impairment or not meeting the basic need, and application of the nursing process. Specific needs discussed include:

- Chapter 8: Skin Integrity
- Chapter 9: Activity and Mobility
- Chapter 10: Sensory and Cognition

- Chapter 11: Sleep and Comfort
- Chapter 12: Oxygenation
- Chapter 13: Nutrition
- Chapter 14: Fluid, Electrolyte, and Acid–Base Balance
- Chapter 15: Urinary Elimination
- Chapter 16: Bowel Elimination
- Chapter 17: Psychosocial Needs
- Chapter 18: Mental Health Nursing

Author Bennita Vaughans' initial motivation for writing this textbook was derived from a sincere desire to assist students in understanding this most important foundational information. The desire to undertake this project was initially ignited by her reminiscing back to her own days as a student and the many sleepless nights that she spent reading and rereading, yet still feeling frustrated by how difficult it was to digest this great mountain of information. This burning desire was further fueled by the numerous similar encounters that she has had, during her teaching career, with students who are dedicated, yet just as frustrated as she was when she was a nursing student.

The authors sincerely hope that this textbook will help each reader to gain a better understanding of this most important information in an easier manner. The authors also hope that this resource will become a permanent part of the reader's reference library to be used over and over again for many, many years.

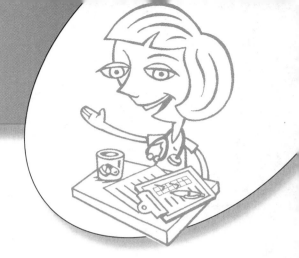

Acknowledgments

Thank you to Susan Barnes for the boundless support you provided during this journey and thank you also for your patience and understanding.

Thank you to Kim Davis for your guidance and assistance with the preparation of this manuscript.

Thank you to Peggy Hall and Dr. Joyce Johnson for your contributions to this manuscript.

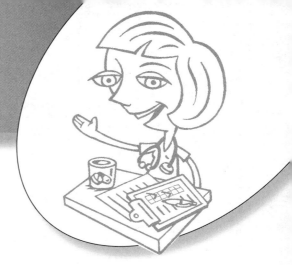

Part I

Introduction to the Nursing Profession

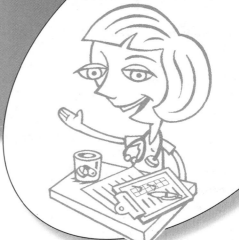

Chapter **1**

Nursing—An Evolving Profession

LEARNING OBJECTIVES

At the end of the chapter, the reader will be able to:

1. Discuss individual contributions made to the historical development of the nursing profession.
2. Discuss key events that influenced the historical development of the nursing profession.
3. Discuss the relationship between the art and science of nursing.
4. Identify the four concepts that are central to the theoretical foundation of nursing.
5. Differentiate between grand nursing theories and midrange nursing theories.
6. Give examples of roles that nurses assume in today's healthcare workforce.
7. Discuss how legal boundaries are set for nursing practice.
8. Discuss the role of nurses in promoting ethically sound decision making in healthcare.
9. Discuss the impact of culture on the provision of healthcare.
10. Describe current challenges that may impact the future of the nursing profession.

KEY WORDS

Culture
Evidence-based nursing practice
Grand theory
Midrange theory

Narrow range theory
Nurse Practice Act
Research

Introduction

Nursing in its most basic form has existed since the beginning of time. It has evolved from an informal act of caring for and nurturing others to a more complex scientific-based profession. Basic tenets of the profession have remained constant. From its infancy, the focus of nursing has been on assisting with meeting basic human needs. Over time, significant changes have occurred to meet the needs of an ever-changing society. Changes in the population make-up, consumer demands, technology, and economics are some of the key factors that have influenced how nursing has evolved. Nursing education, practice settings, and nursing roles have changed significantly. Although nursing has come a long way from the day of strictly providing bedside care, it is by no means anywhere near its full maturity. In fact, nursing will continue to change and evolve as will the world.

Historical Perspective

Understanding how nursing evolved over time is an important part of assimilating and appreciating what nursing is now. So, let's start by looking at nursing's history. The following discussion is by no means all-inclusive but will hopefully provide a basic picture of nursing's origin as well as key influences along the way.

The founder of modern nursing is Florence Nightingale. She developed the first formal training program for nurses. She focused on the role of the nurse in preventing and curing disease through sanitary techniques. Nightingale was responsible for major reform in hygiene and sanitary practices. Even at this early time in nursing, she used evidence-based principles to guide nursing practices. Just as Florence Nightingale made a significant impact on the course nursing has taken, so have many other individuals.

The evolution of nursing in the United States occurred within the context of wartime just as was the case during Nightingale's era. Dorothea Dix, who was not a nurse, is credited with developing the Nurses Corps of the United States Army. Clara Barton founded the American Red Cross, which played a key role in meeting the healthcare needs of soldiers during the Civil War. Linda Richards is credited with being the first trained nurse in the United States, and Mary Mahoney was the first trained African American nurse.

Many other events have contributed in some way to the evolvement of the nursing profession. Two such events were the formation of the American Society of Superintendents of Training Schools for Nurses in the United States, the precursor to today's National League of Nursing, and the Nurses' Associated Alumnae, which eventually became the American Nurses Association (ANA). The National League for Nursing plays a critical role in promoting nursing quality through the accreditation of nursing education programs by the National League for Nursing Accrediting Commission (NLNAC). The ANA is designated as the body that advances the nursing profession through the promotion of nurses' rights and establishment of standards of practice that promotes high-quality nursing practice. The ANA is a member of the International Council of Nurses (ICN). The ICN was founded in 1899, consists of 130 national nurses' associations, and strives to promote quality healthcare through advancing the nursing profession and influencing health policy.

Theoretical Foundation

What is nursing? Several definitions have been proposed (Figure 1–1), but consensus has not been reached on one definition. Perhaps the difficulty lies in how complex nursing is. What there is agreement on is that nursing is an art and a science. The two form a synergistic relationship, the sum of which is much greater than each entity individually. The art that is manifested in the caring and compassionate provision of care cannot stand without the scientific knowledge base that validates nursing actions and vice versa.

It is almost impossible to speak further about what nursing is without addressing the following three subject areas: theory, research, and practice.

Theory, in its simplest form, can be defined as "the general principles or ideas that relate to a particular subject" (Merriam Webster Dictionary); in this instance the subject being nursing. Various theories have been used to explain nursing's purpose. Some theories have been borrowed from other disciplines (eg, psychology and human development), while others have been developed by nurses. Four basic concepts are central elements of most nursing theories: person,

Nursing Then (1955)	Nursing Now
1. "The practice of professional nursing means the performance for compensation of any act in the observation, care, and counsel of the ill, injured, or infirm, or in the maintenance of health or prevention of illness of others, or in the supervision and teaching of other personnel, or the administration of medications and treatments as prescribed by a licensed physician or dentist; requiring substantial specialized judgment and skill and based on knowledge and application of the principles of biological, physical, and social science. The foregoing shall not be deemed to include acts of diagnosis or prescription of therapeutic or corrective measures."	2. Nursing is the protection, promotion, and optimization of health and abilities, prevention of illness and injury, facilitation of healing, alleviation of suffering through the diagnosis and treatment of human response, and advocacy in the care of individuals, families, groups, communities, and populations.
(ANA Board Approves a Definition of Nursing Practice, 1955)	(Source: http://www.nursingworld.org/EspeciallyForYou/ What-is-Nursing)

FIGURE 1–1 · What is nursing? Then and now.

health, environment, and nursing. Nursing theories typically describe the relationship between one or more of these four concepts. Nursing theories are categorized as grand, midrange, or narrow ranged. **Grand nursing theories** are board in scope and are more difficult to apply to practical situations. In contrast, **midrange nursing theories** can be tested in practical situations but are not so narrow in scope that they can only be applied to a particular situation. **Narrow-range theories,** also referred to as situation-specific theories, are narrower in scope (eg, procedural guidelines based on research). An oversimplified example to demonstrate the application level of the three types of theories is as follows:

- **Grand theory:** Certain foods are harmful. (This statement is broad in scope and requires more specificity before it can be tested.)
- **Midrange theory:** Trans fat increases low-density cholesterol and decreases high-density cholesterol. (This statement can be tested yet is broad enough that it can be applied to multiple patients.)
- **Narrow-range theory:** Cindy is allergic to peanut oil. (This statement can be tested but is restricted to this particular patient.)

Research is a tool used to develop new theories and revise or disprove existing theories. The research process contributes to ongoing modification of nursing knowledge. It is an invaluable tool for maintaining current and meaningful knowledge in an ever-changing world.

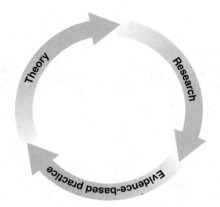

FIGURE 1–2 · The relationship between theory, research, and evidence-based practice.

A somewhat new area of interest in nursing is **evidence-based nursing practice**. We have always talked about the importance of putting theory and evidence originating from research into practice, but we have not talked very much about how the nurse's clinical judgment and the patient's preferences figure into the equation; at least not until now. Evidence-based practice is driven by theory, research, performance improvement, clinical judgment, and patient preferences (Figure 1–2). It involves basing nursing implementation on the best evidence available, combined with nurses' clinical judgment and taking into account patient preferences.

Nursing Roles and Education

Nurses who provide direct bedside care still make up a large portion of the profession's workforce. However, as mentioned previously, practice settings and nursing roles have expanded to keep up with societal demands (Box 1–1). The acuity of patients hospitalized coupled with the need to promote safety and quality of care has led to a need for nurses with more specialized skills. As a result, nurses not only possess licensure but also certification in such areas as gerontological nursing, cardiac and vascular nursing, and prenatal nursing, to name a few. Clinical nurse specialists and clinical nurse leaders are also being used to meet the aforementioned demand. The growing shift toward preventive and patient-centered care as well as the enactment of the Affordable Health Care Act has resulted in nurses being employed more and more in community-based settings, including the home setting. Nurse practitioners are working collaboratively with physicians to meet healthcare needs of patients in both inpatient and outpatient settings.

BOX 1-1
Selected Nursing Career Options

Nursing Roles	Employment Settings
General Registered Nurse	Acute hospitals
Clinical Specialist (numerous specialties)	Long-term care facilities
Clinical Nurse Leader	Doctor offices
Advance Practice Nurse	Outpatient clinics/surgical centers
Nurse Case Managers	Community/home health
Nurse Administrator	Industrial settings
Nurse Educator	Educational institutions (all levels)
Quality/Risk/Patient Safety	Armed forces
Nurse Entrepreneurs	
Nurse Informatics	
Occupational Health	
Nurse Researcher	

Nursing has also established its place at the decision-making table in healthcare organizations, as reflected by nurses assuming roles in such areas as administration and utilization management. Although not considered a component of professional nursing, licensed practical nurses (licensed vocational nurse) also continue to represent a large sector of the nursing workforce. Practical nurses provide technical nursing care usually under the guidance of professional nurses. The practical nursing workforce also serves as an important source for future professional nurses. This discussion of the various nursing roles in healthcare is by no means exhaustive.

NURSING ALERT

Delegation of Responsibilities
A professional Registered Nurse may delegate certain activities to assistive personnel; however, he or she is ultimately accountable for patient assessment and decision making related to nursing care.

Nursing education has also undergone a metamorphosis to equip nurses to assume the changing roles required in the healthcare arena. Over time, nursing education has shifted from a hospital-based apprenticeship model (diploma programs) to college-based models (associate's degree and baccalaureate

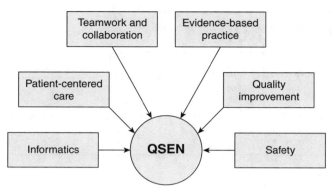

FIGURE 1–3 · QSEN competencies.

degree programs). In 2005 nursing embarked upon yet another transformative journey: "Quality and Safety Education for Nurses (QSEN)" (Cronenwett et al., 2007). The purpose of this initiative was to integrate quality and safety education competencies into nursing curriculums in order to prepare nurses to promote patient safety and continuous quality improvement in healthcare. The initiative was borne out of the recommendation published in the 2003 Institute of Medicine Health Professions Education report. Six preprofessional competencies (Figure 1–3) were identified, forums aimed at preparing faculty to teach the competencies were conducted, curriculums and nursing textbooks are being modified to integrate the six competencies, and work is underway to expand QSEN to graduate education.

Nursing education programs have also changed as a result of recommendations from the 2010 Institute of Medicine report "The Future of Nursing." One key recommendation was to increase the number of baccalaureates prepared registered nurses to 80%. As a result of this recommendation, more nursing programs are offering RN to BSN programs. Beyond entry-level nursing programs are those that offer master's degrees in nursing as well as doctoral degrees (PhD and DNP). Distance learning has also been deployed to expand the nursing workforce.

Legal Perspectives

The Nurse Practice Act provides guidance regarding the legal boundaries of professional nursing practice. Each individual state determines specific regulatory guidelines for the practice of nursing, including the scope of practice, method of governing, and nursing education criteria.

ROUTINE CHECKUP

1. The founder of modern day nursing is _____.
Answer:

2. The majority of the nursing workforce continues to provide direct bedside care. True/false.
Answer:

Licensure is required to practice nursing in all states. All nursing graduates are required to take the NCLEX-RN licensure examination for initial licensure. However, requirements for continuing licensure vary from state to state. For example, some states require completion of continuing education programs for continued licensure, but others do not. The number of continuing education units, if required, also varies from state to state.

NURSING ALERT

Licensure
It is illegal to practice as a nurse without an active license!

Within a broader context of law, nursing practice is measured by standards of care set forth by various bodies (eg, the ANA and The Joint Commission). Nurses may incur legal consequences when it is determined that the nurse did not function within the framework of the Nurse Practice Act or standards of care. Possible charges may include:

- Assault and battery
- Defamation of character
- Fraud
- Invasion of privacy
- False imprisonment
- Negligence
- Malpractice

Consequences may range from fines to imprisonment and may also result in revocation of licensure. Other legally sensitive areas that may involve nurses include informed consent and advanced directives. Nurses should be knowledgeable of the responsibilities related to the aforementioned and practice accordingly.

Ethical Perspective

Providing nursing care that falls within prescribed legal boundaries is much easier to delineate than identifying care that is ethically appropriate. Why? Because what is perceived as morally right or wrong varies from individual to individual and is influenced by a person's religious, cultural, and family beliefs, to name a few. For example, what should a nurse do if a pediatric patient who has a terminal illness asks if he or she is dying? There is not a standard answer for this question. Multiple variables must be considered (eg, parental wishes, religious beliefs, the nurse's values and beliefs, the child's maturity level, the stage of the illness). Professional codes of ethics, to some extent, provide a framework to assist nurses in determining what is ethically acceptable. However, nurses can best equip themselves to effectively handle ethical dilemmas by developing expertise in critical thinking.

Nurses also have a professional responsibility to demonstrate ethically appropriate behavior beyond the confines of individual patient care situations. Advances in technology, spiraling healthcare costs, and staffing shortages all have the potential to trigger ethical dilemmas. Questions surface concerning who gets what care and when (eg, should healthcare be available based on ability to pay or on need?). Nurses can impact the outcome of such questions by being active participants in the decision-making process at the administrative level of their respective organizations, through membership and active participation in state nurses associations, by lobbying local legislatures, and by exercising their individual right to vote.

Cultural Perspective

There are numerous definitions of the word **culture**. *Merriam-Webster's Dictionary* defines *culture* as "the customary beliefs, social forms, and material traits of a racial, religious, or social group." As stated here, it is obvious that culture influences a person's perceptions as well as the decisions he or she makes. Healthcare perceptions and decisions are not excluded. All players in the healthcare process (ie, patients, family members, significant others, nurses, and other healthcare team members) bring cultural beliefs to each healthcare interaction. In recent times, there has been a heightened appreciation of this fact. Nurses and other individuals who interface in various healthcare setting must accept and respect cultural diversity for all parties involved. Doing so promotes patient compliance, satisfaction with healthcare services, and job satisfaction.

The Future of Nursing

Nursing along with the healthcare landscape has changed tremendously over the years. Many positive outcomes have been realized. Healthcare consumers are more informed and more actively involved in making health-related decisions. Nursing roles have extended beyond those of direct patient care. Nurses are respected as autonomous professional members of the healthcare team. Technological advances have significantly improved patient outcomes. However, at the same time, many challenges have surfaced. Healthcare cost is out of control. There is inequality in healthcare access. Staffing shortages threaten the ability to provide high-quality healthcare and, in some situations, safe patient care. The nursing workforce is growing increasingly older. This is compounded by the limited ability of schools of nursing to accept qualified applicants into nursing programs because of faculty shortages. Even though the nursing profession faces many challenges, the profession will prevail. Nursing roles will continue to evolve to meet the needs of the patient population served. Nurses will continue to play active roles in shaping the healthcare landscape. Nurses, being the problem solvers that we are, will also overcome the current issues related to shortages in the profession.

REVIEW QUESTIONS

1. **Which of the following individuals is credited with being the first trained African American nurse?**

   A. Clara Barton

   B. Dorothea Dix

   C. Mary Mahoney

   D. Linda Richards

2. **Which of the following organizations currently serves as the body that oversees the accreditation of nursing programs in the United States?**

   A. American Associated Alumnae

   B. American Nurses Association

C. American Society of Superintendents of Training Schools

D. National League of Nursing

E. B and D

3. **Which of the following can be tested in practical situations such that a generalization can be made to more than just one patient situation?**

A. Conceptual models

B. Grand theories

C. Midrange theories

D. Narrow-range theories

4. **Which of the following BEST assists nurses to make sound ethical decisions?**

A. Baccalaureate nursing education

B. Development of good critical thinking skills

C. Becoming certified as an Advanced Practice Nurse

D. Continuing education related to ethical principles

5. **Which of the following charges may be made against a nurse for not practicing within the legal scope of nursing or according to established standards of practice?**

A. Assault and battery

B. False imprisonment

C. Negligence

D. All of the above

6. **All of the following are considered challenges facing the nursing profession EXCEPT:**

A. Continued large number of nurses providing direct patient care

B. Limited nursing faculty

C. Aging nursing population

D. Rising healthcare cost

ANSWERS

Routine Checkup

1. Florence Nightingale.
2. True.

Review Questions

1. C
2. D
3. C
4. B

5. D

6. A

References

American Nurses Association: ANA board approves a definition of nursing practice. *Am J Nurs.* 1955;55:1474.

Berman A, Snyder SJ, Frandsen G: *Kozier & Erb's Fundamental of Nursing: Concepts, Process, & Practice*, 10th ed. Hoboken, NJ: Prentice-Hall, 2016.

Cronenwett L, Sherwood G, Barnsteiner J, et al: Quality and safety education for nurses. *Nurs. Outlook.* 2007;55:122-131.

Culture. In *Merriam-Webster Dictionary.* Available at https://www.merriam-webster .com/dictionary/culture.

http://www.nursingworld.org/EspeciallyForYou/What-is-Nursing.

Im E: Development of situation-specific theories: an integrative approach. *ANS Adv Nurs Sci.* 2005;28:137-151.

Joel LA: *Kelly's Dimensions of Professional Nursing*, 10th ed. New York, NY: McGraw-Hill, 2011.

Potter PA, Perry AG, Stockert PA, Hall AM, Ostendorf WR: *Fundamentals of Nursing*, 9th ed. St. Louis, MO: Elsevier, 2017.

Wilkinson JM, Treas LS, Barnett KL, Smith MH: *Fundamentals of Nursing Vol. 1: Theory, Concepts, and Applications.* Philadelphia, PA: FA Davis, 2016.

Additional Resources

http://nursingworld.org/

http://qsen.org/competencies/pre-licensure-ksas/

http://www.aacn.nche.edu/media-relations/fact-sheets

http://www.nursecredentialing.org/

https://campaignforaction.org/issue/transforming-nursing-education/

https://www.bls.gov/ooh/healthcare/registered-nurses.htm

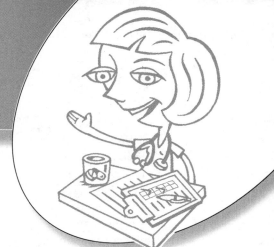

Chapter 2

The Nursing Process

At the end of the chapter, the reader will be able to:

1. Describe the role that critical thinking plays in the nursing process.
2. Discuss key components of the assessment phase of the nursing process.
3. Compare and contrast a medical diagnosis with a nursing diagnosis.
4. Describe the process for developing nursing diagnoses.
5. Describe the components of the North American Nursing Diagnosis Association's nursing taxonomy.
6. Describe key components of the planning phase of the nursing process.
7. State the required components of expected outcomes, outcome criteria, and nursing interventions.
8. Discuss what occurs during the implementation phase of the nursing process.
9. State the purpose of the evaluation phase of the nursing process.
10. Compare and contrast evaluation at the individual patient level to evaluation at the organizational level.

KEY WORDS

Assessment	Independent nursing interventions
Collaborative problem	Interdependent nursing interventions
Comprehensive assessment	Medical diagnosis
Critical pathways	Nursing care plan
Critical thinking	Nursing diagnosis
Data clustering	Nursing interventions
Data validation	Nursing process
Dependent nursing interventions	Objective data
Diagnose	Outcome criteria
Expected outcome	Problem-focused nursing diagnosis
Focused assessment	Risk nursing diagnosis
Formative evaluation	Subjective data
Health promotion diagnosis	Summative evaluation
Implementation	Taxonomy

Overview

The **nursing process** is a five-phase process that includes assessment, diagnosis, planning, implementation, and evaluation. The nursing process helps to define the nursing profession's unique contribution to healthcare and clarify its boundaries. It is a dynamic, adaptive process rather than a static, sequential process. A constant interchange takes place in all directions among the five phases (Figure 2–1).

NURSING ALERT

Evidence-Based Practice
The nurse uses the nursing process as a framework for developing a plan of care that is evidence-based, captures the nurse's clinical expertise, and takes into account the patient/family preferences—QSEN Competency 3: evidence-based practice.

NURSING ALERT

Patient-Centered Care
The patient or designee should take an active role in developing the plan of care, including determining needs, setting goals, selecting interventions, and evaluating whether or not the plan was effective—QSEN Competency 1: patient-centered care.

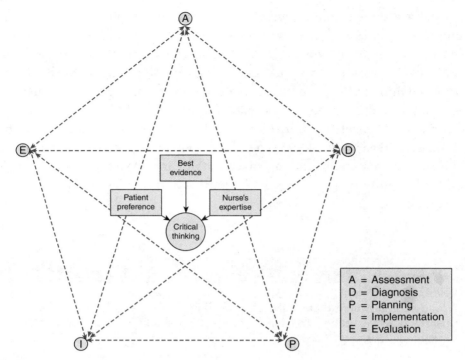

FIGURE 2−1 · The dynamic nursing process.

Critical thinking, "thinking that is purposeful, reasoned and goal directed" (Halpern, 1989), is used to ensure the nursing process continues to be tailored to meet the individual needs of the patient. It prompts nurses to thoroughly analyze information, consider multiple options, and make modifications as appropriate, thus encouraging sound decision making.

Assessment

Assessment is the act of collecting information about the client, organizing the information, and determining its significance. It is the first phase of the nursing process, but assessment actually continues throughout all phases of the nursing process. Effective execution of assessment relies heavily on the presence of a broad knowledge base and good critical thinking skill.

Types of Assessment

The type of assessment performed is dictated by the patient's current health status. A **comprehensive assessment** is performed when the patient presents in a stable state with no immediate life-threatening events. The goal of the comprehensive assessment is to obtain enough information to develop a complete list of nursing diagnoses for the patient. The list can then be prioritized, and a determination can be made of which nursing diagnoses should be addressed initially. If a patient is unstable or is experiencing a life-threatening event, a **focused assessment**, one that has the goal of obtaining only enough information to meet the immediate health needs of the patient, should be performed. Regardless of the type of assessment is performed, it is most important to remember that an inaccurate or incomplete assessment will result in a faulty plan of care for the patient and may even cause adverse outcomes.

NURSING ALERT

Level of Assessment
A focused assessment that can be completed in a short period of time is appropriate when the patient presents with a life-threatening condition—QSEN Competency 5: safety.

Data Collection

Types of Data

The two types of data are subjective data and objective data. **Subjective data** include the patient's report of symptoms and how he or she views his or her health. For example, a client tells you that she has had a fever for 2 days. The patient is the predominant or primary source of subjective information. The patient usually knows better than anyone else what his or her health status is. Family members and significant others are only considered a primary source of information when the patient is a minor, mentally incompetent to make independent decisions, or unable to respond because he or she is in critical condition or unconscious. In all other instances, family members and significant others are considered secondary sources of information. **Objective data** are observable or measurable. An example of objective data is a nurse's observation that a patient's temperature is 101°F. Objective data are obtained from secondary sources such as medical records, other healthcare team members, the nurse's own knowledge base, and literature reviews.

Methods of Data Collection

Health History The nurse interviews the client to obtain the health history and identify the needs of the patient. The following types of information are obtained during the health history:

- Demographic data (eg, name, birth date, employer, insurance information)
- Reason for visit (in the patient's own words)
- Present illness (more detailed information about the current health concern or illness)
- Past illnesses, hospitalizations, surgeries
- Family history
- Social history
- Review of systems (collection of information about all body systems reported by the patient/designee)

Physical Assessment The physical assessment is a significant source of objective information. The nurse uses inspection, auscultation, palpation, and percussion to obtain information about the patient's health status. The physical assessment is also the beginning of data validation. The previous example of a patient stating that she has had a fever for 2 days and the nurse's observation that the patient's current temperature was 101°F demonstrates how the nurse was able to validate that the patient's perception of her health status was probably accurate.

Data Validation

Data validation is the process whereby a nurse filters the facts out from the subjective and objective data that have been collected. One way to do this is by cross-referencing data reported against actual observations made. It is also necessary to verify objective data that at first glance appear to be factual. For example, a nurse obtains the patient's blood glucose level with a glucometer on the nursing unit. The glucose level is high. When reviewing the chart, the nurse notices that this value is out of sequence with previous glucose levels recorded in the patient's medical record. The nurse also checks the log to determine when the glucometer was last calibrated and discovers that the glucometer is due to be calibrated. After calibrating the glucometer, the nurse rechecks the patient's glucose level. The glucose result is within the normal range and is consistent with previous readings. Not all data validation revolves around measurable, objective data; it is also important for the nurse to be aware that his or her own value system may influence how data are interpreted.

Data Interpretation

Assessment is more than mere data collection. It requires that the nurse be able to determine the significance of the information that is being gathered. To do this, the nurse must group data appropriately and make inferences from the data (ie, the beginning step of phase two of the nursing process, nursing diagnoses). The nurse's proficiency in data interpretation increases as his or her knowledge base expands and as he or she gains more practical experience.

Data clustering is grouping data to help the nurse to form a clear picture of the patient's health patterns. There are numerous ways of clustering data, including body systems, nursing theories, non-nursing theories, and so on. Each one of these methods might be appropriate depending on the particular situation. From a more formal standpoint, a nursing school, hospital, or other type of healthcare organization may adopt a certain model as its organizational framework. In such cases, forms, charting systems, and so on would be formatted to reflect that particular model. However, at a more fundamental level, the individual nurse may also use other methods to cluster and make sense of the data that have been collected. For example, the form adopted by the organization for assessment may be laid out by body system. This layout helps to identify problems and potential nursing diagnoses for a particular body system. At the same time, the nurse may use Maslow's hierarchy of needs to determine which body system should be assessed first or even which data within a system are most significant at any given time. It is important to understand that clustering of data is not a one-time activity. Data may have to be regrouped as new information is collected or as the situation changes, and the method of clustering the data may also have to be modified. An example that may help to clarify this is the situation of children being assigned certain seats in class. Initially, the teacher may assign seats alphabetically. Later, the teacher may discover that this arrangement does not meet the learning needs of the students, so the class may

✔ ROUTINE CHECKUP 1

1. _____ is purposeful, goal-directed thinking that encourages sound decision making.

Answer:

2. Data validation is only required for measurable, objective data. True/false?

Answer:

be rearranged using another strategy. The driving factor in this example is meeting the "learning needs" of the students. In the nursing process, the driving factor is meeting the "healthcare needs" of the patient.

Diagnosis

Merriam-Webster's Dictionary defines **diagnose** as "to know." To arrive at the point of knowing, an analysis of the situation must be made. Diagnosing is a part of many different professions—mechanics diagnose what is wrong with a car; meteorologists forecast the weather. Similarly, physicians diagnose diseases and conditions—**medical diagnoses**—related to a person's health. In each of these situations, diagnoses drive the plan for correcting problems and preventing or limiting adverse outcomes. Each of the above professions has set boundaries. Mechanics are not legally authorized to predict the weather or diagnose a disease and vice versa. The same is true for nurses, who are legally authorized to make nursing diagnoses. Nurses are not legally authorized to make medical diagnoses; however, nurses may play a role in managing medical problems that require both interventions prescribed by the physician and independent nursing actions. Problems fitting into this category are referred to as **collaborative problems** (Figure 2–2).

> ## NURSING ALERT
> **Nursing Diagnoses**
> The professional nurse SHOULD NOT, under any circumstances, make a medical diagnosis.

Definition

A **nursing diagnosis** is "a clinical judgment concerning a human response to health conditions/life processes, or vulnerability for that response by an individual, family, group, or community" (Heardman and Kamitsuru, 2014). Nursing diagnoses clarify the scope of nursing practice and allow nurses to have a common language for communicating patient needs (Table 2–1).

Diagnostic Process

The diagnostic process begins during assessment with the clustering of subjective and objective data. The diagnostic process continues with the

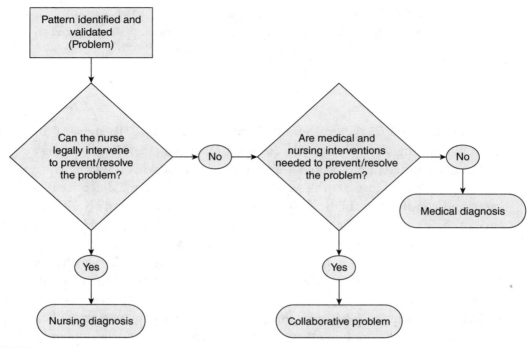

FIGURE 2−2 · Nursing diagnosis versus collaborative problem versus medical diagnosis process flow.

identification of patterns formed from the clustering process and culminates with the validation of patterns.

Pattern Identification

Pattern identification involves correctly grouping data together to determine a patient's response to actual or potential health problems or life processes. It is a process of synthesizing data. Pattern identification can be compared to

TABLE 2−1 Medical Diagnosis Versus Nursing Diagnosis		
Characteristic	Medical Diagnosis	Nursing Diagnosis
Concern with patient's health status	Yes	Yes
Focus on resolving disease and underlying pathology	Yes	No
Focus on patient's responses to diseases and life processes	No	Yes
Includes wellness diagnoses that focus on enhancement of function to a higher level	No	Yes

making a cake. When you make a cake, you may use flour, sugar, eggs, flavoring, milk, and so on. When the cake is baked, you no longer have the individual ingredients; instead, you have a particular type of cake. Also, although different types of cakes may use similar ingredients, how the ingredients are combined, the amount of each ingredient, and the addition or subtraction of a particular ingredient all change the type of cake that comes out of the oven. The same is true of a nursing diagnosis. Various nursing diagnoses may share similar ingredients or defining characteristics, but the omission or addition of a particular defining characteristic will change the nursing diagnosis.

Pattern Validation

Determining whether nursing diagnoses are correct or incorrect occurs during pattern validation. The nurse uses critical thinking skills to make this decision. This involves taking into consideration past clinical experiences, current knowledge base, norms and standards, and research data. The nursing diagnosis **taxonomy** (classification system) developed by the North American Nursing Diagnosis Association (NANDA) serves as a reference for pattern validation as well. The taxonomy identifies supporting evidence that guides nurses to select correct diagnoses.

Validation of the nursing diagnoses with the patient is just as important. There is a greater likelihood of noncompliance with the plan of care if the patient does not agree with the nursing diagnosis (ie, the basis for the plan of care). This does not mean that the nursing diagnoses do not exist or that the nursing diagnoses should not be documented. It does mean that the nurse should take the patient's perceptions into consideration when prioritizing nursing diagnoses and formulating the plan of care.

Diagnostic Statement

The final product of the diagnostic process is the actual nursing diagnostic statement. The diagnostic statement is usually a two-part statement that includes the diagnostic label and the related factors. As stated earlier, NANDA's nursing diagnosis taxonomy serves as a major resource for nursing diagnoses selection.

NANDA'S Nursing Diagnosis Taxonomy

NANDA's nursing taxonomy is a classification system that includes a comprehensive listing of standardized nursing diagnoses. Each nursing diagnosis listed includes the diagnostic label and definition. Defining characteristics, risk factors, and related factors may or may not be included depending on the type of nursing diagnosis.

Diagnostic Label

The diagnostic label is the approved named given for the nursing diagnosis by NANDA. There are three types of diagnostic labels. A **problem-focused nursing diagnosis** describes a current undesirable response to an existing health problem or life process. A **risk nursing diagnosis** describes a vulnerability for developing an undesirable response to a health problem or life process. A **health promotion nursing diagnosis** describes a desire by the individual, family, group, or community to enhance well-being and health potential.

Definition

A definition is assigned to each nursing diagnosis approved by NANDA. The definition describes the characteristic of the human response identified in the diagnostic label.

Defining Characteristics

The defining characteristics are the signs and symptoms (objective and subjective data) that are observed and from which inferences are made. Defining characteristics are only listed for problem-focused and health promotion nursing diagnoses.

Risk Factors

Risk factors are cited for risk nursing diagnoses and describe clinical findings that make the individual family or community vulnerable to developing an actual response to a health problem or life process.

Related Factors

Related factors are variables that contribute to or cause the human response identified in the diagnostic label. The second part of the two-part diagnostic statement is derived from the related factors. The related factors are important because they form the basis for interventions that will be used to resolve the response. Failure to cite related factors will result in treating the symptoms instead of getting rid of the cause of the symptoms. In most cases, the symptoms will reappear if the underlying cause is not eliminated. For example, if you paint over mold, it disappears, but as long as the moisture that causes the mold is not eliminated, the mold will eventually resurface.

Formulating nursing diagnoses is a critical step in the nursing process because the interventions and expected outcomes will be derived from these diagnoses. It is critical that the nurse make sound and valid judgments with input from the patient. Failure to do so can be compared to building a legal case on faulty evidence that leads to conviction and execution of an innocent person.

✔ ROUTINE CHECKUP 2

1. A nursing diagnosis is a clinical judgment about the individual, family, group, or community _____ to actual or potential health problems or life processes.

Answer:

2. _____ are important because they form the basis for interventions.

Answer:

Planning

The third phase of the nursing process is planning. During this phase, diagnoses are prioritized, goals and outcome criteria are established, interventions are identified, and a written plan of care is developed. The planning phase of the nursing process serves the same purpose as starting your day by taking a few minutes at the beginning of the day to reflect on what needs to be accomplished and mapping out a strategy for how to accomplish the tasks ahead. Of course, as the day proceeds, there may be a need to change priorities and make adjustments. The same is true of the planning phases of the nursing process.

Prioritizing Diagnoses

Prioritizing nursing diagnoses is a decision-making process. The type of diagnosis (problem-focused, risk, or health promotion) and whether it is life threatening or not, the healthcare setting, available resources, and patient preferences are some variables that may impact the priority of nursing diagnoses. Life-threatening situations and things that the patient considers very important are classified as high priority. Establishing priorities is not a static activity; adjustments are made as changes in the patient situation occur.

Expected Outcomes and Outcome Criteria

The goal or **expected outcome** (ie, the end toward which interventions are directed) is developed to clearly identify what behavior will indicate a realistic resolution of the nursing diagnoses for the individual patient. It should relate directly to the nursing diagnosis. The goal may be short term, occurring in a matter of hours or days, or long term, occurring over a period of weeks or months. The expected outcome should include who (usually the patient), what, and when. In some instances, it is also appropriate to include how (under what conditions) the outcome will occur.

The **outcome criteria** are specific measurable indicators of progress toward achieving the expected outcomes. They also should include who, what, when, and how (as appropriate).

Expected outcomes and outcome criteria should be patient centered. A common error made by novice users of the nursing process is confusing outcome statements with interventions. The most common mistake is to identify what actions the nurse or support staff will perform. For example, the statement: "The nurse will check the patient's respiratory rate every 4 hours" is different from "The patient will maintain a respiratory rate between 16 and 20 breaths/min during the hospital stay." Remember that as a general rule, the patient will always be the "who" in the outcome statement.

The goal and accompanying outcome criteria should be observable and measurable. In the above example, the respiratory rate is both observable (rise and fall of the chest) and measurable. It is very important to avoid generalized terms such as *normal*, *good*, and *well*. If, for example, we stated: "The patient will have a normal respiratory rate," how then would we define *normal*? Normal for an infant is not considered normal for a geriatric patient.

Last but not least, the goal must be realistic for the particular patient situation and in line with what the patient desires. Ideally, the goal of any plan would be to completely resolve the problem and its underlying cause. However, this is not always possible. For example, a patient who has emphysema may have a diagnosis of an impaired gas exchange. A realistic outcome for this individual may be that effective gas exchange will be maintained with the use of oxygen. An individual who does not have an underlying disease of this nature may be expected to achieve effective gas exchange without the use of oxygen.

A Nursing Outcomes Classification (NOC) system has been developed to standardized outcomes used to evaluate the impact of nursing interventions. This taxonomy of nursing outcomes provides benefits similar to those of the nursing diagnosis taxonomy. It contributes to evidence-based nursing practice, facilitates electronic record documentation, and serves as a resource in nursing education. The classification system is recognized as a standardized language in nursing by the American Nurses Association and is being refined and expanded on a continuous basis (Moorhead, 2013).

Nursing Interventions

Nursing interventions are actions performed by a nurse to achieve the expected outcomes that have been identified for the patient. Generally speaking, nursing interventions may involve assessment, teaching, counseling, or actual hands-on treatments. There are three categories of nursing interventions. **Independent nursing interventions**, also referred to as *nurse-initiated interventions*, fall within the scope of nursing practice and can be performed without orders from other healthcare providers. **Dependent nursing interventions** require a physician or other healthcare provider order before implementation. A nurse may carry out the order but cannot do so without the order (eg, nurse cannot start an intravenous infusion on a patient without an order from a physician). The third category of interventions is **interdependent** (collaborative) **interventions**. Interventions that require the actions of multiple members of the healthcare team fall into this category. For example, a patient who has a nutritional deficit will require interventions from the physician, nurse, and dietician. The physician may request a consultation with the dietician. The dietician will provide expertise regarding dietary requirements, and the nurse will assist with ensuring that the patient follows the prescribed dietary guidelines.

The process of selecting nursing interventions is a deliberate process that requires critical thinking as well as an adequate knowledge base. Nursing interventions, similar to expected outcomes and outcome criteria, should include who, what, when, and how as appropriate for each intervention statement. The following items should be considered before finalizing nursing interventions:

- Associated nursing diagnosis and expected outcomes
- Competency of the provider (nurse, family member, other support staff)
- Benefits versus risks
- Patient preferences
- Standards of care (state boards, The Joint Commission)
- Research (evidenced-based practice)
- Available resources

A variety of resources can be used to assist with the development of interventions (eg, standardized care plans, policy and procedure manuals, nursing journals and textbooks). The University of Iowa's Centers for Nursing Classifications and Clinical Effectiveness has also developed a Nursing Interventions Classification (NIC) taxonomy. Each intervention has an assigned code and includes the name of the intervention, its definition, activities required to carry out the intervention, and background readings. The interventions can be linked to a NANDA nursing diagnosis and NOC outcomes. The NIC system includes interventions that are designed to achieve a wide variety of outcomes. This standardized classification system allows for effective clinical documentation, continuity of care, reimbursement for nursing care, curricular development, and competency and productivity evaluations (Bulechek et al, 2013).

Nursing Care Plans

The **nursing care plan** is a documented outline of the nursing care to be provided for an individual patient. The amount of detail varies depending on the type of care plan. Student care plans are usually very detailed and include documentation of information for all five phases of the nursing process as well as rationales for interventions and citations of resources used. Care plans used in healthcare settings are generally more concise and may only include the nursing diagnoses, expected outcomes, and interventions. How the care plan is formatted varies among healthcare influenced by the nursing theory or model adopted by the school (eg, Roy's adaptation model, Orem's self-care model). There has also been an increase in the use of computerized nursing care plans. The advantages of using computerized care plans are (1) decreased nursing time required to develop the plan of care, thereby increasing the amount of time the nurse has to spend on direct patient care and standardization. Standardization is beneficial but computerized and standardized care plans must be reviewed and revised to ensure that the care plan is individualized for the particular patient (Table 2–2).

Concept Mapping

Concept mapping is used to develop critical thinking skills. Concept mapping is not unique to nursing and is also not limited to application to the nursing process. Concept mapping can be applied to many subject areas and disciplines. The process involves graphically displaying concepts and identifying

TABLE 2–2   Sample Nursing Care Plan

Case Study: Mr. Martin comes to the ED complaining that he burned his hand while cooking a meal at home. The palm of his right hand is red with multiple blisters, some of which are broken and oozing a clear liquid. He is clenching his teeth and has facial grimacing. Mr. Martin says, "It hurts really bad." When asked, he states that his pain is an 8 on a scale of 1 to 10 with 10 being the worst level of pain. He states that he just wants us to "make the pain go away."

Assessment	Diagnosis	Planning Expected Outcomes and Outcome Criteria	Planned Intervention and Rationales
S: Patient states he burned his hand while cooking.	**Acute pain related to burn injury**	I. Patient will verbalize a pain level of 2 at his scheduled return visit 48 hours after treatment.	A. The RN will instruct the patient to take his pain medication when he first begins to experience pain as long as it is not sooner than the recommended time appearing in the directions.
S: Patient makes comment, "It hurts really bad."	Risk for infection related to break in skin	**Outcome Criteria**	**Rationale:** Patients often believe that they should only take medications when they have severe pain and do not know that pain is better control if the medication is taken early on.
S: Patient states pain is an 8 on a scale of 1 to 10.		A. Before discharge, the patient will verbalize that pain medication should be taken at the first sign of pain as long as it is within the prescribed time frame for taking medicine.	B. The RN will ask the patient what his pain level is after he is medicated and before his discharge from the ED.
S: Patient states: "Just make the pain go away."			**Rationale:** Pain is a subjective experience. This information will assist the nurse in determining the effectiveness of the current interventions so adjustments can be made if necessary before discharge from the ED.
O: Clenching teeth		B. Before discharge, the patient will state that the pain level has decreased to 4 on a scale of 1 to 10.	C. The LPN with the assistance of the patient will identify two activities (eg, music or a favorite game show) that can be used as distracters to take the patient's mind off the pain. The LPN will explain that this is to be used in combination, not as a substitute for the pain medication.
O: Facial grimacing			
O: Right palm red		C. Before discharge, the patient will identify two activities that he can use as distracters to help with managing his pain at home.	**Rationale:** Activities that are enjoyable for the patient are most effective in getting the patient's mind off of the pain temporarily. Distracters cannot take the place of pharmacologic methods of alleviating the type pain the patient is experiencing.
O: Blisters on right palm, some broken and oozing clear liquid			

ED = emergency department; LPN = Licensed Practical Nurse; O = objective data; RN = Registered Nurse; S = subjective data.

Before Concept Mapping **After Concept Mapping**

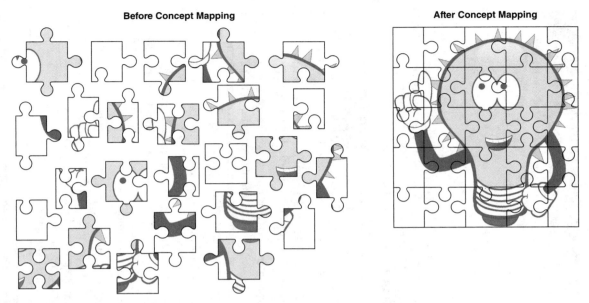

FIGURE 2–3 · Concept mapping. (Source: https://openclipart.org/detail/269989/anthropomorphic-cartoon-light-bulb.)

the relationship between the various concepts. The intended outcome is that the individual will better understand the subject being mapped. It is like putting puzzle pieces together to create a meaningful image (Figure 2–3).

Critical pathways, which integrate interventions for all healthcare disciplines into one care plan, is an alternative approach to nursing care plans. An integrated care plan is just the final product. For this concept to work, there must be an interdisciplinary team approach for the provision of care, and members of the team must meet, communicate, and collaborate to achieve expected outcomes.

Implementation

Implementation is the phase of the nursing process during which the plan is put into action. At first glance, this phase may appear to be the simplest phase to carry out. But a more detailed look at what is involved reveals that this is not true. During implementation, you have to "think on your feet." Implementation of the plan requires a combination of critical thinking skills, psychomotor skills, and communication skills. It also involves continuous assessment of the situation to prioritize appropriately and make modifications when needed. In

✔ **ROUTINE CHECKUP 3**

1. Short-term goals may be achieved within a matter of _____ or _____, but long-term goals may require months to achieve.

Answer:

2. Standardized nursing care plans must be reviewed and revised to ensure that the plan is individualized to meet particular patient needs. True/false?

Answer:

life-threatening situations, there is no time to complete formal planning; instead, implementation must occur immediately. The nurse may be involved in providing direct care or may delegate provision of care to other members of the healthcare team. The model of care that has been adopted for the particular setting usually directs the coordination of care. Examples of care models include primary nursing, team nursing, and case management. Written and verbal communication regarding implementation promotes continuity of care. Written documentation of activities that occur during implementation may be included in the nurse's notes, on various flow sheets, and in the nursing care plan. At a minimum, verbal communication related to implementation should occur any time there is a "hand-off" of the patient from one healthcare member to another (eg, shift changes, when one team member is relieving another team member, patient transfers).

Evaluation

The fifth phase of the nursing process is evaluation. In the nursing process, evaluation is generally the determination of the effectiveness of an individual patient's plan of care. At the organizational level, we evaluate the overall quality of care provided by the organization.

Evaluation at the Individual Patient Level

Two forms of evaluation take place in the nursing process. The first type is **formative evaluation**. This is ongoing evaluation that starts long before reaching the actual evaluation phase in the nursing process. In fact, it begins as early as the assessment phase when the nurse evaluates changes that may be occurring as assessment is taking place as well as the process of validating data. During each phase of the nursing process, some type of evaluation may occur. The feedback obtained during this type evaluation is used to make modifications on an ongoing basis. **Summative evaluation** occurs during the evaluation phase of the nursing process and takes place after the plan of care has been implemented. The ultimate goal of evaluation is to determine if expected outcomes were achieved and nursing diagnoses (including underlying causes) were resolved. As the goals are achieved and the nursing diagnoses resolved, the plan of care is discontinued. Any unresolved nursing diagnoses should be evaluated regularly and the plan of care should be adjusted as the need arises.

Evaluation at the Organizational Level

Organizational evaluation is necessary if we expect to meet the challenge of providing the highest quality and safest care in a cost-effective manner. An important first step for nurses is evaluation of everyday patient care. It is imperative that all nurses, from the novice to the well-seasoned nurse, participate in organizational evaluation and quality improvement. Standards of care set by various accrediting agencies, performance measures, guidelines set forth in evidence-based practice, best practices, and internal benchmarks that have been set within the organization are all used in the process of evaluating the quality of care. Basing your nursing actions on the aforementioned, sharing your observations regarding the effectiveness of your nursing care, accepting responsibility for continuous education and learning, and being receptive to changes are all ways you contribute to ongoing quality improvement.

Conclusion

The nursing process is the organizing framework for providing safe, high-quality nursing care to patients. Although each of the five phases of the nursing process serves a unique purpose in the overall process, the combined dynamic interaction of the five phases most significantly determines the success of the plan of care for the patient. Critical thinking and the nursing process go hand in hand. Desired outcomes would be achieved haphazardly without the integration of critical thinking and evidence-based practice in the nursing process.

Several key points should be noted from the information presented in this chapter:

- The nursing process centers on the patient's responses to actual or potential health problems or life processes.
- Patient involvement is necessary for successful use of the nursing process.
- NANDA, NOC, and NIC classification systems play an important role in establishing the credibility of the nursing process and ultimately the nursing profession's impact on quality healthcare.

REVIEW QUESTIONS

1. **Which of the following individuals would be considered a primary source of information?**
   A. A significant other
   B. The parent of a minor child
   C. The patient
   D. B and C
   E. All of the above

2. **Ms. Lloyd presents at the doctor's office with a complaint of difficulty breathing that began 2 days ago and has progressively worsened. Which of the following data would BEST validate the fact that Ms. Lloyd is having difficulty breathing?**
   A. Oral temperature of 102°F
   B. Patient's report of frequent coughing
   C. Respiratory rate of 30 breaths/min with audible wheezing
   D. Blue nail beds (cyanosis)

3. **Which of the following factors should be considered during the diagnostic process of pattern validation?**
   A. Current knowledge base
   B. NANDA taxonomy
   C. Past clinical experiences
   D. All of the above

4. **A 3-month-old infant is brought to the emergency room by his parents. The mother states that the child has been sleepy all day and has not been breast-feeding well all week. The nurse observes that the child's mucous membranes are dry, the urine in the urine collection bag is dark in color, the skin turgor is**

poor, the "soft spot" (fontanelle) is sunken, and the pulse rate is high. The physician tells the parents that the child is dehydrated. Based on the information that is currently available, which of the following statements represents a correctly stated nursing diagnosis for this client situation?

A. Dehydration related to inadequate breastfeeding
B. Deficient fluid volume related to decreased intake of fluids
C. Imbalanced nutrition—less than body requirement related to insufficient intake of nutrients
D. Risk for ineffective coping related to parental perception of inability to meet role expectations

5. Which of the following expected outcomes is stated correctly?

A. The patient will void 300 cc of urine during each shift.
B. The nurse will feed the patient half of the food on the meal tray at each meal.
C. The patient will feel better by tomorrow morning.
D. The patient will be able to walk with the assistance of a cane.

ANSWERS

Routine Checkup 1

1. Critical thinking.
2. False.

Routine Checkup 2

1. Response.
2. Related factors.

Routine Checkup 3

1. Days, hours.
2. True.

Review Questions

1. D
2. C
3. D
4. B
5. A

References

Alfaro-LeFevre R: *Applying Nursing Process: A Tool for Critical Thinking*, 8th ed. Philadelphia, PA: Lippincott, 2014.

Berman A, Snyder SJ, Fandsen G: *Kozier & Erb Fundamentals of Nursing: Concepts, Process and Practice*, 10th ed. Boston, MA: Pearson, 2016.

Bulechek G, Butcher H, Dochterman J, Wagner C, eds: *Nursing Interventions Classification (NIC)*, 6th ed. St. Louis, MO: Elsevier, 2013.

Diagnosis: In *Merriam-Webster Dictionary*. Available at http://www.m-w.com/dictionary/diagnosis.

Hall A: *Fundamentals of Nursing*, 9th ed. St. Louis, MO: Elsevier, 2017.

Halpern DF: *Thought and Knowledge: An Introduction to Critical Thinking*. Hillsdale, NJ: Lawrence Erlbaum Associates, 1989.

Heardman TH, Kamitsuru S, eds: *Nursing Diagnoses 2015–17: Definitions and Classifications*. Oxford, UK: Wiley Blackwell, 2014:24.

Melnyk BM, Fineout-Overholt E, Stillwell SB, Williamson KM: Evidence-based practice step by step: igniting a spirit of inquiry: an essential foundation for evidence-based practice. *Am J Nurs.* 2009;109:49-52.

Moorhead S, Maas M, Swanson E, eds: *Nursing Outcomes Classifications (NOC)*. St. Louis, MO: Elsevier, 2013.

Potter PA, Perry AG, Stockert P, Hall A: *Fundamentals of Nursing*, 9th ed. St. Louis, MO: Elsevier, 2017.

Wilkinson JM, Treas LS, Barnett KL, Smith MH: *Fundamentals of Nursing Vol. 1: Theory, Concepts, and Applications*. Philadelphia, PA: FA Davis, 2016.

Additional Resources

AHQR Clinical Practice Guidelines Clearinghouse. Available at https://www.guideline.gov/.

Developing a nursing IQ—part 1 characteristics of critical thinking: what critical thinkers do, what critical thinkers do not do. *ISNA Bulletin.* 2014;41:6-14.

Developing a nursing IQ—part III: a picture of thought. *ISNA Bulletin.* 2016;42:7-14.

Evidence-Based Practice. Available at http://guides.mclibrary.duke.edu/c.php?g=158201&p=1036021.

NIH Clinical Practice Guidelines. Available at https://nccih.nih.gov/health/providers/clinicalpractice.htm.

Walton BG: Developing a nursing IQ—part II: the expertise of nursing process. *Ohio Nurse Review.* 2016;91:24-34.

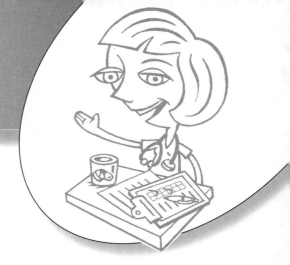

Part II

Fundamental Principles of Nursing Care

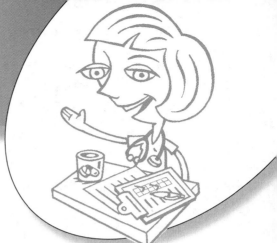

Chapter **3**

Communication and Documentation

At the end of the chapter, the reader will be able to:

1. Describe the five components of the communication process.
2. Discuss variables that may influence the communication process.
3. State the foundational elements of therapeutic communication.
4. Differentiate between therapeutic and nontherapeutic communication techniques.
5. Discuss the purposes of documentation.
6. Describe principles that promote quality documentation.
7. Describe five methods of nursing documentation.
8. Identify situations that require reporting the status of the patient.

Overview

Communication is the process by which messages are relayed between individuals. Life does not exist without communication. Even when no words are exchanged, communication exists. Communication also serves an integral role in the nursing profession. It is the vehicle used by nurses to accomplish the goal of providing quality care to patients. This chapter examines basic principles of the communication process as well as how nurses use the communication process. Documenting and reporting patient care information are also covered.

Communication

Basic Principles

Before you can understand the role that communication plays in nursing, you must understand the general principles of communication. This section describes the components of the communication process and influencing factors.

Components

The five basic pieces to the communication puzzle are the sender, message, channel, receiver, and feedback (Figure 3–1). The **sender** is the person who constructs and sends the message. The **message** is the information that is to be sent. Messages fall into two major categories: (1) **verbal** (spoken or written words) and (2) **nonverbal** (messages communicated by various expressions such as posture, facial expressions, and voice tone). Nonverbal cues significantly impact the meaning of a message. What triggers a person to communicate (eg, anger, stress, happiness, perceived threat) also influences the outcome

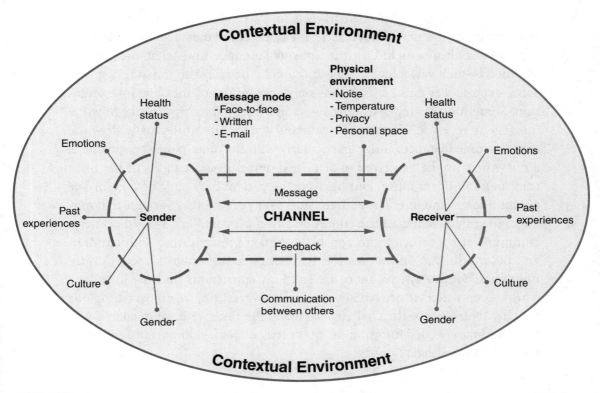

FIGURE 3–1 · The communication process. Items listed in the contextual environment represent only a sample of influencing variables.

of the communication process. The **channel**, or how the message is sent, is another component of the communication process. The channel may be auditory (eg, speaking, singing), visual (eg, written words, pictures), or **kinesthetic** (eg, touch, motion). The recipient of the message is the **receiver**. The receiver, in turn, interprets the message and sends a response or **feedback** to the original sender. No response by the receiver is actually still feedback because the sender will assign a meaning to the nonresponse.

Influencing Variable

In the previous section, we indicated that the receiver interprets the message and responds with feedback. If the receiver interprets the message in a manner that is congruent with what the sender intended the message to be, then the interaction was successful and fairly simple. However, this is not always the case. Congruency of message meaning may not exist, in which case communication becomes more complex.

We already identified that the triggers for communication and the channel of communication may influence the meaning of the messages. Additionally, a person's culture, including the spoken language and what meaning is assigned to such variables as space and touch, may have an impact. Past personal experiences and expectations may also influence message interpretation. Something as simple as how a person is dressed may influence how the message is received. Traditionally, nurses wore white uniforms with white caps. In some instances today, particularly with the older patient population, a nurse may not be perceived to be a "real nurse" because of his or her nontraditional uniform attire, and likewise the patient may alter how he or she communicates and interacts with the nurse. Time is another variable that may affect the effectiveness of the communication process. Box 3–1 lists general communication principles to consider when communicating with children and older adults. Communication is most effective when it occurs under unhurried conditions, yet there are so many constraints on time in today's world. Even when we are having a casual conversation, we are watching our watches. Nurses face the challenge of using the time we have in such a way that we obtain needed information, make the patient feel important, and meet the patient's healthcare needs.

BOX 3–1
Communication and Developmental Consideration

Children	Older Adults
Interview the child as well as the parent unless the parents do not consent. (There are exceptions—**eg**, in situations where child abuse is suspected.) • Speak with not at the child (especially older children/teens) • Begin with nonthreatening topics • Listen attentively • Notice body language and tone of voice • It may be beneficial to speak in third person with younger children • Use games, drawings, and other tools as needed	Normal changes associated with the aging process may impact communication. • Communication in an unhurried manner • Ensure the client can see you • Select a quiet environment • Ensure client has aids (eg, hearing aids/glasses) if appropriate • Do not speak too loud • Allow adequate time for a response • Rephrase if client does not understand • Modify printed material to accommodate cognitive ability and vision impairment • Communicate in a respectful manner

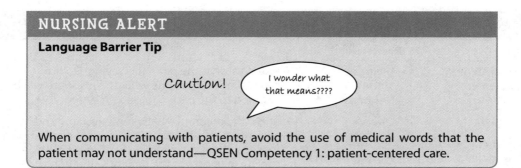

NURSING ALERT

Language Barrier Tip

Caution!   I wonder what that means????

When communicating with patients, avoid the use of medical words that the patient may not understand—QSEN Competency 1: patient-centered care.

Nursing and the Communication Process

Communication is to nursing as air is to life—one cannot exist without the other. Interpersonal relationships that are developed with the patient exist within the context of the communication process. Communication is also the glue that holds together the nursing process. The absence of effective communication leads to faulty data collection, which in turns leads to incorrect nursing diagnoses and the development of a plan of care that will not meet the patient's needs. Furthermore, communication extends beyond nurse–patient interactions. It also occurs between various members of the healthcare team and serves as a tool for care coordination.

Interpersonal Communication

Interpersonal communication is a one-on-one form of communication that occurs between two individuals. Although nurses may engage in interpersonal communication with various members of the healthcare team, nurses' interactions with patients are the most important. **Therapeutic communication**, which is a purposeful communication that produces an established outcome, is used to ensure that effective interpersonal communication occurs with the patient. Therapeutic communication is nonjudgmental and patient centered. It is built on the following foundational elements:

- **Trust and honesty:** Avoid giving false reassurances.
- **Privacy and confidentiality:** Use during both the interaction and away from the interaction.
- **Respect and courtesy:** Use titles and names that are acceptable to the patient. Encourage active participation in the decision-making process.
- **Empathy:** Show a sense of understanding and acceptance of the patient's situation.

TABLE 3–1 Therapeutic Versus Nontherapeutic Communication Techniques

Therapeutic	Nontherapeutic	Tips
• Active listening (restatement, reflection) • Empathy • Exploring (focusing, encouraging elaboration, seeking clarification, giving information, looking at alternatives, using silence, summarizing) • Hope • Self-disclosure • Confrontation	• Giving an automatic response • Offering sympathy • Asking personal questions • Giving false reassurance • Giving personal opinions • Arguing	• Listen to what the patient is saying. Do not stereotype and assume what the response will be or respond to the patient based on stereotypes. • Know the difference between sympathy and empathy. Whereas sympathy focuses on the nurse's feelings about the client's situation, empathy allows the nurse to accept the patient's situation and deals with the issues at hand. • Be honest. Base assurances on facts, not wishes. • Clarify inconsistencies but do not engage in arguing or respond to the patient in a defensive manner. Remember that communication should be nonjudgmental. • Always remember that the focus should be on the patient. Do not allow self-disclosure and sharing of feelings to change the focus to the nurse instead of the patient. It is inappropriate to engage in nonprofessional relationships with the patient (eg, becoming the patient's friend).

Active listening, touch, and silence have also proven to be beneficial components of therapeutic communication. Avoiding pitfalls in the communication process (eg, false reassurance, arguing, sympathy) is just as important as knowing what to include in the communication process. Table 3–1 provides a summary of therapeutic and nontherapeutic communication techniques and tips.

Other Communication Forums

In addition to communicating with the patient, the nurse communicates in other forums. Below is a brief discussion of each type of communication.

Intrapersonal communication. One type of communication that we give very little thought to is **intrapersonal communication**. Intrapersonal communication is communication that occurs within the individual. It is also called self-talk. It can be compared to a dress rehearsal. The nurse can use this as a tool to work through stressful situations (eg, performing a new skill, interacting with a difficult colleague). This type of communication is also helpful for dealing with negative stereotypical thoughts that may yield ineffective communication with others. Additionally, nurses should be aware that patients and other persons they interact with use this same technique. This knowledge may be used to understand human responses during interactions and may be used as an intervention with patients.

Group communication. Group communication involves communication between more than two individuals. Nurses are most often involved in goal-oriented small group communication. Examples include group meetings with a limited number of patients, committee meetings, and interdisciplinary team meetings. Group communication is more complex because it includes multiple recipients of the message, which means there may be the potential for multiple interpretations.

Nurses may also have the opportunity to interact in larger groups. A nurse manager may have staff meetings, nurses who work in community settings may offer classes to the public, and nurses who are active in professional organizations may serve as guest speakers on specific topics. Although large group communication is important and appropriate in certain situations, a drawback is having limited opportunities to validate whether the intended message was received by the audience.

✔ ROUTINE CHECKUP

1. List the five components of the communication process.

Answer:

_____

_____

_____

_____

_____

2. Therapeutic communication is purposeful, nonjudgmental communication that produces an established outcome. True/false?

Answer:

Documentation

Documentation is a written form of communication. It is the evidence that healthcare delivery has occurred. Traditionally, handwritten records were the only means of documentation. However, technology has changed this, and now computerized documentation is available. With this option comes not

---

BOX 3–2
QSEN Spotlight

The Electronic Health Record transcends most of the QSEN standards. It supports patient-centered care, makes team work and collaboration easier, supports safe delivery of care as a result of information sharing, provides data for quality improvement, and improves information management through the use of technology.

Benefits	Risk
• Easy access to a wide range of information (eg, progress notes, orders, test results) • Information sharing across healthcare organization • Patient access to their medical record • Less time spent documenting	• Risk of privacy violation • Legal risk • Format may limit nurse's ability to capture important information that would tell the story of the patient's medical history/status • Potential unintended increase in errors due to repetitive task (eg, checklist) versus critically thinking about what is being documented

only the advantage of increased accessibility to patient information but also there is the added responsibility of protecting the patient's right to privacy. Box 3–2 provides a list of some other benefits and risk associated with computerized documentation. This following section presents information about the purpose, principles, and methods of documentation.

NURSING ALERT

Protecting Patient Health Information
Always create and use a strong password to access the electronic health record. It is equally important to protect the password—QSEN Competency 6: informatics.

Purpose of Documentation

Documentation is a critical part of healthcare delivery and serves multiple purposes, including:

- **Communication:** The nursing process is documented via the nursing care plan. The nursing care plan is the tool that nurses use to direct patient care. Some organizations use a **case management** healthcare delivery approach to providing patient care. This is a multidisciplinary team approach that usually includes input from physicians, social workers, nurses, and staff members working in other disciplines as appropriate. The **critical pathway**, which is a multidisciplinary treatment plan, is a documentation tool used for this mode of healthcare delivery. In each of the above-mentioned cases, documentation is the tool that is used to communicate the plan of care and promote continuity of care.

- **Quality assurance:** Documentation is one of the tools used to evaluate and improve the quality of care. The quality or performance improvement department usually coordinates internal reviews, and external reviews conducted by such agencies as The Joint Commission. In either case, the goal is to identify opportunities for improvement and make positive changes on a continuous basis.

- **Reimbursement:** Information documented in the medical record is used by federal agencies (eg, Medicaid and Medicare) and private insurance companies to determine whether an agency is eligible to receive reimbursement for services provided.

- **Legal evidence:** The medical record may be used as evidence in legal proceedings. It is important for nurses to remember that "if it is not documented, it did not occur." On the other hand, well-documented patient assessment and care provide the best assurance that nurses will not be subjected to legal consequences.

- **Research and education:** Chart reviews provide valuable information that can be used for research purposes. Data may be collected about the presence of a particular sign or symptom (eg, pain, elevated blood pressure, cyanosis) for a certain population of patients. This information may yield information about whether a pattern exists in the occurrence of the particular symptom. Policy and practice changes may in turn be made as a result of the findings. The medical record may also be used as an educational tool. Staff and students alike can learn how to anticipate the care requirements of a particular population of patient based on patterns identified from documented signs, symptoms, and treatment responses.

Principles of Documentation

It is clear that documentation is an essential part of healthcare delivery. However, what is more important is that the documentation is of good quality. Principles that promote quality documentation include accuracy, completeness, and clarity.

Accuracy

Information entered into the medical record should be factual. The nurse should make every effort to provide an objective description of observations made. Behavior should be described versus being labeled. For example, the nurse should not say that a patient is anxious but should instead describe the behaviors that suggest that the patient is anxious.

NURSING ALERT

Documentation Tip

Describe the behavior; do not label it!	
Correct	**Incorrect**
Patient "X" entered the clinic speaking in a loud voice, using profanity, and making verbal threats of bodily harm.	Patient "X" appeared very angry at this clinic visit.
QSEN Competency 1: patient-centered care.	

Significant patient statements should be placed in quotes, and the use of words that require a judgment on your part (eg, "appears," "seems," "good," "appropriate") should be avoided. To avoid errors, it is best to document in an unhurried manner. If an error is made, it should be indicated by drawing a single line through the entry, writing the word "error," and initialing above the erroneous entry.

NURSING ALERT

Error Correction
When correcting an error, do not use correction fluid or otherwise obscure errors; instead, follow the example below:

0510 B. Purifoy, a 12-year-old male was admitted to
error B. V.
room 724 via ~~stretcher~~ wheelchair. B. Vaughans, RN.

QSEN Competency 2: teamwork and collaboration & QSEN Competency 5: safety.

Completeness

Although it is neither necessary nor desirable to document every single thing that occurs during the course of patient care, leaving out significant assessment data, patient responses, and information about interventions may lead to adverse patient outcomes. The nurse should aim to document all pertinent patient care information in a clear and concise manner. Doing so will minimize adverse outcomes and free up more time for direct patient care. To best accomplish this, the nurse should:

- Document pertinent information as close to the time of occurrence as is possible. Doing so increase accuracy as well as the likelihood of including all relevant information.
- Use accepted abbreviations (with caution) and use short phrases that communicate complete thoughts.
- Use late entries when necessary but not excessively.

Clarity

The clarity of documentation is affected by whether the information is logically organized, systematically presented, and legible. Documenting in chronological order is one way to facilitate logical organization. This method requires that entries include a date and time. The sequencing of information within a particular entry also impacts its clarity. To best facilitate systematic documentation and clarity, the steps of the nursing process should be followed. The nurse should first document assessment data and then document patient needs, followed by the intervention, and finally the patient response to treatment or interventions. Entries in the medical record should also be legible. Major errors may occur as a result of entries not being legible. Illegible entries involving numbers and decimals may result in medication errors. Spelling errors may result in misdiagnosis and inappropriate treatments.

Methods of Documentation

Nursing documentation comes in various forms. The method of documentation varies according to the healthcare delivery approach (eg, primary, modular, case management), medical record model (Box 3–3), care setting (eg, hospital, long-term care setting, patient's home, outpatient clinics, doctor's office), organizational policies, and specific circumstances (eg, direct care, incident). Common methods of documentation are described further.

Narrative

Narrative documentation is the traditional method of documentation used by nurses to make entries about nursing care in the medical record. This method of documentation requires that the nurse describes the patient's condition and care

---

BOX 3–3
Medical Record Examples

Source Oriented	Problem Oriented
Medical record organized by disciplines: • Medicine • Nursing • Social work • Others	Medical record focuses on the patient's problems or diagnoses. All disciplines document information for each problem as appropriate. Includes the following components: • Database • Problem list • Care plan • Progress notes

---

provided. Although the advantage to narrative documentation is that the nurse can describe the exact situation, the disadvantages are that the descriptions are sometimes wordy, redundant, and unclear and can consume a significant amount of the nurse's time, detracting from valuable direct patient care time.

Charting by Exception

Charting by exception has replaced narrative documentation in many healthcare organizations. This method of charting requires that the organization establish standards of care. The identified standards of care are used to develop a form that will allow nurses to simply use a check mark to indicate that the standard has been met. With this type of documentation, narrative descriptions of the patient's status and the care provided are only required when there is a deviation from the established norm. Charting by exception requires a lot less time than traditional narrative documentation; however, it is critical that when there are deviations that the nurse provides a detailed description of the deviation. Failure to do so jeopardizes the continuity of patient care and presents a legal risk if the quality of care is challenged.

SOAP

SOAP or SOAPIER is the acronym used for progress notes entered into problem-oriented medical records. Each entry focuses on one problem. The progress note begins with a statement of the problem followed by:

- **S**ubjective data: patient input
- **O**bjective data: observations, labs, and so on

- **A**ssessment: interpretation of meaning of subjective and objective data
- **P**lan: what action is to be taken to resolve problem
- **I**mplementation: specific interventions
- **E**valuation: effectiveness of the plan
- **R**evision: recommended changes

PIE

PIE stands for problem, intervention, and evaluation. This form of documentation is also problem oriented; however, there are several differences. Problem-oriented documentation is based on a medical model and integrates the documentation of multiple disciplines into the progress notes. Thus, although a doctor, nurse, social worker, or staff member working in any other discipline involved in patient care may make an entry in the progress notes, PIE refers specifically to nursing progress notes. This system of documentation includes a nursing assessment flow sheet and nursing progress notes. The nurse documents the problem, interventions to address the problem, and the outcome in the progress notes.

Focus

The central theme of focus documentation is the client's concerns, not just problems. The acronym DAR (data, action, and response) is used to represent information documented in the progress note. Both subjective and objective data are obtained and documented. The interventions or actions taken as well as the patient's response to the interventions are documented.

Reporting

Reporting is a process used for handing off critical information about the patient to other individuals who will be involved in the care of the patient. Situations require that a report of the patient's condition and care be given include:

- Shift changes during which a different group of healthcare team members will assume responsibility for the patient's healthcare
- When one nurse turns over the care of the patient to another nurse (eg, during a lunch break or when leaving the floor for an in-service program)
- Transfers, both in house and to external facilities (eg, surgery to intensive care, acute care setting to long-term care setting)
- Transport for test, treatments, and procedures (eg, radiography, dialysis, physical therapy)

- Telephone updates to physicians (eg, change in patient's status, laboratory results)
- Interdisciplinary team meetings during which information about the patient's current health status and plan of care are discussed

The information included in the report may vary depending on the situation. For example, whereas very comprehensive information should be provided when a patient is being transferred from one facility to another facility, the patient's name and laboratory results may be all that is needed when calling the patient's doctor's office to report recent laboratory finding. Regardless of the situation, it is important that the information is accurate, easy to understand, and concise.

Conclusion

This chapter included a general discussion of communication principles as well as specific instances of the use of communication in nursing. Key points presented include:

- The basic components of the communication process are the sender, message, channel, receiver, and feedback.
- Communication is a dynamic process that is influenced by multiple variables within the contextual environment of the interaction (eg, culture, gender, past experiences, emotions).
- Successful implementation of the nursing process is significantly influenced by the integration of effective therapeutic communication skills.
- Documentation is a written form of communication that is valuable for numerous reasons, including continuity of care, quality assurance, legal evidence, reimbursement justification, research, and education.
- Reporting is a verbal form of communication that facilitates the sharing of critical information about the patient among various members of the healthcare team.

REVIEW QUESTIONS

1. **To promote therapeutic communication with the patient, the nurse should:**
   A. Avoid confronting the patient for clarification of inconsistencies.
   B. Show a sense of understanding and acceptance of the patient's situation.

C. Ensure that the environment is suitable for maintaining privacy during interactions with the patient.

D. B and C

E. All of the above

2. **Which of the following variables may influence the communication process?**

A. Personal appearance

B. Emotional state of the sender and receiver

C. Environmental temperature

D. A and B

E. All of the above

3. **Which of the following documentation entries best promote accuracy, clarity, and completeness?**

A. Patient fell out of bed because side rails were down. A bruise was noted on the right shoulder. The doctor was called for orders. The patient was assisted back to bed and instructed to always call for help to get out of bed.

B. Mr. X, a 75-year-old black male with a diagnosis of Alzheimer disease, fell out of the bed last night and bruised his right shoulder. He is known to have periods of confusion, but he stated that he fell while trying to go to the bathroom. The side rails were down on the bed. The nurse put the patient back to bed and instructed him not to get up by himself anymore. The doctor was informed of the incident.

C. Patient found on floor next to bed. Two-inch diameter, reddish blue, circular area noted on right shoulder. No complaint of pain at the site by the patient. Patient states that he fell out of the bed while trying to go to the bathroom. Side rails were noted to be down. Patient accompanied back to bed by nurse without further incident. Instructed to use call bell for assistance to get out of bed. Call bell placed in reach of patient. Doctor M. notified of fall and patient's condition. X-ray ordered as requested by doctor.

D. Patient states that he fell out of bed while trying to go to the bathroom. Small reddish blue area noted on right shoulder. Dr. notified of patient's status. X-ray ordered as requested by doctor. Patient assisted back to bed, and call bell placed within his reach. Instructed to call for assistance to get out of bed. The side rails were down when the patient fell. Also, the patient did not complain of pain.

4. **Which of the following methods of nursing documentation only requires the nurse to provide a narrative description of the patient's condition when there is a deviation from the accepted norm?**

A. Charting by exception

B. Focus charting

C. Narrative charting

D. PIE charting

E. SOAP notes

5. **Which of the following situations requires the nurse to provide a report of the patient's status?**

   A. Change of shift
   B. Patient transport to another department for test, procedures, or treatment
   C. Before the nurse takes a lunch break
   D. A and B
   E. All of the above

ANSWERS

Routine Checkup

1. Sender
   Message
   Channel
   Receiver
   Feedback
2. True.

Review Questions

1. D
2. E
3. C
4. A
5. E

References

Berman A, Snyder SJ, Fandsen G: *Kozier & Erb Fundamentals of Nursing: Concepts, Process and Practice,* 10th ed. Boston, MA: Pearson, 2016.

Levetown M: Communicating with children and families: from everyday interactions to skill in conveying distressing information. *Pediatrics.* 2008;121:1441-1460.

Potter PA, Perry AG, Stockert P, Hall A: *Fundamentals of Nursing,* 9th ed. St. Louis, MO: Elsevier, 2017.

Wilkinson JM, Treas LS, Barnett KL, Smith MH: *Fundamentals of Nursing Vol. 1: Theory, Concepts, and Applications.* Philadelphia, PA: FA Davis, 2016.

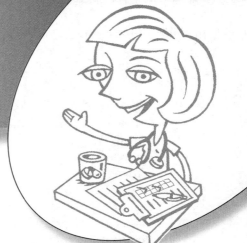

Chapter 4

Vital Sign Assessment

LEARNING OBJECTIVES

At the end of the chapter, the reader will be able to:

1. Discuss variables that may alter a patient's vital signs.

2. Describe how the body conserves and loses heat.

3. State the correct placement of the thermometer for each route of temperature assessment.

4. Describe the procedure for determining a pulse deficit.

5. Describe respiratory characteristics that are assessed during routine vital sign assessment.

6. Describe influencing factors that may affect the accuracy of oxygen saturation measurements.

7. Discuss procedural errors that may alter the accuracy of blood pressure readings.

8. Describe the correct procedure for obtaining a blood pressure that reflects an accurate systolic reading.

KEY WORDS

Apnea	Metabolism
Arrhythmia	Orthostatic hypotension
Bradycardia	Pulse
Bradypnea	Pulse deficit
Core body temperature	Pulse oximetry
Cyanosis	Sphygmomanometer
Diastolic blood pressure	Stethoscope
Dyspnea	Sublingual
Dysrhythmia	Systolic blood pressure
Eupnea	Tachycardia
Expiration	Tachypnea
Frenulum	Thermoregulation
Hypertension	Tympanic
Hypotension	Vasoconstriction
Inspiration	Vasodilation
Korotkoff sounds	Ventilation

Overview

A basic tool that nurses use in caring for patients is vital sign assessment. Vital signs answer basic questions about the patient's health status. The absence of a pulse, respirations, or blood pressure literally means that life has ceased to exist. Temperatures that are at either extremes of high or low may also result in death.

Many variables affect a patient's vital signs, including age, activity level, environment, stress levels, medications, health status, and so on. Nurses must use critical thinking skills and take into consideration all variables when interpreting the significance of vital sign findings (Table 4–1). When possible, influencing factors should be eliminated or minimized. If this is not possible, their presence should be documented.

The patient's baseline vital signs should also be reviewed. Doing so helps to determine whether intervention is required. For example, if a patient has had a temperature ranging from 101.8°F to 103°F over the past 24 hours and the current temperature reading is 101.4°F, the nurse would be correct to interpret this finding as a continued improvement in the patient's temperature. But if the nurse did not take into consideration the previous temperature data, he or she may erroneously interpret the significance of the current temperature (eg,

TABLE 4–1	Critical Thinking Applied to Vital Sign Interpretation			
	Vital Signs			
Influencing Factors	**Temperature**	**Pulse**	**Respirations**	**Blood Pressure**
Age	• Greater variation during infancy • ↓ Temperature related to increase surface loss for infants and elderly people	↓ Pulse with increased age	↓ Respirations with increased age	↑ BP with increased age
Activity and stress	• ↑ Activity or stress ↑ Temperature	↑ Pulse with increased activity	↑ Respirations with increased activity	↑ BP with increased activity
Environment temperature	↑ Environmental temperature ↑ Body temperature ↓ Environmental temperature ↓ Body temperature	↑ Environmental temperature ↑ pulse ↓ Environmental temperature ↓ pulse	↑ Environmental temperature ↑ body temperature, which may ↑ respiratory rate	
Medications	↑ Temperature related to hypersensitivity reaction to medication	Stimulants ↑ pulse Depressants ↓ pulse	Narcotics, sedatives, hypnotics, and general anesthetics ↓ respiratory rate	Antihypertensives and opioids ↓ BP Decongestants, certain illicit drugs, oral contraceptives may ↑ BP
Disease and others	↑ Temperature with infections, hyperthyroidism ↓ Temperature with hypothyroidism	↑ Pulse with acute pain, hemorrhage, infection Cardiovascular disease cause irregular pulse	↓ Respiratory rate with acute pain, anemia, smoking, altitude ↑ Respiratory rate with head trauma injury involving brain stem	Kidney disease, cardiovascular disease, pain may all ↑ BP BP may ↓ hemorrhage, heart attack, and change to upright position (orthostatic or postural hypotension)

BP = blood pressure.

notify the doctor that patient has started running a fever or possibly order laboratory work that was only required at the first evidence of a temperature elevation). The remainder of this chapter is devoted to taking a closer look at each one of the vital signs.

Temperature

Thermoregulation

Proper functioning of life-sustaining body processes rests on maintaining an optimal environment. This includes maintaining the **core body temperature** (ie, temperature deep inside the body) within a narrow range. Regulation of the core body temperature, **thermoregulation**, is achieved by maintaining a balance between heat production and heat loss. To warm the body, the hypothalamus sends out a signal that causes shivering. Shivering in turn increases **metabolism** (energy production), which in turn increases body heat. **Vasoconstriction**, narrowing of the blood vessels, occurs simultaneously. The combined effect is heat conservation or heat production depending on the needs of the body. When the body is too hot, the hypothalamus sends out a signal that triggers sweating. Additionally **vasodilation**, expansion of the blood vessels, occurs to increase the flow of blood to vessels close to the body surface. The blood is then cooled through the processes of radiation, conduction, convection, and evaporation (Table 4–2).

Behavioral factors also influence thermoregulation. It is almost instinctual to add or remove covers and adjust the thermostat controls to achieve a

TABLE 4–2 Heat Loss Mechanisms

Mechanism	Definition	Example
Conduction	Heat loss by transfer from a warmer surface to a cooler surface via direct contact	Warm baby on a cool scale
Radiation	Heat loss by transfer from a warmer surface to a cooler surface that is not in direct contact	Bed occupied by a patient positioned close to an outside window during a cold month
Convection	Heat loss that occurs when cool air blows across a warmer surface	Fan blowing on a patient who has an elevated temperature
Evaporation	Heat loss that occurs when liquid such as sweat or water on the body surface changes to a gas	Cooling effect of lukewarm water as it dries from the surface of the body

comfortable environmental temperature range. Having the ability to sense the need to make such adjustments should be taken into consideration when conducting the health assessment. Nurses should not assume that all individuals will have the resources or cognitive ability to make adjustments that most people often take for granted.

Temperature Variations

The normal temperature range is influenced by the patient's activity level, age, environmental temperature, hormones, route of assessment, stress level, and time of day the temperature is taken. Other variations in the body may be the result of actual disease processes. Table 4–3 includes a brief description of selected temperature deviations.

Procedural Tips

Sites

The four commonly used routes for temperature measurement are the oral, tympanic, axillary, temporal, and rectal routes. Other less commonly used routes include the esophagus, pulmonary artery, and urinary bladder. The oral route can be used for adults and older children. However, in some situations, the oral route is contraindicated, such as when a patient has had oral surgery

TABLE 4–3 Temperature Deviations	
Terms	**Description**
Fever, hyperthermia, or pyrexia	Elevated temperature outside of the normal range
Malignant hyperthermia	Serious inherited condition characterized by rapid increase in temperature up to ≤105°F and muscle contraction when the individual receives general anesthesia
Heat exhaustion	Condition that occurs over the course of several days as a result of exposure to extreme heat in the absence of adequate fluid intake
Heat stroke	Emergent condition in which the temperature regulation fails and the temperature rises quickly to high level; the end result may be permanent disability or death
Hypothermia	Decreased temperature outside the normal range
Frostbite	Condition in which there is damage to the skin as result of exposure to extreme cold; the most common sites for frostbite are the fingers, toes, ears, and nose

or is having difficulty breathing. The **tympanic** (eardrum) temperature, which is obtained by inserting the probe of the tympanic thermometer into the external ear canal, is also a commonly used route. This method is minimally invasive, readings can be obtained rather quickly, and some sources suggest that tympanic readings closely reflect the core body temperature. It would not be appropriate to use the tympanic route if the patient has any type inflammatory ear condition or ear surgery. The axillary route is sometimes used as well; however, it is not the preferred route because it requires a significantly longer period of time to assess, and it reflects the body surface temperature instead of the core body temperature. The rectal route is the most reliable method of obtaining the core body temperature, but it is more invasive than the oral, tympanic, temporal, and axillary routes. Rectal temperature assessment is contraindicated when the patient has diarrhea, certain cardiac conditions, or rectal bleeding or has undergone rectal surgery.

Correct placement of the thermometer during temperature measurement is required without exception. Incorrect placement may result in an inaccurate reading or injury in some instances. The oral thermometer should be placed under the tongue in the posterior **sublingual** (under the tongue) pocket on either side of the **frenulum** (strip of tissue that attaches the underside of the tongue to the floor of the mouth in the midline) (Figure 4–1). The rectal thermometer should be inserted into the anal opening. The insertion distance varies depending on the age of the patient. The nurse should ensure that the tip of the thermometer is in contact with the skin of the armpit when placing a thermometer for axillary temperature measurement. The nurse should inspect the patient's ear canal, carefully remove excess earwax, or choose an alternate route

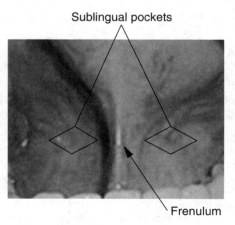

FIGURE 4-1 · Oral thermometer placement.

if removing earwax is not possible (the patient's ear may require ear irrigation). Additionally, the ear lobe should be gently pulled up and back for adults and children 3 years of age and older and down and back for children younger than 3 years of age to ensure correct placement of the tympanic thermometer.

Equipment

Traditionally, the temperature was assessed using a glass thermometer. This is no longer the case; in fact, the use of glass thermometers is discouraged because of the danger of mercury poisoning and injury from glass breakage. Instead, electronic thermometers, including tympanic thermometers, are more commonly used in healthcare settings today. One-time disposable strips are also available for use but are more often used in the home setting. In each of these cases, the correct disposable covering should be placed over the thermometer probe to prevent the transmission of microorganisms. Additionally, when assessing the rectal temperature, a water-based lubricant should be used on the probe cover.

NURSING ALERT

Infection Connection
Never assume that a thermometer color coded blue has only been used orally and that a thermometer color coded red has only been used rectally—QSEN Competency 5: safety.

NURSING ALERT

Infection Connection
When providing care to patients in the home setting the nurse should discourage the use of glass thermometers and teach the patient and caregivers about the danger of mercury poisoning—QSEN Competency 5: safety.

✔ ROUTINE CHECKUP 1

1. _____ of blood vessels conserves heat, and _____ of blood vessels causes heat loss.

Answer:

2. Tympanic temperature readings are thought to closely reflect core body temperature. True/false?

Answer:

Pulse

Have you ever been standing along the beach shore and saw a boat past by in the distance. A little while later, you see waves come in that begin to hit the seashore. A similar process occurs when the heart contracts. The contraction causes pulsations to radiate out to the aorta and all the blood vessels that extend off the aorta. As a result, we are able to feel the pulsations at various points on the patient's body (Figure 4–2). We refer to this as the patient's **pulse.**

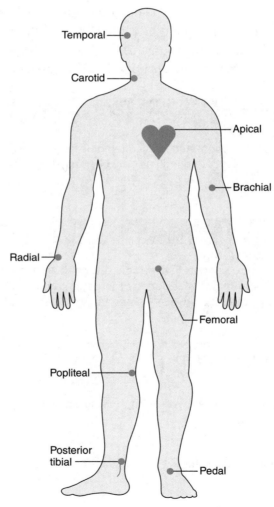

FIGURE 4–2 · Pulse points.

Pulse Characteristics

An assessment of the pulse includes a determination of the rate of the pulse as well as an evaluation of the quality of the pulse.

Rate

The normal pulse rate varies depending on the age of the individual. Typically, the younger the patient, the faster the pulse; for example, a pulse rate of 120 bpm is perfectly normal for an infant but would raise concern if present in an adult. A pulse that is too slow is called **bradycardia**, and a pulse that is too fast is called **tachycardia**.

Quality

The quality of the pulse includes the rhythm and strength of the pulse. The pulse is usually regular in rhythm. A **dysrhythmia** or **arrhythmia** occurs when the interval between beats is irregular. The strength of the pulse is affected by the volume of blood pumped from the heart with each contraction in combination with the elasticity of the blood vessels. Picture in your mind water streaming from a water hose. If you place your hand at the end of the hose, you can feel an increase in the pressure of the water as you increase the flow of water through the hose (the same as increasing the volume of blood pumped from the heart). If you add a sprayer (which is a metal and has no elasticity) to the end of the hose, the pressure increases even more (the same as the increased volume of blood flowing through hardened arteries). When describing the strength of the pulse terms such as *weak*, *firm*, *full*, and *bounding* may be used or a numerical scale may be used.

Procedural Tips

Sites

The most common site used to assess the pulse for routine vital sign assessment is the radial pulse. The radial pulse is located on thumb side of the inner wrist. A watch with a second hand is the only equipment required to assess the pulse. In emergency situations such as when a patient is believed to be experiencing a cardiac arrest, the carotid pulse, which is located in the neck, is assessed. The carotid arteries should be palpated one at a time. Palpating both carotids at the same time may significantly impair the flow of blood to the brain. During the physical assessment, other pulses—such as the temporal, femoral, pedal, and apical pulses—may be assessed. If the apical pulse is assessed, a stethoscope is needed.

Technique

To assess the radial pulse, place the first two to three fingers in the groove located on the thumb side of the patient's inner wrist. Apply light but firm pressure. Initially, you may not be able to feel the pulse; release the amount of pressure applied until you feel the pulse. Evaluate the strength, rhythm, and rate of the pulse. If the pulse is irregular, note whether there is a pattern to the irregularity. If the pulse is regular, determine the rate by counting the number of beats palpated in 30 seconds and multiply that number by 2. The pulse should be counted for 1 full minute any time it is irregular or there is a deviation in the quality of the pulse. To fully assess the adequacy of a specific pulse, it may be necessary to compare the pulse at one site with the pulse at another site. For example, comparing the pedal pulse on the top of both feet may reveal that one is stronger than the other. This information may assist with determining if the circulation to the foot with the weaker pulse is impaired. In some instances, the **pulse deficit**, which is the difference between the apical pulse and radial pulse, may need to be determined. Two people are required to obtain the pulse deficit. One individual counts the apical heart rate, and the other counts the radial pulse beats. Both start and stop counting at the same time.

Respirations

Breathing is the body's way of taking in oxygen and getting rid of carbon dioxide. It also assists with maintaining acid–base balance on a short-term basis. Accurate assessment of the respiratory status is very important because it provides information that, if acted on in a timely manner, could save a person's life. In contrast, failing to recognize cues provided in respiratory assessment data could be deadly.

Respiratory Characteristics

The act of breathing involves taking oxygen into the lungs, or **inspiration**, and expelling carbon dioxide from the lungs, or **expiration**. One respiration or **ventilation** is equivalent to one inspiration plus one expiration. When assessing respirations during vital sign assessment, the nurse counts the number of respirations and observes the rhythm and depth.

Rate

The respiratory rate is measured by counting the number of respirations (inspiration/expiration cycles) occurring in a certain time interval. If the rate falls within the normal range for the patient, the term **eupnea** is used. **Tachypnea** refers to a respiratory rate that is too fast, and **bradypnea** describes an abnormally slow rate of breathing. The complete absence of breathing is referred to as **apnea**.

Rhythm

The rhythm is assessed by observing the pattern of the rise and fall of the chest. Normally, there are equal intervals between the rise and fall of the chest or a regular rhythm. Symmetry should also be noted. Symmetry is evaluated by comparing the movement of the right side of the chest with the movement of the left side of the chest; both sides should move at the same time.

Depth

Depth is evaluated by looking at how much the chest expands. Does it expand a little or a lot? During routine vital sign assessment, the nurse makes a subjective evaluation of the depth of breathing. Minimal expansion of the chest on a consistent basis signifies shallow breathing. Deep breathing is signified by consistent overexpansion of the chest wall. Table 4–4 provides a summary of common variations in breathing patterns.

TABLE 4–4 Breathing Pattern Variations

Variation	Description
Apnea	Absence of breathing
Bradypnea	Slow breathing rate
Tachypnea	Fast breathing rate
Kussmaul	Fast, deep gasping breathing as seen with diabetic ketoacidosis
Biot's	Shallow breathing with variable intervals of apnea
Cheyne-Stokes	Cycle in which respirations gradually increase in rate and depth, peak, and then decrease followed by a period of apnea

Procedural Tips

A watch with a second hand is required to count the respiratory rate. The patient should not be aware that the respiratory rate is being evaluated because he or she may alter the pattern of breathing. It is important to position the patient so that chest and abdominal movement are easily visible. The type of clothing that the patient is wearing sometimes impairs visualization of chest and abdominal movement. Therefore, it is a good idea to also place your hand in contact with the chest wall or abdomen to feel the fall and rise of the chest. When possible, it is also a good idea to have the neck, chest, and abdominal areas exposed so you can visualize the pattern and depth of chest movement. To determine the respiratory rate, count the number of inspiration/expiration cycles (1 respiration) for 30 seconds and multiply by 2. To ensure accuracy, begin counting with the first inspiration within the 30-second time period and end counting with the last expiration within the 30-second time frame. Count respirations for 1 minute if the patient has an irregular respiratory rhythm or respiratory difficulty. While counting the respirations, also observe the rhythm, depth, symmetry of chest movement, and breathing effort.

NURSING ALERT

Patient Privacy
When assessing the breathing pattern, ensure that adequate privacy is provided during visualization of the patient's chest!—QSEN Competency 1: patient-centered care.

It is also important to observe whether the patient has any apparent signs of **dyspnea** (difficulty breathing) or inadequate oxygenation. Is the patient gasping for breath or experiencing **cyanosis** (bluish discoloration resulting from decreased oxygen), especially in and around the mouth? What position is the patient assuming? Is there noisy breathing?

Pulse oximetry, which provides an indirect measurement of the oxygen level in the blood (SpO_2), may be included as a part of the respiratory evaluation when the patient is at risk for or actually experiencing respiratory distress. A pulse oximeter and the correct probe are needed if oxygen saturation is to be measured. The most common sites for oxygen saturation measurement are the earlobe, finger, and sole of the foot. The site must be free of moisture and have good circulation. Nail polish must be removed if a digit (finger or toe) is used. An alternate site must be chosen if the patient has acrylic or gel nails. Other variables that influence the accuracy of the SpO_2 include the hemoglobin level, the temperature of the site (hypothermia causes vasoconstriction), and the oxygen use. If pulse oximetry is included, apply the probe to the site, ensure that pulse reading on the oximeter is consistent with the patient's actual pulse, and record the reading from the display when the value is stable.

✔ ROUTINE CHECKUP 2

1. A pulse that is too fast is called _____, and a pulse that is too slow is called_____.

Answer:

2. The respiratory rate should be counted for _____ if the patient has an irregular breathing pattern or difficulty breathing.

Answer:

Blood Pressure

The blood pressure is a measurement of the pressure exerted by blood flowing through the arteries at two points—when the heart is contracting, which is the **systolic blood pressure**, and when the heart is relaxing, which is the **diastolic blood pressure**. The same two factors that determine the strength of the pulse—the volume of blood circulating and the elasticity of the blood vessels—affect the blood pressure. As the volume of blood increases or the elasticity of the blood vessels decreases, the blood pressure increases. The blood pressure decreases when the volume of blood flow decreases or the elasticity of the blood vessels increases.

Blood Pressure Variations

Various factors influence the blood pressure. Some factors can be controlled, and others cannot. Controllable factors include stress, diet, smoking, and medications. Uncontrollable variables include the person's age, gender, and race. **Hypertension** (high blood pressure) and **hypotension** (low blood pressure) are the two main blood pressure deviations that may occur. Hypertension occurs most often as a result of the controllable and uncontrollable variables mentioned previously. Diseases affecting the heart, blood vessels, and kidneys contribute to the development of hypertension. Consequences of persistent hypertension include stroke and heart attack. Hypotension occurs less frequently than hypertension. Hypotension may occur when there is a significant blood loss or dehydration and in some cases with sudden changes in positioning (**orthostatic hypotension**). Some medications may also cause hypotension.

Procedural Tips

The blood pressure is usually measured while the patient is sitting or lying down. The environment should be quiet, and the patient should be calm and relaxed. The equipment required to assess the blood pressure includes a **stethoscope** (instrument that transmits sounds through a rubber tube from the source to the listener's ears) and a **sphygmomanometer** that includes a cuff and measuring component for determining the arterial blood pressure. The arm size should be determined, and the appropriate cuff size should be selected. A cuff that is too big will result in a false low reading, and a cuff that is too small will result in a false high reading. The cuff should also be checked for proper functioning (gauge and bladder). The end piece of the stethoscope should be checked for damage, and the earpieces should be the right fit for the listener's ears. The most common site for assessing the blood pressure is the arm. If the arm is used, it should be positioned at the level of the heart. After the blood pressure cuff is appropriately applied to the arm, the brachial or radial pulse should be located and palpated while the blood pressure cuff is being inflated. The point at which the pulse is no longer palpable should be noted, and the cuff should be inflated 30 mm Hg above this point. While the nurse is still palpating for the pulse, the cuff should be slowly deflated until the pulse reappears. The cuff should then be completely deflated, and the arm should be allowed to rest for 1–2 minutes. When the cuff is reinflated, it should be inflated 30 mm Hg above the number where the pulse was last felt during palpation. Doing so will assist the examiner in obtaining an accurate systolic reading (Box 4–1). The cuff is then gradually deflated while the examiner listens for the **Korotkoff sounds** (pulsating sounds heard during blood pressure assessment). The first sound heard represents the systolic blood pressure, and the last sound heard represents the diastolic blood pressure.

Vital Sign Documentation

Methods of documenting the vital signs vary depending on the type of healthcare setting. In a doctor's office, the vital signs may simply be included in the narrative note in the patient's medical record. In the hospital setting, the vital

BOX 4–1
Procedure Tip: Blood Pressure Auscultatory Gap

In some patients, the Korotkoff sounds temporarily disappear. This is called an auscultatory gap. In patients with an auscultatory gap, the true systolic blood pressure may be missed if the blood pressure cuff is not inflated above the gap. The following procedure is used to prevent obtaining a false low systolic blood pressure.

While palpating the brachial or radial pulse inflate the cuff until the pulse disappears	Inflate the cuff an additional 30 mm Hg
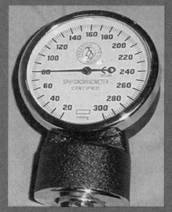	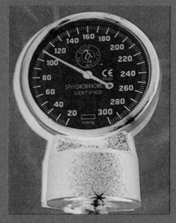
Pulse last palpable at 80 mm Hg	Inflate the cuff to 110 mm Hg (80 mm Hg +30 mm Hg)

Then slowly deflate the cuff. You should feel the reappearance of the pulse at approximately the same point as it disappeared during inflation. This serves as a double check of the point where the pulse disappeared.

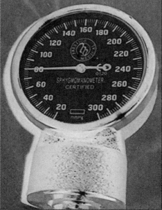

The pulse is palpable again at 80 mm Hg. This finding lets you know that you correctly identified the disappearance point for the pulse during inflation.

BOX 4–2
Temperature Scales

- Fahrenheit to Celsius (larger to smaller; thus use the smaller fraction and subtract)
  $C = (F - 32°) ´ 5/9$ ex: $C = (97.1 - 32°) \times 5/9$: $65.1 \times 5/9 = 36.2°C$
- Celsius to Fahrenheit (smaller to larger; thus use the larger fraction and add)
  $F = (C \times 9/5) + 32$ ex: $F = (38° \times 9/5) + 32$: $68.4 + 32 = 100.4°F$

signs, especially the temperature, are usually recorded on a graph. This method allows for easy visualization of trends and patterns. The site or route used, unit of measurement (Fahrenheit or Celsius) (Box 4–2), and position of the patient are also documented. The vital signs should be documented in the patient's medical record as soon as possible after they are obtained to minimize faulty recall of measurements. Consistency is very important. The same units of measurement and the same route/site should be used when possible.

Qualitative information about the vital signs, such as the rhythm, depth, signs of distress, and influencing variables, is documented in the narrative notes. Any time there is a deviation that has not occurred previously, the finding should be documented and verbally reported in a timely manner. Many facilities are also moving toward the use of electronic medical records. Some electronic records are kept at the patient's bedside, which promotes accurate documentation and ready access to previously recorded measurements. Additionally, electronic records sometimes allow remote access to vital signs by other healthcare team members in a very timely manner.

NURSING ALERT

Avoid Calculated Guesses
Rectal temperature 1° > Oral temperature
Axillary temperature 1° > Oral temperature
Caution! Leave the adding and subtracting to the mathematicians. Record just what you assess and document the route (eg, 99.1°F orally)—QSEN Competency 5: safety.

Just as there are electronic medical records, we also are relying increasingly more on electronic equipment for vital sign measurement. In most instances, this is advantageous, but we must always be mindful that equipment can malfunction and be prepared to manually assess vital signs when necessary.

Conclusion

It was no arbitrary decision that the name *vital signs* was chosen to describe the temperature, pulse, respiration, and blood pressure because each one of these measurements gives clues about the status of a person's life. Thus, it is critical for nursing students to master the techniques for obtaining and interpreting these measurements. Key points presented in this chapter include:

- Assessment of influencing variables and baseline data is critical in determining the significance of current vital sign findings.
- Proper patient preparation and equipment use are required to ensure accurate measurement data.
- Qualitative data, such as rhythm, depth, strength, and so on, are just as significant as quantitative data.

REVIEW QUESTIONS

1. **A patient is being seen in the doctor's office for an ear irrigation. You are preparing to obtain the vital signs. Which route of temperature assessment should you avoid using?**
   A. Axillary
   B. Oral
   C. Rectal
   D. Tympanic

2. **Which of the following describe(s) the technique(s) that should always be included when assessing the pulse?**
   A. Palpate the pulse for 1 minute.
   B. Place two or three fingers on the thumb side of the patient's inner wrist and apply firm but light pressure.
   C. Evaluate rate, rhythm, depth, symmetry, and strength.
   D. B and C
   E. All of the above

3. **All of the following breathing patterns would cause concern EXCEPT:**
   A. Apnea
   B. Bradypnea
   C. Dyspnea
   D. Eupnea

4. **You are counting the respiratory rate for a patient with a regular breathing pattern and no respiratory distress. To correctly assess the respiratory rate, you should:**

A. Begin counting with the first inspiration and end counting with the last expiration within the 30-second time frame. Multiply the total number of complete inspiration/expiration cycles by 2.

B. Begin counting with the first inspiration and end counting with the last expiration within the 60-second time frame. Add up the total number of complete inspiration/expiration cycles.

C. Begin counting with the first inspiration or expiration and end counting with the last inspiration. Add up the total number of inspirations and expirations within the 30-second time frame and multiply by 2.

D. Begin counting with the first inspiration or expiration and end counting with the last inspiration. Add up the total number of inspirations and expirations within the 60-second time frame.

5. **Which of the following factors may alter the accuracy of pulse oximetry readings?**

A. Anemia

B. Acrylic or gel nails

C. Hypothermia

D. A and C

E. All of the above

6. **When assessing a patient's blood pressure, the nurse last palpates the brachial pulse at 90 mm Hg. When the nurse reinflates the cuff to auscultate the blood pressure, it should be inflated to:**

A. 60 mm Hg

B. 90 mm Hg

C. 120 mm Hg

D. 160 mm Hg

ANSWERS

Routine Checkup 1

1. Vasoconstriction, vasodilation.
2. True.

Routine Checkup 2

1. Tachycardia, bradycardia.
2. 1 minute.

Review Questions

1. D
2. B
3. D
4. A
5. E
6. C

References

Berman A, Snyder SJ, Fandsen G: *Kozier & Erb Fundamentals of Nursing: Concepts, Process and Practice,* 10th ed. Boston, MA: Pearson, 2016.

Potter PA, Perry AG, Stockert P, Hall A: *Fundamentals of Nursing,* 9th ed. St. Louis, MO: Elsevier, 2017.

Venes D, ed: *Taber's Cyclopedic Medical Dictionary,* 23th ed. Philadelphia, PA: FA Davis, 2017.

Wilkinson JM, Treas LS, Barnett KL, Smith MH: *Fundamentals of Nursing Vol. 1: Theory, Concepts, and Applications.* Philadelphia, PA: FA Davis, 2016.

Additional Resources

www.cdc.gov

https://medlineplus.gov/videosandcooltools.html

UpToDate. Available at http://patients.uptodate.com/topic.asp?file=othr_inf/21242.

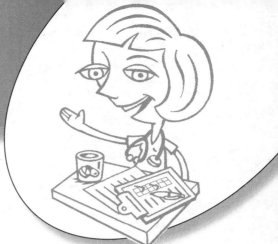

Chapter 5

Health Assessment

At the end of the chapter, the reader will be able to:

1. Discuss the purpose of performing a health assessment.
2. Identify two factors that influence the effectiveness of the interview process while obtaining a health history.
3. Briefly describe information that is usually collected for each category of the health history.
4. Describe each of the four general techniques used when performing a physical assessment.
5. Describe what environmental, equipment, and patient preparation are required before and during the physical examination.
6. Briefly describe each of the major components of the physical examination.

> ## KEY WORDS
>
> | | |
> |---|---|
> | Auscultation | Palpation |
> | Deep palpation | Percussion |
> | Dorsal recumbent | Supine |
> | Inspection | Turgor |
> | Light palpation | Visual acuity |

Overview

Health assessment is the data collection part of the assessment phase in the nursing process. It includes the nursing health history, vital sign assessment, and the physical assessment. It serves as the foundation for the patient's plan of care and is a very important piece of the overall process of providing quality care. The end result of a faulty health assessment will be a faulty plan of care. This chapter includes a discussion of the nursing health history and the physical assessment. Vital signs assessment is covered in depth in Chapter 4.

Nursing Health History

The nursing health history provides a snapshot of the patient's perception of his or her health status and healthcare needs. The nurse interviews the patient to obtain the nursing health history. The nurse must have good interpersonal skills to obtain sufficient and accurate information about the patient. The nurse must also know what types of questions to ask to obtain the desired information. When the goal is to obtain a brief and direct answer, closed-ended questions should be asked. On the other hand, open-ended questions should be used when the patient needs to expand on the topic being discussed. For instance, during the interview, the nurse may ask the patient if he or she is happy (closed-ended question). If the patient's response is yes, there may be no further need for additional information. However, if the patient's response is no, the nurse may ask the patient to tell why he or she is not happy (open-ended question). The amount of information gathered is dictated by the circumstances. Whereas more emergent situations only allow for the collection of the most essential information, routine visits for annual physical examinations allow for the collection of more comprehensive information.

> **NURSING ALERT**
>
> **Health History Tip**
> Be aware of the impact of your nonverbal gestures on what information the patient will be willing to share with you. If the patient perceives disapproval, openness may be diminished, and information disclosed may be limited—QSEN Competency 1: patient-centered care.

Components of the Health History

Headings for the various categories of information collected during the health history may vary from form to form or text to text, but the content is usually very similar and includes the following:

- **Biographical and demographical data:** Include data such as the patient's name, age, gender, birth date, employment information, and insurance information at a minimum.

- **Reason for seeking healthcare:** This is the patient's statement of his or her reason for seeking healthcare at this particular time. The statement should be documented as a direct quotation from the patient. This is a very important component of the health history and should not be omitted because it identifies just how the patient perceives the problem as well as what is most significant about the situation.

- **Present illness or health concern:** After the patient states his or her reason for seeking healthcare, the nurse should probe further to gather additional information about the present illness. Questions about when the problem or concern first occurred, whether or not it is continuous or intermittent, what makes it better, and what makes it worse should be asked.

- **Past illnesses, surgeries, and hospitalizations:** Information about the patient's past illnesses, including those that are chronic in nature and continue to exist as well as previous hospitalization and surgeries, may yield information that explains current issues with the client's health as well as current health practices. For example, a client may reveal that he or she had leukemia as a child and received radiation therapy. This information may provide a valuable piece to the puzzle for an adult who is now suspected of having cancer given the fact that radiation treatment during childhood has been associated with the occurrence of certain types of cancers seen in adults.

- **Medications:** Information about the patient's use of prescribed medications, over-the-counter medications, herbal preparations, and recreational drugs (including tobacco use) should be gathered. Collection of information related to the patient's use of medications can create a very touchy situation. Patients often fear being judged by nurses and other healthcare team members and may withhold information because of this. It is important for the nurse to establish a trusting relationship with the patient and explain just how important it is to gather complete and accurate information. The use of examples may be one way the nurse can convey the importance of the information provided. Examples should not be used as a scare tactic but only to help the patient understand why the information is needed.

- **Allergies:** The patient should be asked to list any known medication allergies (prescribed as well as over the counter) and food allergies. Many times when patients are asked this question, they only think of medication allergies; thus, important that the nurse ensures that the patient understands that information about all allergies, including food, animal, and environmental ones, is needed.

- **Current health and lifestyle patterns:** The client's health practices (eg, eating habits, exercise patterns, self-examination practices, use of preventive health resources) should be explored. Information obtained often provides the foundation for patient teaching. It is important to reinforce positive practices and discourage practices that may be harmful to the patient's health (Box 5–1).

- **Family history:** The family history provides information about the health status of the patient's immediate blood relatives (grandparents, parents, siblings). This information helps to identify the patient's risk for having certain health problems that tend to run in families.

- **Environmental history:** It is important to find out what type of community, work, and home environment the patient is accustomed to.

BOX 5–1
Health Promotion Tip

- Avoid being judgmental.
- Include the patient in identifying alternatives to harmful practices.

Example:

It is easy to tell a patient to stop eating high-fat foods, but will telling the patient be enough to change the behavior? It is usually not enough. There is a greater likelihood of a behavior change if you explore the patient's likes and dislikes and the resources available to the patient and then mutually identify alternatives to the high-fat foods.

Information about the community including but not limited to healthcare facilities, grocery stores, recreation resources, crime/safety should be gathered. Physical characteristics of the home (type of dwelling, utilities, location, number of people living in the home) and workplace (type work, use of chemicals, noise level) should be included as well. Additionally, information should be collected about the psychosocial impact of the community, work environment, and home environment.

- **Psychosocial history:** The psychosocial history provides information about the patient's beliefs and support system. Questions are asked about:
  - Family make-up (eg, single parent, traditional [husband, wife, children], blended, extended)
  - Religious beliefs
  - Other beliefs and values
  - Coping mechanisms
- **Review of systems:** The review of systems portion of the health history allows the nurse to collect subjective information about the various body systems (eg, skin, head, neck, eyes). The review of systems can focus on one or two systems or can include all systems. The nature of the healthcare visit and the type of healthcare issues the patient is experiencing influence how detailed the review of systems is. The information collected during the review of system serves as a valuable guide to determining how to proceed with the physical examination portion of the health assessment (Box 5–2).

ROUTINE CHECKUP 1

1. A successful interview is facilitated by good _____.

Answer:

2. An elaboration on the patient's reason for seeking healthcare is included in which of the following sections of the health history?

   a. Current health and lifestyle patterns
   b. Review of systems
   c. Reason for seeking healthcare
   d. Present illness or health concerns

Answer:

3. The review of systems provides objective information about each one of the patient's body systems. True/false?

Answer:

BOX 5–2
Healthy Community Design Checklist

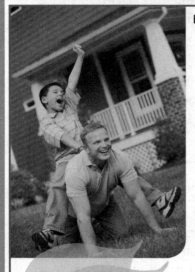

Health starts where you live, learn, work, and play

Your address can play an important role in how long you live and how healthy you are. The physical design of your community affects your health every time you step out your front door. Sometimes making healthy choices is not easy—getting enough exercise is difficult if parks are far away and sidewalks don't exist; eating right is hard when healthy food choices are hard to find. **You** can help make the healthy choice the easy choice. Attend community meetings where decisions are made about how land will be developed, talk with your elected officials, and support policies that make your community healthier.

Your actions can help:

- Reverse the trend in adult and childhood obesity
- Reduce your risk of heart disease, high blood pressure, and diabetes
- Improve air quality
- Reduce traffic injuries
- Make streets safer for people who walk, bike, and drive
- Make the community stronger and more enjoyable for everyone
- Increase safety and reduce crime

A simple checklist is on the back of this sheet. The checklist can help you make decisions about land use in your community that will make everyone happier and healthier. For more information on healthy community design, go to the following Web sites:

Centers for Disease Control and Prevention
Healthy Places
www.cdc.gov/healthyplaces

LEED-ND and Healthy Neighborhoods
www.cdc.gov/healthyplaces/factsheets/LEED-ND_tabloid_Final.pdf

Physical Activity and Health
www.cdc.gov/physicalactivity/everyone/health/index.html

Community Guide to Preventive Services. Environmental and Policy Approaches to Increase Physical Activity: Community–Scale Urban Design Land Use Policies
www.thecommunityguide.org/pa/environmental-policy/communitypolicies.html

U.S. Environmental Protection Agency Smart Growth
www.epa.gov/smartgrowth

University of Minnesota Design for Health
www.designforhealth.net

New York City Department of Design+Construction
www.nyc.gov/html/ddc/html/design/active_design.shtml

National Association of City and County Health Officials
www.planning.org/research/healthy/pdf/electedofficialsfactsheet.pdf

National Center for Environmental Health
Division of Emergency and Environmental Health Services

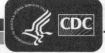

BOX 5–2 (*Continued*)

Health starts where you live, learn, work, and play

I want more options to help me get outside and be more active.
- ❑ Sidewalks
- ❑ Bike lanes
- ❑ Parks/trails/open spaces
- ❑ All my daily needs within walking and biking distance

Other:_____

I want to have healthier and more affordable food choices.
- ❑ Healthier food choices in grocery stores
- ❑ Community gardens
- ❑ Farmers market
- ❑ Fewer liquor/fast food/convenience stores

Other:_____

I want to get around in my community more easily without a car.
- ❑ Better access to public transportation
- ❑ Safer and easier to bike and walk to my daily activities

Other:_____

I want to feel safer in my community.
- ❑ More street lighting
- ❑ Well-marked crosswalks and bike lanes
- ❑ Reduced vehicle speeding on residential streets
- ❑ More "eyes on the street" day and night

Other:_____

I want to have more chances to get to know my neighbors.
- ❑ Pleasant public spaces to gather

Other:_____

I want my community to be a good place for all people to live regardless of age, abilities, or income.
- ❑ Housing for all income levels and types of households
- ❑ Easy for people to get around regardless of age or abilities

Other:_____

I want to live in a clean environment.
- ❑ Reduced air and noise pollution from sources like freeways
- ❑ Clean water supply and proper sewage treatment facilities
- ❑ Soil that is free of toxins from past uses

Other:_____

CS235536-A

Source: https://www.cdc.gov/healthyplaces/factsheets/healthy_community_checklist.pdf.
Centers for Disease Control/National Center for Environmental Health/Division of Emergency and Environmental Health Services.

Physical Examination

The physical examination is the primary source of objective data. It is also a way to collect additional information about concerns and problems that the patient identified during the health history. Additionally, the physical examination helps the nurse to validate information reported by the patient and others. The physical examination may be comprehensive and include all of the body system or may focus only on certain body systems. The following discussion highlights key components of the physical examination and associated techniques. However, it is not intended to provide a comprehensive review of procedures for assessing each body system.

General Techniques

The four basic techniques used throughout the physical assessment are inspection, auscultation, palpation, and percussion. Each one of the techniques allows the nurse to collect valuable information about the patient's health status.

Inspection

Inspection involves using the senses to make observations regarding the patient's health status. A multitude of information can be obtained using this technique. Inspection begins at first contact with the patient and continues throughout the assessment process. General observations during conversation as well as more specific observations made during the examination of specific body systems contribute valuable information about the patient's health status. When inspecting specific parts of the body, it is important to take note of the size, shape, and symmetry as appropriate. Additionally, to maximize the benefit of information obtained, the examiner should have knowledge of normal characteristics as they relate to the particular observation being made. For example, if the examiner does not know that the normal color of the sclera of the eye is white, then observing a sclera that is yellow would not be considered a significant finding to the examiner. The conditions under which inspection take place are just as important as the skillfulness of the examiner. Good environmental lighting, adequate exposure of the body part being examined, and an unrushed approach yield the best results.

Auscultation

Auscultation involves listening to sounds produced by the body with or without the assistance of aids. Auscultation is usually the last of the four basic

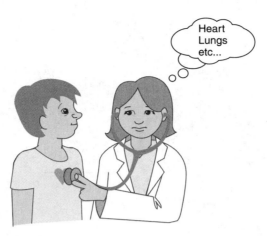

FIGURE 5–1 · Auscultation tip.

techniques to be performed. However, when examining the abdomen, auscultation should be performed prior to palpation and percussion. The order change prevents alterations in the bowel sounds that may occur with manipulation of the abdomen. The examiner needs to have knowledge of what sounds are normal in order to evaluate the significance of findings during auscultation. Although a novice examiner may not be able to determine what specific abnormal sound is being heard, he or she will be able to at least report the presence of a sound that deviates from what is normally heard. To facilitate successful auscultation, the examiner should also:

- Listen for the loudness, frequency, duration, and quality of sounds.
- Picture underlying body structures (eg, heart, liver, stomach) for area being examined (Figure 5–1).
- Listen in a quiet environment.
- Practice listening as much as possible.
- Know how to properly use a stethoscope (Figure 5–2).

Palpation

Palpation is the act of using touch to obtain data during the health assessment. During palpation, the examiner assesses the **turgor** (skin elasticity), temperature (using the back of the hand), texture (using the finger pads), size, and shape of the area being examined (Figure 5–3). During palpation, the examiner should also observe the patient for signs of tenderness (verbal reports as well as nonverbal cues such as grunting and facial grimacing). Known tender

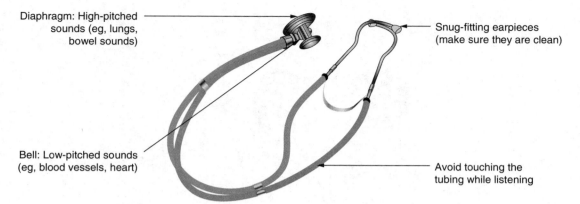

Diaphragm: High-pitched sounds (eg, lungs, bowel sounds)

Snug-fitting earpieces (make sure they are clean)

Bell: Low-pitched sounds (eg, blood vessels, heart)

Avoid touching the tubing while listening

FIGURE 5–2 · Tips for using a stethoscope.

areas should be palpated last. The patient should be relaxed. The examiner should have warm hands and short nails. Two types of palpation may be performed—**light palpation**, which requires the examiner to apply sufficient pressure to palpate structures 1/2 inch (1 cm) below the skin surface, and **deep palpation**, which requires enough pressure to palpate underlying organs

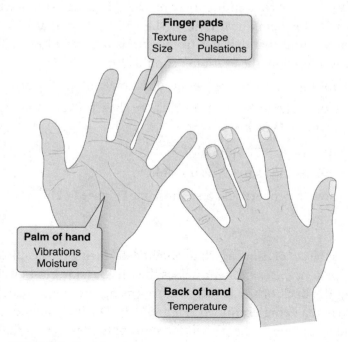

Finger pads
Texture   Shape
Size   Pulsations

Palm of hand
Vibrations
Moisture

Back of hand
Temperature

FIGURE 5–3 · Palpation tips.

1–2 inches (2–4 cm) below the skin surface. Deep palpation can be performed using a single hand or both hands (bimanual). Light palpation should precede deep palpation. Novice examiners should always be supervised when performing deep palpation.

Percussion

Percussion requires touching or tapping an area of the body with the fingertips to evaluate the size, shape, and make-up of the underlying structures (ie, air filled, solid, or liquid). There are two types of percussion. Direct percussion involves tapping the skin surface directly with the fingertips. Indirect percussion requires the use of both hands. The finger of one hand is placed against the skin surface of the area to be percussed while the fingertip of a second finger from the opposite hand is used to tap the skin at the base of the nail bed of the first finger (Figure 5–4).

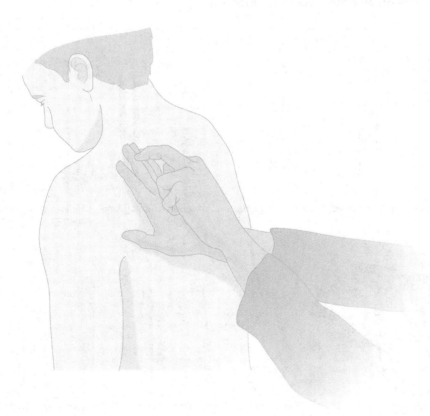

FIGURE 5–4 • Percussion technique. Note: For best results, only the finger (not the hand) should make contact with the area being percussed.

Preparing for the Examination

Before performing the physical examination, the nurse should gather any equipment that may be required, prepare the environment, and prepare the patient.

Equipment and Environmental Preparation

The examination should be performed in a quiet, private setting. The lighting should be checked to ensure that it is adequate for the type of examination being performed.

The type of equipment that will be required will depend on how comprehensive the examination will be (Figure 5–5). Regardless of which equipment is being used, the nurse should make sure it is properly functioning (eg, good batteries or available electrical source, clean if reusable, appropriately sized for the patient and safe for patient use). Additionally, the nurse should use good body mechanics and infection control precautions during the preparation phase and during the actual examination.

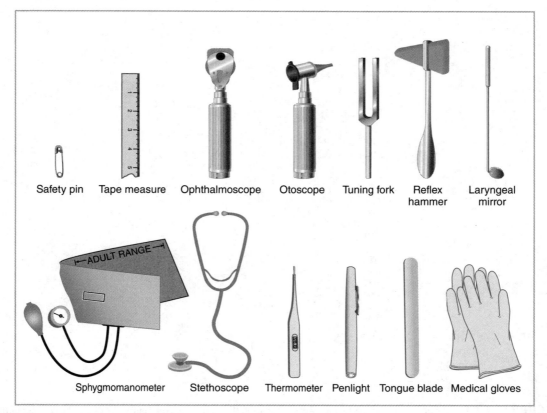

Safety pin   Tape measure   Ophthalmoscope   Otoscope   Tuning fork   Reflex hammer   Laryngeal mirror

Sphygmomanometer   Stethoscope   Thermometer   Penlight   Tongue blade   Medical gloves

FIGURE 5–5 · Common equipment used during the physical examination.

Patient Preparation

The first thing the nurse should do as a part of preparing the patient for the examination is to introduce him- or herself and give a general overview of what will take place during the examination.

Other pertinent information (eg, what will take place at a particular point of the examination, patient teaching information) should be given to the patient as the examination is performed. All instructions and information should be given in terms the patient will understand. The nurse should be sure to take into account the influence of cultural beliefs on the patient's perception of the examination process. Additionally, the nurse should:

NURSING ALERT

Cultural Influences
Before initiating the nursing history and physical examination, the nurse should obtain information about the person's cultural background and beliefs. Doing so will assist the nurse in obtaining the patient's cooperation during the assessment process—QSEN Competency 1: patient-centered care.

- Provide a gown and drape as appropriate to promote privacy (Figure 5–6).
- Promote comfort:
  - Check room temperature.
  - Offer the opportunity to use the bathroom (collect a specimen if needed).
- Evaluate whether the patient can assume the required position(s).
- Always show respect for the patient (do not talk about patient as if he or she is not there).

✔ ROUTINE CHECKUP 2

1. List the four basic techniques used during the physical examination.

Answer:

_____

_____

_____

_____

2. To promote safety, the nurse should use _____ and _____ throughout the examination.

Answer:

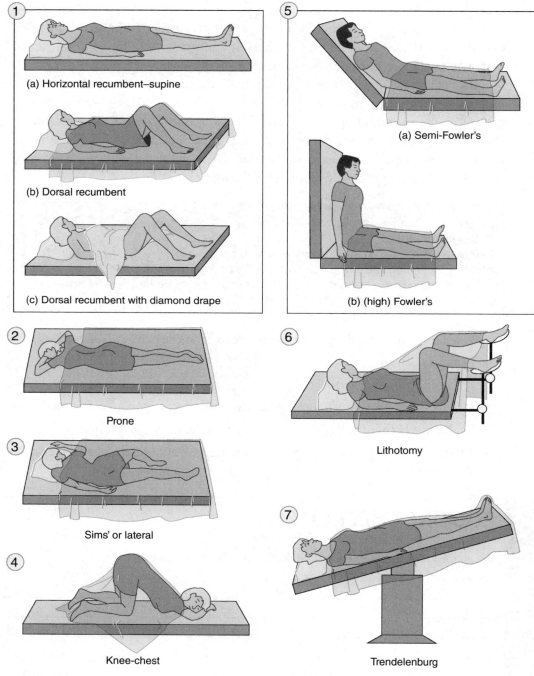

FIGURE 5–6 · Positions and drapes.

Performing the Examination

The depth of the examination should be relevant to the nature of the visit. A systematic approach should be followed to prevent omitting parts of the examination. The examination usually begins with a general survey and proceeds in a head-to-toe order. However, the order may be adjusted depending on the situation. For example, with children, the format may be adapted so that least invasive parts of the examination are performed first and more invasive parts are saved for last. A brief description of each specific component of the physical examination is provided in Table 5–1.

General Survey

Information is gathered about the overall appearance and behavior of the patient. Personal hygiene, signs of distress, and emotional state are examples of specific information that is obtained. Body measurements, such as the height, weight, and body circumferences, may also be gathered at this point in the examination.

Hair, Skin, and Nails

An examination of the hair, skin, and nails may provide cues about the patient's circulation, oxygenation, nutritional status, local skin damage, and certain diseases (eg, liver—jaundice, kidneys—uremic frost).

- **Hair:** The nurse should note the distribution of the patient's hair. Is there any balding? Is there hair located in unusual places? What is the texture of the hair?
- **Skin:** The skin's color, texture, and integrity should be assessed. Also, the nurse should observe for the presence of calluses and corns. Any skin lesions should be examined closely because they may be indicative of serious disorders such as skin cancers or a methicillin-resistant *Staphylococcus aureus* (MRSA) infection.
- **Nails:** The color, thickness, and shape of the nails as well as any signs of nail biting should be noted during the examination. This information may cue the nurse to the presence oxygen deficits, fungal infections, and the presence of stress.

Head and Neck

The head and neck examination include an examination of the patient's eyes, ears, nose, mouth, and throat.

TABLE 5–1 Physical Examination Tips

Category	Equipment Needed	Tips
General survey	Tape measure Scale	Continue observations throughout the entire examination.
Hair, skin, nails	Gloves if there are skin breaks or lesion	May be done all at once or with each body system
Head and neck (also include eyes, nose, mouth, throat, and ears)	Pen light, ophthalmoscope, vision charts, otoscope, tuning fork, tongue blade	During ophthalmoscopic examination, check the patient's right eye with your right eye and vice versa. Perform in a dark room. Clean cerumen (wax) from the ear. Pull the ear up and back for patients 3 years of age and older and down and back for patients younger than 3 years of age.
Chest (include lungs, heart, breast tissue)	Stethoscope	Lung auscultation order: 1→2 ↓ 4→3 Use a systematic process for examining the breast to prevent skipping an area of breast tissue. Use a small pillow or folded towel to distribute tissue evenly. Used the opportunity to teach the patient about self-examination.
Vascular system	Stethoscope	Do not under any circumstances occlude both carotid pulses at the same time. Place the patient in the semi-Fowler position during carotid artery and jugular vein assessment.
Abdomen	Stethoscope	Nine-region assessment may be appropriate for a client who presents with abdominal symptoms.
Musculoskeletal system	Tape measure	Take safety precautions, especially for patients suspected of having muscular weakness.
Nervous system	Reflex hammer, pen light	Give simple clear instructions. Take into consideration the patient's language and cultural influences.
Reproductive system and rectal examination	Gloves, lubricant, vaginal speculum	Patient preferences for the gender of the examiner should be taken into consideration.
Anus and rectum	Gloves, lubricant	Easier to inspect with the patient in the side-lying position. Care should be taken when examining the patient who has hemorrhoids.

- **Head:** The size and shape of the head as well as the symmetry of facial features should be noted.

- **Eyes: Visual acuity**, which is how well the patient can see, is evaluated. Tests to determine eye muscle strength, visual field adequacy, and pupillary response are performed. The nurse should also assess the position and color of the eyes. The ophthalmic examination is performed at this time to evaluate the condition of the internal eye cavity.

- **Nose:** The symmetry of nose placement on the face is noted. Each nostril is inspected with a penlight. The color of the mucous membranes is noted as well as the presence of any lesions, drainage, or swelling. The nurse may also palpate for the presence of tenderness over the sinus areas (just above the eyebrows and on both sides of the nose).

- **Mouth:** The color and symmetry of the lips are noted. The nurse must keep in mind that normal color variations of the lips exist depending on the race of the patient. The inside of the mouth and posterior throat are observed, including the tongue and its undersurface, teeth, tonsils, roof of the mouth (hard and soft palate), and uvula.

- **Neck:** Neck muscle strength, thyroid size, size and shape of lymph nodes, and pulsations of the neck blood vessels are assessed during the neck examination. It is very important that the nurse *does not* examine both carotid arteries in the neck at the same time because this may significantly compromise blood flow to the brain.

Chest

The chest examination includes an assessment of the external chest as well as the lungs, heart, and breast tissue. The nurse should inspect the anterior and posterior chest wall, noting the symmetry of chest movement and the presence of any lesions or discolorations.

- **Lungs:** Lung sounds should be auscultated over the anterior and posterior chest wall with the stethoscope. The chest wall should be percussed and palpated for the presence of abnormal vibrations and to determine the degree of chest expansion. The nurse should make note of the specific location of any abnormal breath sounds. The order of the examination should proceed from one side of the chest to the same location on the opposite side of the chest, then down, and then back to the other side of the chest directly across from the last area auscultated. This allows for comparisons between the various lung fields.

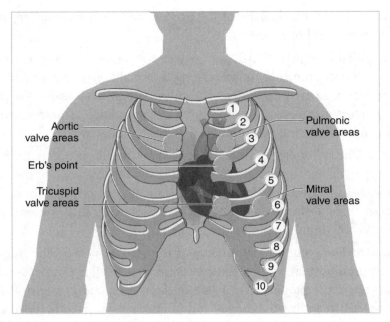

FIGURE 5–7 · Heart assessment: anatomical landmarks.

- **Heart:** The nurse should auscultate over each of the five areas of the heart (aortic, pulmonic, Erb's point, tricuspid area, and mitral area) (Figure 5–7). The rate, quality, and rhythm of the heartbeat should be observed. Novice examiners may not be able to definitively identify abnormal sounds but should be able to identify that a sound is deviating from the normally expected heart sounds and report findings accordingly.

- **Breasts:** Examination of breast tissue is usually performed as a part of the physical examination of female patients. The breasts are examined with the patient standing, bending over, and **supine** (ie, lying on the back). The nurse should observe the vascularity and texture of the skin and palpate the breast tissue and underarm area for the presence of masses or nodules.

Vascular System

The vascular examination consists of assessment of the carotid artery, jugular vein, and peripheral blood vessels. Assessment of the peripheral blood vessels may be done as a part of the examination of the body extremities during the musculoskeletal examination. Information regarding the assessment of peripheral pulses is presented in Chapter 4. In addition to the pulses, the temperature and color of the skin should be evaluated because deviations may suggest the presence of compromised peripheral circulation.

Abdomen

The order of the abdominal examination is modified so that auscultation is performed before palpation and percussion because bowel sounds may be affected by both of these techniques. To successfully perform this portion of the examination, the patient must be relaxed. Placing the patient in the **dorsal recumbent** position (lying on back with knees bent and feet flat on the examination table surface) facilitates relaxation. The abdomen is divided into four regions using the umbilicus as the center point. The nurse should listen for bowel sounds in all four areas of the abdomen, visualize the underlying organ content of the abdominal cavity during the examination, and observe the patient during the examination for signs of pain.

Musculoskeletal System

The musculoskeletal examination is conducted to assess muscle strength and joint mobility. The spine is also inspected, and any abnormal curvatures are noted. If the patient is unable to perform active range of motion, then the examiner should carefully perform passive range of motion to determine just how much mobility the patient has. Throughout the examination, the nurse should observe for any indications of pain.

Nervous System

Central nervous system function and peripheral reflexes are assessed during this portion of the physical examination. The level of consciousness and cognitive ability are evaluated. The cranial nerves are tested, and the reflex responses are assessed. The patient must be in a relaxed state in order for the reflex responses may be accurately assessed. Portions of the neurologic examination may be performed during the assessment of other body systems. For example, the optic nerve assessment may be performed during the eye examination. As the nurse becomes more comfortable with performing physical examinations, he or she may integrate more flexibility in the order of performing the examination and will be guided more by the particular patient situation.

Reproductive System and Anal Examination

The reproductive examination is often combined with the rectal examination. The components of the examination vary depending on the gender of the patient.

- **Female:** Examination of the female reproductive system includes an inspection of the external genitalia, including the pubic hair, clitoris, urethral and vaginal openings, labia, and perineum. The nurse observes for vaginal discharge and odor and for lesions such as warts, chancres, and blisters. The anal area is assessed for external hemorrhoids. Examination of the internal genitalia and rectum is restricted to physicians and advance practice nurses. The nurse may, however, assist with the rectal and internal genitalia examination.

- **Male:** The nurse examines the penis, scrotum, and anal area during this portion of the physical examination. The absence or presence of foreskin is noted. If the foreskin is intact, it is gently retracted, and the head of the penis is observed for lesions and discharge. The scrotum is also examined for any signs of irritation, swelling, or lesions. The testicles are palpated, and the size, shape, and presence of any masses are noted. The anal area is inspected for hemorrhoids just as in the female examination. The nurse should take this opportunity to educate the patient about self-examination of the reproductive tract and hygiene requirements, always doing so in a respectful manner.

Conclusion

The role of the nurse in completing the health assessment has changed from that of being an assistant to an active participation in the process. Thus, it is more important than ever for nurses to master the skills of obtaining a health history and performing a physical examination. The information obtained during the health assessment is not only shared with other members of the healthcare team but is also used as the foundation for the nursing plan of care for the patient. Key points presented in this chapter include:

- The health history provides information about the patient's health practices and how the patient views his or her health status.

- The accuracy of information obtained during the health assessment is affected by multiple human variables, including the nurse's ability to articulate questions in a simple and clear manner, the ability of the nurse to be nonjudgmental, and the patient's trust of the nurse.

- The amount of information obtained during the health assessment is dictated by the nature of the health visit. Visits for emergent care usually do not allow for comprehensive health assessments.

- The nurse is responsible for preparing the examination room, equipment, and the patient for the physical examination.

REVIEW QUESTIONS

1. **When collecting the health history, the nurse should:**
   A. Have the patient give a statement of his or her reason for seeking healthcare at this visit.
   B. Gather information about all allergies, including environmental, food, and medicine allergies.
   C. Gather information about prescription, over-the-counter, and recreational drug use.
   D. All of the above

2. **To accurately assess skin temperature, the nurse should use which part of the hand?**
   A. Back of the hand
   B. Fingertips
   C. Finger pads
   D. Palm

3. **When examining the abdomen, it is BEST to use which of the following orders?**
   A. Inspection, palpation, percussion, auscultation
   B. Inspection, percussion, auscultation, palpation
   C. Inspection, auscultation, palpation, percussion
   D. Auscultation, inspection, percussion, palpation

4. **The nurse should use the bell of the stethoscope to auscultate:**
   A. Blood vessels
   B. Bowel sounds
   C. Lung sounds
   D. All of the above

5. **During the health assessment, the nurse notes that the patient has a history of hypertension, smokes, and is overweight. The nurse can be MOST effective in influencing the patient to adopt positive health practices by:**
   A. Discussing the consequences of hypertension, obesity, and smoking with the patient.
   B. Collaborating with the patient to identify changes he or she is willing to make to control the blood pressure.

    C. Giving the patient a list of healthy foods to eat.

    D. Giving the patient the name, meeting times, and location of a smoking cessation support group.

ANSWERS

Routine Checkup 1

1. Interpersonal skills.
2. d.
3. False.

Routine Checkup 2

1. Inspection
   Palpation
   Auscultation
   Percussion
2. Good body mechanics and infection control precautions.

Review Questions

1. D
2. A
3. C
4. A
5. B

References

Berman A, Snyder SJ, Fandsen G: *Kozier & Erb Fundamentals of Nursing: Concepts, Process and Practice*, 10th ed. Boston, MA: Pearson, 2016.

Potter PA, Perry AG, Stockert P, Hall A: *Fundamentals of Nursing*, 9th ed. St. Louis, MO: Elsevier, 2017.

Venes D, ed: *Taber's Cyclopedic Medical Dictionary*, 23th ed. Philadelphia, PA: FA Davis, 2017.

Wilkinson JM, Treas LS, Barnett KL, Smith MH: *Fundamentals of Nursing Vol. 1: Theory, Concepts, and Applications*. Philadelphia, PA: FA Davis, 2016.

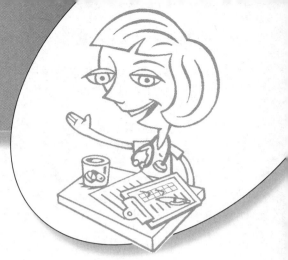

Chapter 6

Medication Administration

LEARNING OBJECTIVES

At the end of the chapter, the reader will be able to:

1. Describe the roles of each of the three key players in the medication administration process.

2. Describe the four pharmacokinetic processes that occur when a medication is administered.

3. Differentiate between a drug action and a drug effect.

4. Describe federally mandated requirements that should be included when administering controlled substances.

5. Describe critical components of each of the six rights of medication administration.

6. Describe the main activities that should take place during each of the five phases of the nursing process.

7. Describe the nurses' role in handling medication errors.

KEY WORDS

Absorption
Distribution
Drug
Drug action
Drug effect
Elimination ˙
Half-life
Intended effect

Medication
Medication reconciliation
Metabolism
Pharmacodynamics
Pharmacokinetics
Pharmacology
Polypharmacy
Unintended effect

Overview

Various plants, animals, and minerals from the earth have been used for their medicinal effects almost since the beginning of time. Our most primitive thought of this activity probably takes us back to the age of the medicine man. Moving to a more recent time in history, we probably think of the doctor who made visits to the home and either gave the patient medications or gave instructions to the family or patient on how to take the medication. Things have changed quite a bit since those times. Although some medications still are derived from plants and animals, others are synthesized in a laboratory or genetically engineered. There are literally thousands of medications available for use. With the increase in the number of medications available comes the increase in the possibility of unwanted interactions and side effects as well as chances for medication errors, some of which can be deadly. Safe medication administration is a shared responsibility. The physician is responsible for prescribing the appropriate medication for the patient, the pharmacist is responsible for dispensing the medication ordered, and the nurse administers the medication to the patient or ensures that the patient understands how to self-administer the medication. To administer medications in a safe and effective manner, the nurse must have the knowledge of basic pharmacological principles as well as medication administration principles. Additionally, the nurse's practice should be guided by the law (federal, state, and local) and by organizational policies. It is imperative that the nurse uses the nursing process as the framework for medication administration and integrates well-developed critical thinking skills throughout the medication administration process. This chapter is devoted to highlighting information relevant to each one of these requirements.

BOX 6–1 Drug Names	
Chemical	Gives description of chemical ingredients and molecular structure. Not commonly used in the clinical setting.
Generic name	Simpler name than the chemical name. Assigned to the drug by the United States Adopted Names Council.
Brand (trade) name	Assigned by the manufacturer. Indicates that the drug is registered by the manufacturer and therefore cannot be used by anyone other than the manufacturer.

Example:
Generic name: Acetaminophen
Brand name: Tylenol

Basic Pharmacological Principles

Pharmacology is the study of drugs and their effects on living organisms. A **drug** is a substance that changes the function of a living organism in some way (Box 6–1). Drugs can be used for pleasure (recreational) or as treatment. A drug that is used for a therapeutic purpose is called a **medication**. Medications are used to diagnose, prevent, and treat various illnesses.

Pharmacokinetics

Pharmacology is broken down into several subcomponents, one of which is pharmacokinetics. **Pharmacokinetics** is the branch of pharmacology that describes what the body does to medications after they enter the body. The four events that occur after a medication enters the body are absorption, distribution, metabolism, and elimination.

- **Absorption** occurs from the time the medication enters the body until the medication enters into circulating body fluids (lymph and blood). The route of administration (Figure 6–1) and the medication form are the two main factors that influence medication administration (Table 6–1).

- **Distribution** occurs when the medication is absorbed into the body fluids. From this point, the medication is taken to its site of action via the circulatory system. Medications that are administered intravenously

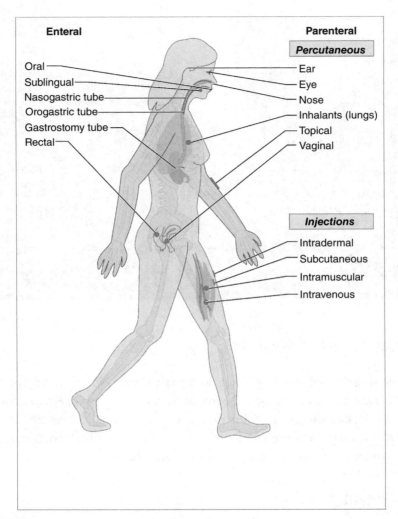

FIGURE 6-1 · Common routes of medication administration.

skip absorption and are immediately available for distribution to the target site.

- **Metabolism** is the process whereby medications are inactivated. The primary site of medication metabolism is the liver. Thus, a person who has liver disease may be given a smaller dose of medication than the person who does not have liver disease because a damaged liver will take longer to complete the inactivation process.

TABLE 6–1 Common Medication Forms		
Category	**Forms**	**Description and Tips**
Solids and semi-solids	Tablets • Enteric coated • Layered • Scored	• Tablets are administered via the oral, sublingual, and vaginal routes. • Many medications come in tablet form. Do not rely on the appearance of a tablet in identifying a medication. • Do not crush enteric-coated or time-released tablets. Doing so may alter the action of the medication or cause stomach irritation. • Partial doses of a tablet may be given *only* if the tablet is scored. Tablets are usually scored in 1/2 or 1/4 parts.
	Capsules	• Capsules consist of a gelatin outside casing that contains the actual medication inside which may be liquid or solid in form. • Do not remove and administer the contents of a time-released capsule. Doing so may alter the medication's action.
	Suppositories	• Semi-solid medication that dissolves when inserted into the prescribed body cavity.
	Creams and ointments	• Semi-solid medication that is most commonly administered topically. Creams are usually rubbed into the skin and do not leave any type of residue. Ointments usually have an oil base.
Liquids	Syrups Elixirs Suspensions Emulsions Lotions	• Syrups are sugar-based medications. Avoid shaking syrups to prevent bubble formation, which may alter the accuracy of the dosage. • Elixirs are usually alcohol-based or water-based medications. • Suspensions must be shaken before being administered because the drug and liquid parts usually separate after the medication stands for a while. • Lotions are for topical use and are usually rubbed into the skin and do not leave any type of residue.
Others	Transdermals Inhalants Sprays	• Transdermals deliver the medication through the skin over a set period of time. • Inhalants are administered either nasally or orally via small particles that allow for easy absorption into the mucous membranes of the respiratory tract.

- **Elimination** is the means by which the body gets rid of the medication. The kidney is the primary site of medication elimination. The rate of elimination of the medicine from the body may impact how often the medication is ordered. The amount of time it takes 50% of the medication to be eliminated from the body is called the medication's **half-life**. A medication that has a long half-life, meaning it will take longer for 50% of the medicine to leave the body, may be given over longer intervals (eg, every 12 hours vs. every 4 hours) and vice versa. The nurse who has an understanding of this principle emphasizes to the patient the importance of taking medications at the prescribed intervals. For example, a patient may be tempted to take a pain medication more often than ordered by the doctor. The nurse should explain to the patient that taking the medication more frequently than prescribed may result in complications associated with an overdose. The nurse should instruct the patient to notify the doctor if the pain medication is not effective in controlling his or her pain.

Pharmacodynamics

Pharmacodynamics explores a drug's action and its effect on the body. The **drug action** includes changes that are occurring at the cellular level (what is going on inside the body that you cannot see). The **drug effect** is the response you are able to see as a result of the drug action. For example, an antihypertensive medication may exert its action by binding to a site, thereby preventing another chemical from attaching to the site. The effect that is produced by this action is that the blood pressure decreases. If the antihypertensive medication had not been given, then the chemical would have attached to the site, and the blood pressure would have gone up. In this example, the **intended effect**, what you want to occur, was that the blood pressure remained in the normal range. Sometimes the patient experiences **unintended effects**, which are effects that you do not want to occur for various reasons. Thus, it is very important for the nurse to be familiar with possible unintended effects of medications (Box 6–2). In some instances, the doctor may have to change the patient's medications because the unintended effects outweigh the benefits of administering the medication.

Legal Guidelines for Medication Administration

The federal government sets guidelines to ensure that medications are safe for use and that they do what the manufactures says they will do. Also, the federal

BOX 6–2
Unintended Drug Effects

Side effect or adverse reaction	Known unintended effects of a medication that you can monitor for and inform the patient to monitor for. Usually can be controlled by a dosage adjustment.
Idiosyncratic reaction	Unpredictable response that most often occurs when a medication is first administered. Thought to have a genetic link.
Allergic reaction	Hypersensitivity to a medication. Can range from mild (itching and hives) to severe (wheezing and respiratory distress or arrest).
Carcinogenic	Medication causes development of cancerous cells.
Teratogenic	Medication causes birth defects.

government sets guidelines for the distribution and use of controlled substances (Table 6–2). Laws at the state and local level may be more stringent than federal laws but cannot require less than what is prescribed by federal laws. The same is true of organizational policies. The policies may be stricter but must, at a minimum, meet the requirements of local, state, and federal laws. Additionally, each state's Nurse Practice Act defines the role of the Registered Nurse and the Licensed Practical Nurse, including boundaries related to medication administration. While each state's Nurse Practice Act is different in some aspects, all define the nurse's role as that of administering medications and require that nurses assume total responsibility for their actions. It is not acceptable for a nurse to administer a medication just because it is prescribed. Instead, the nurse must have complete knowledge of medications he or she administers (eg, recommended amount and frequency, contraindications, side effects) and be familiar with the patient's health history as it may relate to the prescribed medications.

TABLE 6–2 Controlled Substance Schedule

The Controlled Substance Act of 1970 classifies drugs according to their abuse potential. The Drug Enforcement Agency (DEA) is the enforcing agency.

Schedule and Examples	Dependence Potential	Things You Should Know
I • Heroin • Lysergic acid diethylamide (LSD) • Marijuana • Methaqualone	High potential for dependence	• Not approved for medical use • Research use only • Vault or safe storage required • Separate record keeping required
II • Morphine • Phencyclidine (PCP) • Cocaine • Methadone • Methamphetamine	High potential for dependence	• Separate record keeping required • Vault or safe storage required • Written prescription required; no refills allowed
III • Anabolic steroids • Codeine • Hydrocodone with aspirin or acetaminophen	Lower potential for abuse; may lead to moderate to low physical dependence and high psychological dependence	• Readily retrieval records required but do not have to be separate • Secure storage area; does not require a vault or safe • Requires written or oral prescription; refill allowed
IV • Darvon • Talwin • Equanil • Valium • Xanax	Low potential for dependence	
V • Cough medicines with codeine	Low potential for dependence	• Readily retrieval records required but do not have to be separate • Secure storage area; does not require a vault or safe • Some schedule V drugs require a prescription, and those that do not require a prescription still have stricter guidelines for distribution than the non-narcotic over-the-counter drugs

Data from the Department of Justice's Regulatory Requirements Controlled Substances Table. Available at http://www.usdoj.gov/dea/pubs/ abuse/1-csa.htm.

✔ ROUTINE CHECKUP 1

1. Medications that are administered _____ skip absorption and are immediately available for distribution to the target site.

Answer:

2. The drug effect includes changes that occur at the cellular level, whereas the drug action is the response you are able to see as a result of the drug effect. True/false?

Answer:

3. The nurse's role in medication administration is legally defined by the _____.

Answer:

Medication Administration Principles

Although safe medication administration is a shared responsibility of the person ordering the medication, the pharmacist, and the person administering the medication (Table 6–3), the person who actually administers the medication

TABLE 6–3 Key Players in the Medication Administration Process

Role	Cast Member	Responsibility
Prescribe	• Physician • Advance Practice Nurse • Physician assistant	Provides the medication order, including the name of the medication, dosage, route, and frequency verbally (via telephone or face-to-face) or in writing. Written medication orders are entered in the medical record on the physician order form or on a legal prescription pad.
Dispense	• Pharmacist	Accurately labels and dispenses the correct medication, including the correct dosage strength and form. Usually a set amount is dispensed and replenished according to agency policy or what is written on the legal prescription.
Administer*	• Registered Nurse • Licensed Practical/Vocational Nurse	Ensures that the right medication in the right amount and by the right route has been prescribed and dispensed for the right patient. The nurse is also responsible for administering the right medication in the right amount by the right route and at the right time to the right patient. If the nurse does not administer the medication to the patient, he or she is responsible for ensuring that the patient understands how to safely self-administer the medication.

*The medication is usually administered by a Registered Nurse or Licensed Practical Nurse, but in some instances, other members of the healthcare team (eg, physician, nurse practitioner, medical assistant) may assume this role.

BOX 6–3
General Guidelines for Safe Medication Administration

- Wash your hands.
- Prepare medications in a well-lit area.
- Always check medication label against order three times (name, dosage strength, route and form, and so on).
- Always check for allergies.
- Consistently follow the six rights of medication administration.
- Give only medications prescribed by a legally authorized person.
- Only give medications you have prepared; do not leave medications unattended.
- Never give a medication with an altered appearance.
- Never give a medication that you have concerns about (better to be safe than sorry; check with the pharmacist or prescriber).
- Shake medications if required.
- Measure medications at eye level.
- Use universal precautions and sharps precautions as appropriate.
- Safely store medications (separate look-alike, sound-alike medications; label high-alert medications).
- Avoid taking shortcuts and performing work-arounds.
- Always be honest!

can ultimately prevent an unsafe and possibly deadly situation from occurring (Box 6–3). The administration step represents the last chance to ensure that the right person receives the right medication in the right amount by the right route at the right time.

Right Patient

It is absolutely necessary without exception that the nurse makes sure that the right patient is given the ordered medication. The current requirement is that two patient identifiers be used when administering medications. The determination of which two identifiers to use is left up to the organization and should be standardized throughout the organization. Examples of patient identifier combinations include requesting that the patient state his or her full name and full social security number or full name and full date of birth. Additionally, in an inpatient setting, the nurse will also check the name on the patient's identification armband against the name appearing on the medication order. In outpatient settings, such as a physician's office and or clinic, the patient may not be wearing an identification armband; in this case, the patient may be asked to provide some form of identification such as a driver's license. In the home setting, after each individual nurse establishes the patient's identity, then he or she may be allowed to use facial recognition as one of the two patient identifiers. Again, whether this is allowed is an organizational decision.

Right Medication

The right medication can only be given if the prescriber's order is correct, the pharmacist dispenses what the prescriber ordered, and the nurse gives the medication that the prescriber ordered. Mistakes can be made by any of the key player in the medication administration process. Thus, it is crucial that the nurse not make any assumptions. The nurse should:

- Check for inconsistencies between what has been ordered and the patient's medical history, including contraindications, allergies, medical diagnoses, and laboratory values. It is very important that the nurse verify any medication order that is unclear or inconsistent with assessment information obtained during the preparation process.

- Check for discrepancies between what is ordered and what is dispensed. There are numerous look-alike, sound-alike medications (eg, Xanax and Zantac) that could result in the wrong medication being dispensed and given.

- Check the medication label three times to ensure that you have the right medication before giving the medication to the patient.

- If the patient disputes whether or not he or she should be taking the medication that has been ordered, verify that the prescriber has ordered the correct medication.

NURSING ALERT

Prohibited Abbreviations

Abbreviations once accepted for use are now prohibited from being used because of associated safety risk, especially regarding medication administration.

- U or u: Write "unit"
- IU: Write "international unit"
- Q.D., QD, q.d., qd: Write "daily"
- Q.O.D., QOD, q.o.d., qod: Write "every other day"
- Do not use a trailing zero (eg, 0.10); instead, write 0.1
- Always include a leading zero (eg, write 0.1, not .1)
- MS, MSO$_4$, MgSO$_4$: Write out "morphine sulfate" or magnesium sulfate"

QSEN Competency 5: safety.

Right Dose

Giving the patient the right amount of medication is just as important as giving the right patient the right medication. Giving an amount that is less than what has been prescribed may result in the patient's not being adequately treated and may delay recovery from illness and prevent optimal health. It may also cause a resistance to the medication in the future. Giving the patient a dose that is more than what was ordered may create new problems for the patient, some of which could be deadly. Steps to ensure that the right dose is given include:

- Checking the label for the dosage strength
- Performing dosage calculations accurately to ensure that the amount ordered is consistent with what is recommended in drug information sources (eg, the *Physician's Desk Reference*, recommended dosages on the medication label, drug books) and to determine the amount required in the form of the medication that is on hand (Box 6–4)

Right Route

We have already established that the route of medication administration affects how the body processes a medication. To ensure that the intended effect is achieved, the nurse must ensure that the medication route prescribed is appropriate and ensure that the ordered route is used if there are no contraindications. For example, a medication that is ordered by mouth may be contraindicated if the patient has had oral surgery or may not be effective if the patient is experiencing vomiting. Thus, it would not be appropriate to proceed with giving the medication without first consulting with the prescriber or checking to see if the medication has also been ordered by an alternate route. Another example of the significance of giving the medication by the right route can be demonstrated in the situation when the route of administration dictates the amount of medication ordered. Case in point, Toradol, a nonopioid analgesic can be given by mouth (PO), intramuscularly (IM), or intravenously (IV). The recommended amount to be given to adults by mouth should not exceed 40 mg/day. The recommended amount for this same population when given IV should not to exceed 120 mg/day. Thus, if you gave the recommended IV dose to a patient by mouth, you could potentially give the patient three times the prescribe amount per day, which could in turn result in the patient's experiencing increased side effects.

BOX 6–4
Dosage Calculations Crash Course

Basic Steps
- Convert different units to the same units (eg, ounces/milliliters or pounds/kilogram).
- Convert like units to the same size (eg, grams/milligrams).
- Think: Reason for the logical answer. For example, if the doctor ordered 500 mg and you have 250-mg tablets on hand, it is logical that you would give two tablets. Or if the doctor ordered 100 mg of medication and you have 1000 mg/10 cc, you would give 1 cc.
- Calculate the dosage.

Method 1
Dosage ordered (D) over dose on hand (H) times the quantity (Q).

$$\frac{D}{H} \times Q$$

Critical Point: the unit of measurement for D and H must be the same.

Hint: Q represents form amount (eg, mL, tablets, capsules) and should be the label that is attached to your answer.

Example:
Ordered: 500 mg. **(D)**
On hand: 1 g **(H)**/4 mL **(Q)**
Convert 1 g to equivalent of 1000 mg:
1000 mg **(H)**/4 mL **(Q)**

$$\frac{\overset{1}{\cancel{500\ mg}}}{\underset{2}{\cancel{1000\ mg}}} \times 4\ mL = \frac{\overset{2}{\cancel{4\ mL}}}{\underset{1}{\cancel{2}}} = 2\ mL$$

Method 2
Ratio/or proportion: the amount on hand (H) over quantity on hand (Q) is equivalent to the amount ordered (D) over X quantity. Solve for X:

$$\frac{H}{Q} \diagdown \frac{D}{X} \text{ (cross-multiply)}$$

Critical Point: unit of measurement for H and D must be the same.

Hint: Q represents the form amount (eg, mL, tablets, capsules) and will be the label that should be attached to your answer.

Example:
Ordered: 500 mg. **(D)**
On hand: 1 g **(H)**/4 mL **(Q)**
Convert 1 g to equivalent of 1000 mg:
(H)/4 mL **(q)**

$$\frac{\overset{250}{\cancel{1000\ mg}}}{\underset{1}{\cancel{4\ mL}}} = \frac{500\ mg}{X\ mL} \text{ (cross - multiply)}$$

$$250X = 500 \qquad \frac{\overset{1}{\cancel{250}}X}{\underset{1}{\cancel{250}}} = \frac{\overset{2}{\cancel{500}}}{\underset{1}{\cancel{250}}} = 2\ mL$$

- Think again: Is my calculated answer consistent with my logical answer? If not, critique both. Also ask yourself if the amount is reasonable. For example, if you came up with an answer of 10 tablets, is it unusual for you to give a patient 10 tablets at once?

Additional Things to Consider
- Only give a partial tablet if it is scored for the amount calculated!
- Rule of thumb when rounding: ≥0.5 rounds up and <0.5 rounds down. Be careful when rounding and consult with prescriber if there is any question (eg, pediatric patients, elderly patients, patients with liver or kidney disorders).
- In some situations, it may be a good idea to have another person double check your calculations (eg, for high-risk medications such as insulin and heparin).

Right Time

The right time includes the right interval as well as the right time of day. Giving a medication more frequently or less frequently than prescribed has the potential to impact the intended effect of the medication. Also, some medications should be given at a particular time of day. For example, diuretics (medications given to remove excess fluid from the body) are typically given in the morning. Scheduling administration of this class of medication for the evening may prevent the patient from getting adequate rest. Another example of why the time of administration is important can be demonstrated when laboratory tests are ordered in relation to when a medication is given. Altering the time of medication administration without also notifying the laboratory may result in inaccurate laboratory results. This could result in unnecessary dosage adjustments with subsequent negative outcomes.

Right Documentation

Documenting medication administration has been added to the traditional five rights of medication administration, and rightly so. It is critical that other healthcare team members involved in the care of the patient know the amount, time, and route of medications administered to the patient. It is also important for the other healthcare team members to know how the medication is affecting the patient. Were the expected results achieved? Were there any unintended effects? This information is communicated to others via documentation in the medical record. Key points to keep in mind when documenting medication administration include:

- Remember that initialing a medication on the medication administration record (MAR) indicates that the nurse gave the medication just as it was prescribed and according to the organization's policy.
- When deviations are required, such as a time change, medication form change, or route change, then appropriate actions as dictated by policy should be followed, and the changes should be clearly communicated in writing and verbally if necessary. Remember that a new medication order may be necessary when deviations are required.
- The effectiveness of the medication or lack of effectiveness should be documented according to the organization's policy (usually documented on the MAR or in the nurse's notes). This information helps the next person administering the medication to effectively meet the patient's needs.

✔ ROUTINE CHECKUP 2

1. _____ patient identifiers must be used when administering medications.

Answer:

2. The nurse should not administer a medication that the patient questions until he or she verifies the medication order with the prescriber. True/false?

Answer:

3. List the six rights of medication administration.

Answer:

a. _____

b. _____

c. _____

d. _____

e. _____

f. _____

Nursing Process and Medication Administration

Medication administration is a routine activity performed by nurses probably more than any other skill outside of vital sign assessment. But it is more than a skill. A nurse can easily slip into a robotic mode when giving medications to patients, especially if the same types of medications are used for the population being cared for. To avoid costly mistakes, nurses should always use the nursing process as the backdrop for medication administration—assessing the situation, identifying what the patient needs are, planning how medications will be given, taking the appropriate precautions when giving the medications, and evaluating the process and outcomes.

Assessment

During assessment, the nurse should review the patient's history, including the medication history, to determine if the medications ordered are appropriate for administration to the particular patient. Allergies should be reviewed. Medication history should be reviewed and evaluated to prevent duplications (overdoses) and unintended interactions. Developmental variations (geriatric and

BOX 6–5
Pediatric and Geriatric Tips

Pediatric Tips	Geriatric Tips
• Children usually require smaller doses because of immature body processes. • Assistance may be required, especially for injections. • When possible, offer the child a choice, but do not offer a choice if there is no alternative. • Elicit information from the parents regarding how to best administer medications to the patient. • Be careful in selecting sites of injections. Certain muscle groups may not be large enough to accommodate the prescribed dosage. • Syringes without the needles and spoons, especially designed for liquid medicines, may facilitate administration of accurate doses of medications to children. • A spacer, which is a device that can be attached to an inhalant medication, may improve the accuracy of dosage administration for inhalants.	• Dosage adjustments may be required for older adults because of deteriorating function of body systems. • Take extra precautions during the patient identification process because the elderly client may have altered mental status or altered hearing. • Assess the swallowing capability of patient. • Determine if the patient is capable of safe self-administration of medication or if he or she will require assistance. • Use assistive devices when appropriate (eg, a pill box). • Plan for additional time when providing patient teaching. Make instructions as simple as possible. • Carefully review medical record and question the patient to determine all medications that the patient is taking because complications associated with polypharmacy are a real danger for the geriatric population.

pediatric) should also be taken into consideration (Box 6–5). For example, a geriatric patient is more susceptible to drug interactions, adverse reactions, and overdosage as a result of **polypharmacy** (ie, taking many medications at the same time). Information about the patient's current health status should be reviewed. For example, a patient's liver and kidney function and nutritional status may affect his or her ability to metabolize and excrete the medication(s) ordered. Just as important is the assessment of the patient's cultural beliefs and value system. The patient's beliefs may influence whether or not she/he complies with the prescribed medication regime. The nurse who is equipped with this information will be better prepared to discuss concerns and educate the patient so that he or she can make an informed decision about the proposed medication regime.

> ### NURSING ALERT
>
> **Medication Reconciliation**
> An accurate medication list should be obtained when the patient is admitted to the hospital, when there is a patient transfer (internal and external) and at the time of discharge—QSEN Competency 2: teamwork and collaboration & QSEN Competency 5: safety.

Nursing Diagnosis

An accurate assessment will lead to the identification of patient needs related to medication administration. Possible diagnoses that the patient may have include:

- Noncompliance (eg, related to lack of knowledge, lack of financial resources)
- Ineffective swallowing (impacts ability to take medications by oral route)
- Impaired urinary elimination (impacts excretion of medications)
- Fluid volume deficit (impacts distribution of medications)

Not only will the nurse identify patient needs and nursing diagnoses but he or she will also begin to prioritize the care provided. For example, the first priority for a patient who has impaired urinary elimination may be to consult with the physician to verify whether the prescribed medications in the amount ordered need to be modified. Noncompliance because of financial difficulties, although important, may take a lower priority during the initial hospitalization period because medications are being supplied by the hospital.

Planning

Planning for medication administration is a critical piece of the puzzle. During this phase of the nursing process, the nurse has the opportunity to eliminate the occurrence of potential errors; make efficient use of time by ensuring that all required equipment, supplies, and medications are available; prepare for teaching the patient and family about safe medication administration; and determine what outcomes are expected.

Implementation

The implementation phase is the time for putting the nursing plan into action. Although the main action is to administer medications, the nurse should also use this last opportunity to review the "rights" (right patient, right medication, right amount, right time, right route). Adjustments should be made as necessary. Patient and family education should also be integrated. Box 6–6 includes medication safety considerations in the home setting. Documentation begins during the planning phase when medications are being prepared (inpatient settings) and continues during this phase.

> **NURSING ALERT**
>
> **Safe Medication Administration**
> Do not leave the medications at the bedside for the patient to take. Remain with the patient and confirm the medication is taken—QSEN Competency 5: safety.

> **NURSING ALERT**
>
> **Safe Medication Disposal in the Home**
> Teach patients about proper disposal of medications. Flushing medications down the toilet or throwing them into the regular trash may lead to contamination of our water supply—QSEN Competency 5: safety.

Evaluation

The evaluation phase is the time to review the process and determine if the expected outcomes were achieved. Questions that should be asked include:

1. Was the medication administered as prescribed, or did you run into problems?
2. Was the patient's response to the medication as expected, or did the patient experience adverse reactions or unintended effects?

Box 6–6
Home Care—Medication Safety Consideration

Instruct patient as follows:
- Do not share medications
- Consult pharmacist before taking over-the-counter medications in combination with prescription medications
- Take all medications as prescribed; do not deviate from the instructions provided
- Use a pill container (weekly/monthly) to assist with taking medication at the right time
- Do not take expired medication
- Use childproof lids if children are members of the household

3. Did the patient or family understand how to safely and effectively take or administer the medications?

Adjustments are made accordingly, and this information is documented as well as communicated verbally as necessary. Although the goal is to administer medications in a safe and effective manner, medication errors do occur. In fact, medication errors rank as one of the highest categories of errors in patient care. Although there may be many contributing factors, ultimately it is the nurse (in most instances) who administered the medication. The nurse should handle all medications errors with integrity. Actions should be taken to minimize adverse outcomes that could result from the error. Also, the error should be documented according to organizational policy. Documenting the error is important because it provides evidence that actions were taken to ensure the safety of the patient as well as provide data critical to ensuring overall improved quality of care for patients.

NURSING ALERT

Handling Medication Errors
- Recognize the error
- Stay calm
- Report the error immediately
- Follow the prescriber's orders for correcting the error
- Document the error according to organizational policy (usually on an occurrence report, not the nurse's notes)—QSEN Competency 5: safety.

Conclusion

Nurses play a critical role in the medication administration process. Although medication administration is a part of the nurse's daily routine, it is far from being a routine skill. With this in mind, the following key points were presented in this chapter:

- Medication administration requires knowledge of basic pharmacologic principles, legal requirements, and medication administration principles.
- Critical thinking along with the nursing process provides for a safe, effective, systematic approach to medication administration.
- A review of the medication rights (right patient, right medication, right dose, right route, right time, and right documentation) should always be included during medication administration.

- Medication actions and effects are influenced by how the medication is absorbed, distributed, metabolized, and excreted by the body.

- Medications have intended effects and unintended effects. The goal of medication therapy is that the patient receives medications that provide the best benefit without unintended effects or with minimal unintended effects. The nurse provides valuable information to the prescriber for the determination of how this balance can best be achieved.

- The nurse is totally accountable for his or her actions as it relates to medication administration, including responsible reporting of medication errors in a timely manner so as to ensure the safety of the patient.

REVIEW QUESTIONS

1. **The subcategory of pharmacokinetics that deals with inactivation of a medication is called:**

   A. Absorption

   B. Distribution

   C. Metabolism

   D. Elimination

2. **The doctor ordered 300 mg of a medication to be given by mouth every 8 hours. On hand you have 200 mg scored (1/2 portions) tablets. The nurse should:**

   A. Consult the doctor to see if he or she should give one tablet because two tablets would be more than the dose ordered.

   B. Give one whole tablet and half of a second tablet.

   C. Contact the pharmacy to determine if the medication is available in a different dosage strength so the exact amount of the medication can be given.

   D. Crush the medication, add water, and prepare an amount equal to the exact dosage ordered.

3. **A nurse is preparing to administer oral medications to an 80-year-old client who was admitted to the hospital with a medical diagnosis of dehydration. To ensure safe medication administration, the nurse should:**

   A. Before administering a dose of the medication, carefully assess the patient's hydration status and report to the prescriber any findings that may alter the medication's distribution.

   B. Consult a drug reference resource and give the lowest recommended dose identified to prevent overdose and adverse reactions.

   C. Assess the patient's ability to swallow.

D. A and C

E. All of the above

4. **A pediatric patient is being discharged home in a couple of days. The doctor has left orders for the patient to continue taking oral medications at home. The nurse is preparing to teach the parents how to administer the medication to the patient. To ensure that the parents understand how to safely administer the medications, the nurse should:**

A. Provide the parents with clear and simple written and verbal instructions on how to give the medication.

B. After providing a demonstration, leave the medication at the bedside for the parents to administer all doses until discharge.

C. Read the information from the prescription to the parents and ask if they have any questions.

D. A and B

5. **To ensure that patient safety is maintained, the nurse who commits a medication error should:**

A. Notify the doctor during the next regularly scheduled rounds.

B. Take appropriate corrective action as prescribed by the doctor.

C. Document the occurrence in the nurse's notes.

D. A and B

E. All of the above

ANSWERS

Routine Checkup 1

1. Intravenously.
2. False.
3. Nurse Practice Act.

Routine Checkup 2

1. Two.
2. True.
3. (a) Patient
   (b) Medication
   (c) Route
   (d) Time
   (e) Dose
   (f) Documentation

Review Questions

1. C
2. B

3. D
4. A
5. B

References

Berman A, Snyder SJ, Fandsen G: *Kozier & Erb Fundamentals of Nursing: Concepts, Process and Practice*, 10th ed. Boston, MA: Pearson, 2016.

Fulcher EM, Fulcher RM, Solo CD: *Pharmacology: Principles & Applications*, 3rd ed. St. Louis, MO: Elsevier, 2017.

Potter PA, Perry AG, Stockert P, Hall A: *Fundamentals of Nursing*, 9th ed. St. Louis, MO: Elsevier, 2017.

Wilkinson JM, Treas LS, Barnett KL, Smith MH: *Fundamentals of Nursing Vol. 1: Theory, Concepts, and Applications*. Philadelphia, PA: FA Davis, 2016.

Additional Resources

www.dea.gov/pr/multimedia-library/publications/drug_of_abuse.pdf#page=8

http://ismp.org/Tools/default.aspx#lists

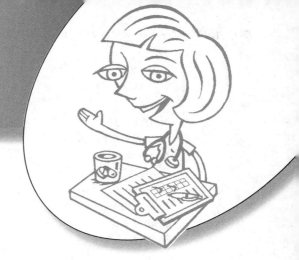

Chapter 7

Safety

At the end of the chapter, the reader will be able to:

1. Describe the components of the infection cycle.

2. Discuss key characteristics of an effective infection control plan.

3. Differentiate between medical asepsis and surgical asepsis.

4. Differentiate between standard precautions and transmission-based precautions.

5. Identify health promotion intervention that the nurse can implement to help patients remain free of infection.

6. Identify two variables that increase the risk that an individual will experience a particular type of injury.

7. Identify nursing actions that can be taken to prevent injuries in the healthcare setting.

Overview

Nurses share the responsibility of maintaining a safe and secure environment of care for themselves, the patient, and other members of the healthcare team. Nurses are also responsible for teaching patients and their families how to maintain safety outside of the patient care setting. To achieve this end, two key areas should be targeted—infection control and injury prevention. This chapter takes a closer look at the nurse's role in effective management of the two identified target areas.

Infection Control

We coexist in a world filled with microorganisms; some of which contribute in a positive way to our existence and others that may cause harm. Microorganisms that have the potential to cause infectious diseases are called **pathogens**. Nurses who are equipped with an understanding of the infection cycle will be better prepared to implement a plan to break the cycle, thereby preventing or minimizing the occurrence of infectious diseases.

Infection Cycle

The infection cycle includes six components: the pathogen or infectious agent, the reservoir, the portal of exit, the mode of transmission, the portal of entry to host, and the susceptible host. Characteristics of each one of the components influence the pathogen's ability to produce an infectious disease as well as its ability to spread from one source to another (Figure 7–1).

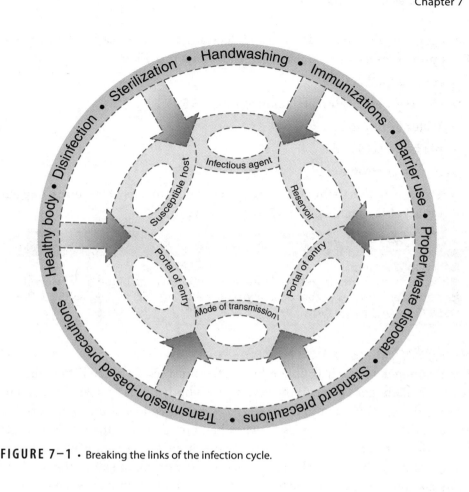

FIGURE 7–1 · Breaking the links of the infection cycle.

Infectious Agent

Bacteria, fungi, viruses, and protozoa are all microorganisms that may cause an infection. Characteristics of the pathogen that influence whether an infection will occur include the number of pathogens present, their **virulence** or ability to cause disease, their ability to enter a host successfully, and their ability to survive inside the host.

Reservoir

The **reservoir**, or source, is the place where the pathogen lives until a **susceptible host** (capable of being infected by the pathogen) becomes available. Nonliving objects such as cutting boards for food preparation, food, and soil can serve as reservoirs just as living organisms such as plants, animals, and humans can serve as reservoirs. Humans and animals that serve as reservoirs for a pathogen but who do not develop an infectious disease are said to be **carriers**. The optimal reservoir for a pathogen is one that provides:

- A good food source
- The right environmental temperature (~95°F)
- Water or moisture
- pH between 5 and 8
- A dark environment
- Oxygen if the pathogen is **aerobic**, which means it requires oxygen (**anaerobic** organisms do not require oxygen)

> **NURSING ALERT**
>
> **Infection Warning!**
> The dark, moist environment inside the human body is one of the best reservoirs for pathogens; thus, we must do everything we can to KEEP PATHOGENS OUT!— QSEN Competency 5: safety.

Portal of Exit and Mode of Transmission

For a pathogen to reach a susceptible host, it must have a means of exiting the reservoir. Pathogens can exit the reservoir via body fluids such as blood, genital secretions, urine, wound drainage, feces, emesis, and sputum. The portal of exit and the mode of transmission work hand in hand. For the infection cycle to continue, the pathogen has to be transmitted to a location where it can access a susceptible host. The relationship of the portal of exit to the mode of transmission can be compared to a situation in which individual has the money to make a desired purchase but can only do so if transportation (eg, bus, car, bicycle) is available to get to the store where the merchandise is located. The three main methods of transmission are direct, indirect, and airborne.

- **Direct transmission** occurs when there is physical contact between the reservoir or source and the susceptible host. In other words, it occurs when a susceptible host has physical contact with reservoirs such as the skin and various body secretions.
- **Indirect transmission** occurs by one of two means. In the first instance, the susceptible host comes into contact with a **fomite**, which is an inanimate object (eg, dressings, contaminated needles, surgical instruments, eating utensils, used tissue, toys) that is contaminated with the pathogen. The second means of indirect transmission is referred to as **vector** transmission. It occurs when an animal such as a mosquito, flea, or tick transports (usually via a bite) the pathogen to a susceptible host.

- **Airborne transmission** occurs when pathogens are carried via droplets (eg, cough or sneeze) that are suspended in the air to the susceptible host. Without a barrier in place, droplets can travel far distances.

Portal of Entry

The portal of entry is how the pathogen enters a susceptible host. The pathogen can enter a susceptible host through any body opening (eg, eyes, ears, mouth, urinary meatus, rectum, vagina) as well as through the skin, especially when there is a break in the skin.

Susceptible Host

Characteristics of the targeted host also influence whether the pathogen can cause an actual infectious disease. Very young and very old individuals tend to be more susceptible to infectious agents because they either have an immature immune system (very young) or a weakened immune system (very old). A person's nutritional status, stress level, and overall health status also influence his or her susceptibility to the harmful effects of pathogens.

Infection Control Strategies

An effective infection control program is multifaceted and includes a diverse group of team members ranging from top administrators to housekeeping staff. The organization must be committed to developing an agency-wide infection control plan. In addition to general infection control interventions, the plan should include a program that specifically addresses healthcare-associated infections (HAIs).

HAIs may occur secondary to treatments/interventions administered in the healthcare setting. There are four main types of HAIs:

- Central line-associated bloodstream infections (CLABSIs)
- Catheter-associated urinary tract infections (CAUTIs)
- Ventilator-associated infections
- Surgical site infections

Healthcare organizations are required to monitor for HAIs and to have programs in place to prevent this group of infections (Box 7–1). Additionally, an effective infection prevention program includes an employee health program, identification and control of work-related infection risk, and treatment of actual infection exposure.

Nurses spend a significant amount of time providing direct patient care. As a result, nurses serve as key players in the prevention of infection. The most

BOX 7–1
EBP Spotlight—Prevention of Catheter-Associated Urinary Tract Infections

Evidence show past practices, once thought to be prudent, in fact increase the likelihood of the occurrence of urinary tract infections. The following recommendations are based on evidence:

- Only catheterize patients when appropriate. Monitoring urinary output and urinary incontinence, in and of itself, are not appropriate reasons for indwelling catheterization. Exception: when patient has stage 3 or 4 perineal/sacral wound and is incontinent.
- Use appropriate catheterization insertion and maintenance techniques:
  ✓ Consider having two people present for insertion
  ✓ Wash hand
  ✓ Do not routinely change catheter/drainage system without cause
  ✓ Position drainage bag below level of patients bladder and ensure drainage is unobstructed.
  ✓ Avoid irrigating the catheter system
  ✓ Clean port when obtaining a sample
  ✓ Routine perineal cleansing with soap and water daily (increased frequency not supported by the evidence
  ✓ Remove catheter as soon as possible
- Avoid excessive urine cultures (asymptomatic patients who are catheterized should not be cultured)
- Avoid inappropriate use of antibiotics (patients should not be treated for asymptomatic bacteriuria)

Source: AHRQ Safety Program for Reducing CAUTI in Hospitals—Toolkit for Reducing CAUTI in Hospital Units: Implementation Guide at https://www.ahrq.gov/sites/default/files/publications/files/implementation-guide_0.pdf.

effective and efficient way for nurses to facilitate infection control is through the implementation of the nursing process. Using the nursing process ensures that all variables that place an individual patient at risk for infection are considered. Assessment of the total impact of an infectious disease on the patient and the risk of spreading infection should also be included. Nursing diagnoses unique to the individual patient can then be identified and a plan of care can be tailored to meet the patient's needs (Table 7–1).

Asepsis

Interventions aimed specifically at infection control in the healthcare setting fall into two categories: **medical asepsis**, or clean technique, which is used to control the number of microorganisms, and **surgical asepsis**, or sterile technique, which requires the complete removal of microorganisms and spores. Some techniques fall into both categories of asepsis. For example, gloves can be used for the purpose of medical asepsis as well as surgical asepsis. The difference between the two is that gloves for surgical asepsis must be donned in

TABLE 7–1 Infection Control and the Nursing Process

Assessment	Potential Nursing Diagnoses (Examples)	Planning (Goals and Outcomes)	Implementation	Evaluation
Risk Factors • Defense mechanisms • Age • Heredity • Stress • Current health status • Medication or procedures • Nutritional status **Clinical Findings** • Signs and symptoms of infection • Laboratory and diagnostic test results • Impact of existing infection on patient or family functioning	• Infection, risk for • Knowledge, deficient • Skin integrity, impaired • Social interaction, impaired • Caregiver role strain, risk for	• Prevention or control of infection • Patient or family knowledge of preventing and controlling infection • Maintenance of skin integrity • Social interaction through means that do not interfere with infection control • Adequate resources to prevent caregiver role strain	• Medical and surgical aseptic techniques • Monitor for signs, symptoms, and laboratory and diagnostic results that suggest the presence of infection • Teach the patient and family how to prevent infection and how to recognize early signs of infection • Provide means for social interaction (visitor using appropriate infection control precautions, telephone interactions, and written communication) • Assist the patient or family to identify resources that will minimize caregiver role strain	• Determine progress toward achieving goals and outcomes • Determine the effectiveness of interventions • Modify the plan of care as needed

such a way as to maintain sterility of the gloves. Failure to use sterile technique in donning sterile gloves may result in the introduction of microorganisms into the susceptible host (ie, the patient).

Medical Asepsis

Handwashing is the most important way to maintain medical asepsis. When the hands are not visibly soiled, an antiseptic handwashing solution is recommended. It is important to use the correct amount of antiseptic handwash and to continue to rub the hands together until they are dry. Handwashing using an antimicrobial soap, water, and vigorous friction for a minimum of 15 seconds should be used when the hands are visibly soiled (Box 7–2). Special attention should be given to the nail beds and under the fingernails. The fingernails should be kept short. Acrylic nails and chipped nail polish should be avoided because both are major culprits for microorganism growth.

NURSING ALERT

Infection Warning!
Artificial nails, chipped nail polish, and long nails may all serve as host sites for organisms associated with hospital-acquired infections—QSEN Competency 5: safety.

Personal protective equipment (PPE), such as gloves, gowns, mask, goggles, and face shields, may also be used to achieve medical asepsis. Recommendations for hand hygiene and the use of PPE are provided in standard precaution guidelines (Table 7–2) and transmission-based precaution guidelines (Table 7–3) outlined by the Centers for Disease Control and Prevention.

BOX 7–2
Handwashing Tips

Wash your hands:

- Upon arriving to work
- Between patient contacts
- Before and after performing invasive procedures
- After removing soiled gloves
- After handling contaminated equipment
- After coming in contact with body secretions
- Before eating
- After using the bathroom
- Before leaving work

TABLE 7-2 Standard Precautions (To Be Used with All Patients)

Component	Recommendations
Hand hygiene	After touching blood, body fluids, secretions, excretions, contaminated items; immediately after removing gloves; between patient contacts
Personal Protective Equipment (PPE)	
Gloves	For touching blood, body fluids, secretions, excretions, contaminated items; for touching mucous membranes and nonintact skin
Gown	During procedures and patient care activities when contact of clothing or exposed skin with blood, body fluids, secretions, or excretions is anticipated
Mask, eye protection (goggles), face shield*	During procedures and patient care activities likely to generate splashes or sprays of blood, body fluids, secretions, especially suctioning, endotracheal intubation
Soiled patient care equipment	Handle in a manner that prevents transfer of microorganisms to others and to the environment; wear gloves if visibly contaminated; perform hand hygiene
Other	
Environmental control	Develop procedures for routine care, cleaning, and disinfection of environmental surfaces, especially frequently touched surfaces in patient care areas
Textiles and laundry	Handle in a manner that prevents transfer of microorganisms to others and to the environment
Needles and other sharps	Do not recap, bend, break, or hand-manipulate used needles; if recapping is required, use a one-handed scoop technique only; use safety features when available; place used sharps in puncture-resistant container
Patient resuscitation	Use a mouthpiece, resuscitation bag, and other ventilation devices to prevent contact with the mouth and oral secretions
Patient placement	Prioritize for single-patient room if patient is at increased risk of transmission, is likely to contaminate the environment, does not maintain appropriate hygiene, or is at increased risk of acquiring infection or developing an adverse outcome after infection
Respiratory hygiene and cough etiquette (source containment of infectious respiratory secretions in symptomatic patients, beginning at the initial point of encounter, eg, triage and reception areas in emergency departments and physician offices)	Instruct symptomatic persons to cover their mouth or nose when sneezing or coughing; use tissues and dispose in a no-touch receptacle; observe hand hygiene after soiling of hands with respiratory secretions; wear surgical mask if tolerated or maintain spatial separation (>3 feet if possible)

*During aerosol-generating procedures on patients with suspected or proven infections transmitted by respiratory aerosols (eg, SARS), wear a fit-tested N95 or higher respirator in addition to gloves, gown, and face and eye protection.

Adapted from Siegel JD, Rhinehart E, Jackson M, Chiarello L, Healthcare Infection Control Practices Advisory Committee: 2007 Guideline for Isolation Precautions: Preventing Transmission of Infectious Agents in Healthcare Settings, June 2007:129-130. Available at http://www.cdc.gov/ncidod/dhqp/pdf/guidelines/Isolation2007.pdf.

TABLE 7–3 Transmission-Based Precautions

Category	Suggested Precautions
Contact precautions	• Single-patient room preferred • ≥3 feet separation in multi-patient room • Gown and glove for all interactions requiring patient contact or contact with contaminated areas in patient's environment • Put on PPE upon entry to patient's room • Discard PPE before exiting patient's room
Droplet precautions	• Single-patient room preferred • >3 feet separation in multi-patient room with curtain drawn between patients • Wear a mask (respirator not necessary) when in close contact with infectious patient • Put on a mask upon entry to patient's room • When transport is required, a mask should be worn by the patient if tolerated
Airborne precautions	• Airborne infection isolation room (AIIR) preferred (room equipped with special ventilation features) • When an AIIR is not available, mask the patient and place in a private room with the door closed until the patient can be transferred to an AIIR • Healthcare employees should wear masks or respirators depending on disease-specific recommendation • Mask or respirator should be put on *before* entering the patient's room • Nonimmune healthcare employees should not be assigned to provide care for patients with vaccine-preventable airborne diseases (eg, chickenpox, measles, small pox)

Note 1: Transmission-based precautions are used in addition to standard precautions when standard precautions are not adequate for preventing the transmission of infectious agents.

Note 2: Transmission-based precautions should not be delayed until test results confirm the presence of pathogens; instead, precautions should be initiated at the first sign of clinical signs and symptoms.

Data from Siegel JD, Rhinehart E, Jackson M, Chiarello L, Healthcare Infection Control Practices Advisory Committee: *2007 Guideline for Isolation Precautions: Preventing Transmission of Infectious Agents in Healthcare Settings,* June 2007:69–72. Available at http://www.cdc.gov/ncidod/dhqp/pdf/guidelines/Isolation2007.pdf.

Cleansing and disinfection are two medical aseptic techniques used to remove microorganisms from equipment and supplies used in patient care. **Cleansing** is the process whereby visible soiling is removed; it does not ensure that all microorganisms are eliminated. On the other hand, **disinfection** requires the use of chemicals and results in the elimination of most, if not, all microorganisms with the exception of spores.

Surgical Asepsis

Sterile technique or surgical asepsis is required whenever there is a need to have a microorganism-free environment. Providing care using sterile technique requires the use of sterile supplies, including gloves (Box 7–3), a gown,

BOX 7–3
Procedure Spotlight

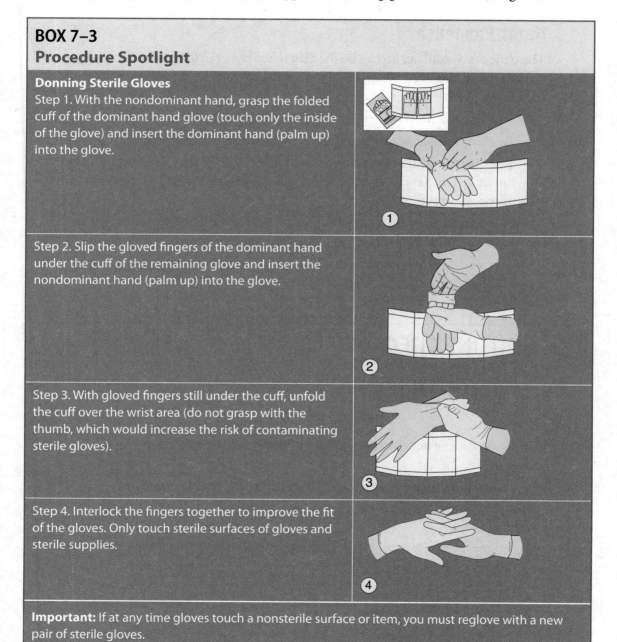

Donning Sterile Gloves

Step 1. With the nondominant hand, grasp the folded cuff of the dominant hand glove (touch only the inside of the glove) and insert the dominant hand (palm up) into the glove.

Step 2. Slip the gloved fingers of the dominant hand under the cuff of the remaining glove and insert the nondominant hand (palm up) into the glove.

Step 3. With gloved fingers still under the cuff, unfold the cuff over the wrist area (do not grasp with the thumb, which would increase the risk of contaminating sterile gloves).

Step 4. Interlock the fingers together to improve the fit of the gloves. Only touch sterile surfaces of gloves and sterile supplies.

Important: If at any time gloves touch a nonsterile surface or item, you must reglove with a new pair of sterile gloves.

a facemask, a cap, and shoe covers. Additionally, a sterile field for equipment to be used may be required. Specific items required depend on the specific procedure being performed. All equipment used for sterile procedures should be either disposable or sterilized after use.

Health Promotion

The patient's overall health can be the difference between there being a risk for infection and the occurrence of an actual infection. The nurse can help the patient avoid infection in several ways, including:

- Stressing the need to keep immunizations up to date
- Teaching the patient or family correct handwashing techniques
- Teaching the patient or family about the infection chain and how to break the chain (eg, handwashing, coughing and sneezing into elbow-bend area, proper food storage)
- Teaching the patient or family how to perform procedures using clean technique in the home setting (eg, catheterization, dressing changes)

When teaching the patient, it is important to communicate information in a way that the patient can understand and validate that he or she understands the instructions given.

✔ ROUTINE CHECKUP

1. Humans and animals that serve as reservoirs for infection but who do not develop an infection are said to be _____.

Answer:

2. The most important way to prevent the spread of infection is _____.

Answer:

3. List four health promotion strategies for preventing the spread of infection:

Answer:

_____

_____

_____

_____

Injury Prevention and Security

Injury prevention is twofold—the nurse is responsible for teaching patients how to prevent injury occurrences in their everyday living environments and for promoting injury prevention in the healthcare setting. The nurse also plays a role in providing a secure patient care environment and maintaining a safe workplace.

Injury Prevention: General Guidelines

Every individual runs the risk of being the victim of an injury, but developmental characteristics increase the risk for certain types of injuries (Table 7–4). For example, infants in the oral stage of development often put unsafe objects in their mouths that may cause poisoning or choking. To counter this, the nurse should teach the parents to be alert for this risk and provide the parents with examples of unsafe objects to keep out of the infant's reach. Personal lifestyle choices may also contribute to the occurrence of certain types of injuries. An adult may choose to drink alcohol. If the individual drives under the influence of alcohol, he or she will be more prone to having a car accident. Although the nurse cannot force the individual to stop drinking alcohol, he or she can inform the person of associated risk and identify resources that may help the individual to stop drinking.

The list of injuries that may occur as a result of developmental characteristics and lifestyle choices exceeds the scope of this text. However, the examples provided will hopefully raise the nurse's consciousness of her or his role in recognizing risk and educating patients and their families in ways to facilitate optimal safety.

Injury Prevention in the Healthcare Setting

There are many opportunities for injuries to occur in the healthcare setting. Some of the injuries that may occur include:

- Falls
- Patient care errors (medication, fluid overload, faulty equipment leading to burns or shocks)
- Fires
- Assaults (patient and staff)

TABLE 7–4 Development Stage-Specific Injury Risk	
Infants and toddlers	• Unintentional suffocation secondary to choking or strangulation • Motor vehicle accidents (failure to use recommended restraint a factor) • Drowning (bathtubs, buckets, toilets, residential swimming pools) • Falls • Child abuse (blunt head trauma, violent shaking)
Preschoolers and school-age children	• Motor vehicle accidents (inappropriate seat belt positioning a factor) • Drowning • Injury secondary to being hit by a car as a pedestrian • Homicide (firearms a factor) • Falls • Child abuse (sexual abuse a possible factor)
Teenagers	• Motor vehicle accidents (not using seat belts, alcohol intoxication) • Sports-related concussions • Homicides • Suicides
Adults	• Motor vehicle accidents • Homicide • Suicide • Falls • Overexertion
Older adults	• Falls • Motor vehicle accidents (especially among those 65 years of age and older) • Traumatic brain injury • Suicide

Data from Centers for Disease Control and Prevention: *CDC Injury Fact Book*. Available at http://www.cdc.gov/ncipc/fact_book / Injury Book2006.pdf.

The first level of healthcare setting injury prevention is the establishment of sound organizational policies to prevent injuries. Procedural policies as well as policies related to fire safety, security, fall prevention, and disaster response should be in place and should be reviewed by all members of the healthcare team. Nurses as well as other members of the healthcare team are accountable for following organizational policies. Nurses are also responsible for orienting patients to their role in injury prevention. Written information is often provided to patients in the form of patient information booklets. Written instructions should always be reinforced verbally. Additionally, individual patient characteristics (developmental stage, medical therapies) should be taken into consideration when determining the patient's risk for injury. Table 7–5 provides a summary of some actions nurses can take to promote safety in the healthcare setting.

TABLE 7–5 Safety Promotion Nursing Interventions for the Healthcare Setting	
General	• Follow guidelines outlined in safety policies and procedures • Attend safety training programs • Participate in organizational performance improvement activities (eg, root cause analysis, process action teams, safety drills) • Wear name tags • Promptly report injuries and errors according to organization policy
Falls	• Identify patients at risk for falls • Put the call system in easy reach of the patient • Ensure a well-lit, uncluttered environment • Teach patients to change positions slowly • Use restraints only if absolutely necessary (follow monitoring guidelines)
Patient care errors	• Dispose of sharps appropriately • Follow organizational policies regarding electrical safety • Remove faulty equipment from patient use; label and sent it to the appropriate department • Monitor IV infusions closely (use IV pump)
Fires	• Know the locations of fire alarms and extinguishers • Know exit routes • Actively participate in fire drills (do not ignore them) • Know fire evacuation procedures
Assaults	• Monitor visitor traffic • Be aware of behaviors that suggest a potential for violent behaviors • Report potential violent or hostile situations immediately when possible • Diffuse situations when possible (avoid retaliatory actions) • Position yourself for easy escape from assault • Limit the presence of objects that can be used as weapons • Keep patient care equipment and supplies that can be used as weapons in a locked area

Conclusion

Safety is everyone's business—top management, members of the direct care team, auxiliary staff, and patients. An effective safety plan addresses patient safety and employee safety. Key components of a comprehensive safety plan include provisions for promoting infection control, injury prevention, and a secure environment. Nurses are in a unique position to promote safety both within and outside of the healthcare setting. The nursing process is the preferred means for ensuring that individual patient safety needs are met. Additionally, nurses should be familiar with specific infection control intervention, injury risk associated with each development stage, and the potential impact of lifestyle choices on safety.

REVIEW QUESTIONS

1. **Which of the following is NOT one of the six links in the infection cycle?**
   A. Infectious agent
   B. Mode of transmission
   C. Susceptible host
   D. Vector

2. **Which of the following situations would require the nurse to wash his or her hands for a minimum of 15 seconds with an antimicrobial soap?**
   A. After taking a patient's blood pressure
   B. After cleaning an open wound
   C. After coughing into his or her hands
   D. Before preparing medications for a patient
   E. B and C

3. **When educating the patient about ways to prevent exposure to and the spread of infection, the nurse should inform the patient to:**
   A. Dispose of the used tissue and then wash his or her hands.
   B. Cover his or her mouth and nose when coughing.
   C. Use insect repellent when there is a chance of exposure to mosquitoes, fleas, or ticks.
   D. A and B
   E. All of the above

4. Which of the following precautions should be taken for a patient who is admitted to the hospital with an infection that is spread via droplets?

A. Assign the patient to an airborne infection isolation room (AIIR).

B. Put on a respirator before entering the patient's room.

C. Keep the curtains drawn between patients assigned to a semi-private room.

D. All of the above

5. Which of the following actions should be taken to prevent falls for patients who are admitted to inpatient areas (hospital, long-term care facilities)?

A. Maintain a well-lit, clutter-free environment in the patient's room.

B. Keep the patient restrained when a caretaker is not at the bedside.

C. Refrain from administering pain medications to the patient.

D. Require a family member to remain with the patient at all times.

E. A and B

ANSWERS

Routine Checkup

1. Carriers.
2. Handwashing.
3. (a) Stressing the need to keep immunizations up to date.
   (b) Teaching the patient or family correct handwashing techniques.
   (c) Teaching the patient or family about the infection chain and how to break the chain (ie, handwashing, coughing or sneezing into elbow-bend area, proper food storage).
   (d) Teaching the patient or family how to perform procedures using clean technique in the home setting (ie, catheterization, dressing changes).

Review Questions

1. D
2. B
3. E
4. C
5. A

References

Berman A, Snyder SJ, Fandsen G: *Kozier & Erb Fundamentals of Nursing: Concepts, Process and Practice,* 10th ed. Boston, MA: Pearson, 2016.

Potter PA, Perry AG, Stockert P, Hall A: *Fundamentals of Nursing*, 9th ed. St. Louis, MO: Elsevier, 2017.

Wilkinson JM, Treas LS, Barnett KL, Smith MH: *Fundamentals of Nursing Vol. 1: Theory, Concepts, and Applications*. Philadelphia, PA: FA Davis, 2016.

Additional Resources

https://www.cdc.gov/infectioncontrol/tools/index.html

https://www.cdc.gov/handhygiene/

http://www.cdc.gov/ncidod/dhqp/pdf/guidelines/Isolation2007.pdf.

https://www.ahrq.gov/sites/default/files/publications/files/implementation-guide_0.pdf

http://www.cdc.gov/InjuryViolenceSafety/

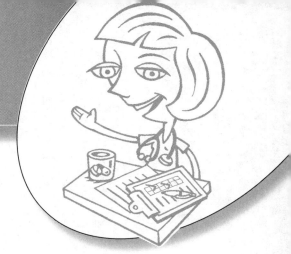

Part III

Meeting Basic Human Needs

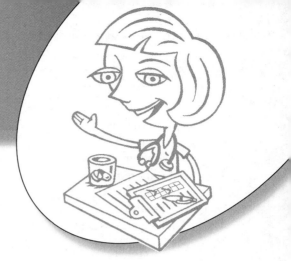

Chapter 8

Skin Integrity

LEARNING OBJECTIVES

At the end of the chapter, the reader will be able to:

1. State the primary functions of the skin.

2. Identify and describe the function of the major structures of the skin.

3. Discuss factors that influence the function of the skin.

4. Describe common types of skin lesions.

5. Identify common pressure points associated with the occurrence of skin breakdown.

6. Discuss key components of the skin assessment.

7. State the three North American Nursing Diagnosis Association (NANDA) nursing diagnoses directly related to alterations in skin function.

8. Discuss nursing interventions aimed at promoting healthy skin, preventing skin impairment in at-risk patients, and treating patients with impaired skin integrity.

Overview

Most people do not think of the skin as an organ, but it is one. In fact, the skin is the largest organ of the body. It is our first line of defense against harmful elements in the environment. The skin along with its appendages (hair and nails) plays a significant role in our outward appearance. We make judgments about how we feel by looking at our skin color and feeling the texture and temperature of our skin. We also rely partially on our outward appearance to establish our self-concept. Others use the same cues that we use in our self-evaluation to make judgments about our health (physiological and psychological) as well as who we are (eg, values, culture).

It should be evident from the discussion up to this point that maintaining skin integrity is as important as maintaining proper function of other organ systems. Nurses play a key role in assisting patients to maintain skin integrity through preventative teaching, protective intervention, and restorative interventions when skin impairment occurs.

The Structure and Physiology of the Skin

The primary functions of the skin are protection, temperature regulation, and sensory perception. The skin consists of an outer layer called the **epidermis** and an inner layer, the **dermis**, which is referred as the true skin (Figure 8–1). Each layer of the skin and its associated structures perform specific functions. **Subcutaneous tissue**, although not actually a part of the skin, is usually discussed when referencing the skin. Subcutaneous tissue underlies the skin and is also referred to as the **hypodermis**. It is composed of fat and connective tissue.

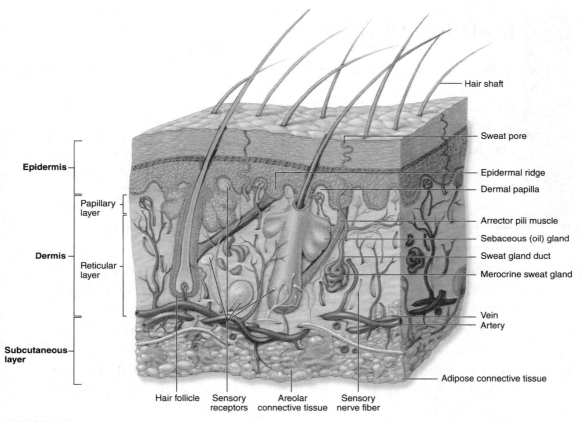

FIGURE 8-1 · The skin is composed of layers with each layer having a purpose. Layers are epidermis, dermis, and hypodermis. (Reproduced with permission from Mescher AL: *Junqueira's Basic Histology: Text and Atlas,* 12th ed. New York, McGraw-Hill, 2010, Fig. 18-1.)

The primary role of the epidermis is protection. It serves as a barrier to fluid loss and protects the internal environment of the body from harmful elements in the external environment. The epidermis contains **keratin**, a protein that functions as a barrier; **melanin**, which gives pigment or color to the skin; and **Langerhans cells**, which provide protection against infections and certain foreign substances.

The dermis provides nourishment to the epidermis. It contains connective tissue, blood vessels, and nerves. The hair, sweat glands, and sebaceous glands, collectively referred to as skin appendages, also arise from the dermal layer of the skin.

- Connective tissue is composed of collagen and elastin, which are responsible for the elasticity and strength of the skin.

- Blood vessels play a key role in temperature regulation. When a person is in a cold environment, the blood vessels constrict to conserve heat. When in a hot environment, the blood vessels dilate to prevent overheating.

- Nerve endings in the skin allow the body to perceive environmental stimuli (eg, hot, cold, sharp, dull, pressure, itching, pain).

- Sweat glands allow a person to sweat or perspire. The sweat produced facilitates cooling of the body through the process of evaporation (see Chapter 4).

- Sebaceous glands produce sebum, which helps to keep the skin lubricated, thereby facilitating skin integrity and preserving the skin's protective function.

Factors Influencing Skin Function

Age, nutrition, hydration, hygiene, the environment, and health deviation all have the potential to alter the integrity of skin function.

Age

- Newborns and infants have thin, fragile, sensitive skin. As a result, they are at risk of developing contact **dermatitis** (inflamed and itching skin) secondary to exposure to irritants. Friction and pressure may cause breaks in the skin and increase the risk for infections. Because the newborn's skin is so thin, topically applied creams, lotions, and medications can be easily absorbed through the skin and may cause an unwanted systemic effect. Significant fluid loss may also occur because of the thinness of the skin. Excessive sun exposure or excessive exposure to cold temperatures both pose significant problems for infants.

NURSING ALERT

Sunscreen for Infants
Parents should be informed that the use of sunscreen products is not recommended for infants younger than 6 months and should be cautioned to limit infants' sun exposure.

- During the adolescent years, the sebaceous glands become more active, increasing the likelihood of acne. Also, adolescents and young adults are more likely to engage in sunbathing and tanning booth use, both of which increase the risk of skin cancer.

- As we age, the skin becomes thin, dry, and wrinkled. There is diminished elasticity, circulation, and immunologic activity. The combined effect of these changes is an increased risk for skin irritation, tears, pressure ulcers, and infection. This is compounded by the fact that wound healing is more difficult in elderly patients because of decreased circulation.

Nutrition and Hydration

A well-balanced diet and adequate fluid intake are important in maintaining healthy skin. Malnutrition results in a loss of subcutaneous tissue as well as a lack of vitamins and minerals that are needed to maintain healthy skin. When a person is malnourished, the skin may be dry and vulnerable to skin breaks; the nails and hair may become brittle and break; and there may also be changes in the color of the skin.

Hygiene

Healthy skin requires routine cleansing. Failure to clean the skin results in the accumulation of sweat, bacteria, and dirt, all of which may clog skin pores and lead to skin infections or infestations. It is just as important to avoid excessive cleaning of the skin. Excessive scrubbing and bathing may cause the skin to become dry and irritated. Lubricating agents should be used to assist with keeping the skin moisturized. When instructing patients about hygiene requirements, the nurse must take into consideration the impact of cultural

---

Box 8–1
Cultural Influences on Hygiene Practices

When cultural practices influence an individual's hygiene practices, the nurse can be most effective by listening and encouraging the patient to be an active participant in identifying alternatives for meeting hygiene needs without compromising cultural requirements. Remember that the ultimate decision to accept or decline care rests with the patient.

---

and socioeconomic factors on hygiene practices (Box 8–1). People with limited income may not be able to afford products required to keep the skin clean. In this case, the nurse has a responsibility to assist the patient in identifying community resources. Individuals with limited ability to perform self-care activities and who are incontinent are also at risk for alterations in skin integrity, especially when the individual is also immobilized or bedridden.

Environment

The sun, the wind, allergens, and infectious agents in the environment as well as chemical irritants (dyes, detergents, creams, lotions, ointments, plants, latex, insects) all have the potential to cause skin damage. Whether a person actually experiences skin damage is highly individualized. What may be very irritating to one person may not cause any problems for another. The overall health of the skin at the time of exposure to the environmental agent, the immunologic status of the individual, and the use or lack of use of protective products (eg, SPF products, certain types of clothing) play a role in the individual's susceptibility to environmental hazards. In some instances, the skin condition may be simple and temporary, but in other situations, such as the case of a **melanoma** (skin cancer), the condition may be deadly.

NURSING ALERT

Skin Self-Examination
Patients should be taught to regularly check their skin for the following. Positive findings should be reported immediately!

A: Asymmetrical lesion (if an imaginary line were drawn to divide the lesion into equal halves, the two halves would not match)

B: Borders of the lesion are irregular

C: Color varies within the lesion

D: Diameter >6 mm (the size of a pencil eraser)

Health Deviations

Allergic reactions secondary to environmental triggers have already been discussed. However, a person may also experience skin changes secondary to systemic allergic responses (eg, medications and autoimmune disorders such as lupus). Infections (bacterial, fungal, or viral) may cause changes in the skin, including itching and the presence of various types of skin lesions (Table 8–1).

Immobility may lead to ulcer formation secondary to friction or prolonged pressure (**pressure ulcers**), especially over bony parts of the body (Table 8–2). Altered circulation may cause pooling of blood, especially in the legs. The area becomes swollen, itchy, and dark in color. At this point, the individual is said to have **stasis dermatitis**. Eventually, the skin will break, and a **stasis ulcer** will develop. Left untreated, the person may develop **gangrene** (death of tissue secondary to poor circulation). Diabetes and atherosclerosis are two underlying disorders that may cause altered circulation.

Skin wounds may also occur as a result of traumatic injuries, either intentional (violent injuries) or unintentional (accidental falls, cuts, scraps, punctures). Another type of intentional wound is a surgical wound. Surgical wounds may be temporary or permanent. For example, a tracheostomy may be temporary or permanent depending on the underlying reason for the procedure.

TABLE 8–1 Skin Lesions		
Lesion Name	**Description**	**Example**
Macule	Flat, nonpalpable discolored area on the skin <1 cm in size	Freckle
Papule	Raised, solid lesion <0.5 cm in size	Mole (raised), wart
Nodule	Raised, solid lesion that may extend deeper into the skin layers; usually 0.5–2.0 cm in size	Sebaceous cyst
Vesicle	Fluid-filled lesion <0.5 cm in size; the fluid contained in a vesicle is clear	Blister
Bulla (plural, bullae)	Fluid-filled lesion that is larger in size than a vesicle (>0.5 cm).	Large blisters seen with second-degree burns
Pustule	Pus-filled lesion	Acne pimples
Wheal	Raised, irregularly shaped area of skin caused by inflammatory response such as with hives or an insect bite; may also be produced as a result of an intradermal injection	Mosquito bite, TB skin test
Fissure	Crack in the skin	Athlete's feet

TABLE 8−2 Pressure Points		
	Position	**Pressure Points**
	Supine (bed-bound)	• Back of head • Shoulder blade • Elbows • Buttocks • Heels
	Side-lying (bed-bound)	• Ears • Shoulder • Elbows • Hips • Inner surface of knees • Inner surface of ankles
	Sitting (bed-bound)	• Back of head • Shoulder blade • Elbows • Buttocks • Heels
	Wheelchair-user	• Shoulder blade • Elbows • Hips • Buttocks • Heels

Additionally, surgical wounds may be clean or dirty (appendectomy with an intact appendix vs. appendectomy with a ruptured appendix).

The Nursing Process and Skin Integrity

Assessment

The assessment of skin integrity should include subjective data obtained from the patient as well as objective data obtained during the physical examination of the patient. During the interview process, the nurse should inquire about the presence of itching and pain as well as the presence of any skin lesions (rashes, bruises, abrasions, cuts, pustules). The nurse should also ask the patient about any recent changes in the skin (skin color and texture). Any reported alterations or concerns should be explored in more detail. The nurse should inquire about recent changes in the patient's diet, skin products (soaps, lotions, and perfumes), and laundering products. The patient's medical history, including the patient's social history as well as the family history, should be reviewed to obtain information about contributing and risk factors associated with impaired skin integrity. During actual inspection of the skin, the color, texture, turgor, perfusion (eg, capillary refill time), and skin temperature should be assessed. Inspection should also include observation for lesions or any other variation other than those considered to be normal variations from individual to individual. To ensure the accuracy of observations, the skin should be inspected in a well-lit environment.

Skin assessments should be performed on a regular basis for patients who are at risk for the development of pressure ulcers (immobilized, bedridden, incontinent, and mentally impaired patients). Multiple formal assessment tools such as the Braden scale have been developed for the purpose of performing systematic skin assessments. Patients with open wounds (eg, surgical wounds as well as wounds caused by trauma) should be monitored for signs of infection such as increased pain, temperature elevations, and **purulent** (containing pus) foul-smelling drainage.

Nursing Diagnosis

As is the case most of the time, numerous nursing diagnoses may be relevant or applicable to the patient at risk for or actually experiencing alteration in skin function. However, the nursing diagnoses that are directly related are limited to impaired skin integrity, risk for impaired skin integrity, impaired tissue integrity. Examples of other diagnoses that may be applicable depending on the specific patient circumstances include:

- Bathing and hygiene self-care deficit
- Chronic confusion
- Chronic low self-esteem
- Deficient fluid volume
- Diarrhea
- Disturbed body image
- Imbalanced nutrition: Less than body requirements

- Impaired mobility (bed, physical, wheelchair)
- Urinary incontinence

Planning and Implementation

Successful development of an effective plan of care for an individual who is at risk for or actually experiencing altered skin integrity depends on the completeness and accuracy of data obtained during the assessment phase. It is critical that patient input is integrated and that the plan of care is collaboratively developed by the patient and/or significant others when appropriate. Goals, outcomes, and interventions fall into two main categories: those directed toward preventing impairment of skin integrity and those directed at correcting alterations that have already occurred.

Health Promotion

Health promotion is the first course of action in preventing alterations in skin integrity. Individuals should be taught the following strategies for promoting healthy skin:

- Eat a well-balanced diet, including an adequate intake of protein, vitamins, and minerals.
- Drink an adequate amount of fluid to promote well-hydrated skin.
- Regularly cleanse the skin with mild, nonabrasive cleansing agents.
- Moisturize the skin with lotions and creams.
- Limit exposure to damaging rays (sun and tanning booths).
- Protect the skin with clothing, hats, and sunscreen (SPF 15 or higher).
- Wear properly fitting clothes and shoes to prevent skin irritation from friction.
- Practice accident prevention strategies to decrease the occurrence of traumatic skin injuries.
- Exercise to promote healthy blood circulation.

Prevention of Skin Impairment in At-Risk Patients

Beyond health promotion, there is also a need to closely monitor and intervene for patients who have an increased risk for impaired skin integrity. Populations most vulnerable to impaired skin integrity include those immobilized for extended periods of time, those who have stool and urine incontinence, and those who are unable to meet basic hygiene needs because of neurologic impairment. Patients with compromised circulation are also at a greater risk for impaired skin integrity. Frequent skin assessment is an important part of the plan of care for patients falling into this high-risk population. Specific interventions aimed at preventing skin breakdown for at-risk patients include:

- Keep the skin (especially over bony prominences and in body creases) clean and free of moisture.
- Keep the skin properly moisturized with lotion.
- Avoid massaging bony prominences as well as reddened or already damaged skin areas.

> ### NURSING ALERT
>
> **Change in Practice for Massage**
> *Do not* massage reddened skin or areas over bony prominences; doing so may cause damage to the skin!

- Frequently reposition the patient (at least every 2 hours) to prevent skin breakdown secondary to excessive pressure, friction, and shearing force (Figure 8–2).
- Use assistive devices to reposition the patient if needed. Do not pull or tug on the patient. Doing so may cause shearing force injuries.
- Maintain a 30-degree angle to the bed when the patient is in the sidelying position.

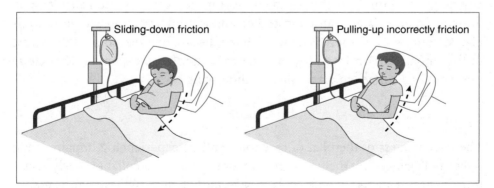

FIGURE 8–2 · Shearing force. Shearing force damage occurs as a result of the friction against skin produced as the patient slides down in the bed and when the patient is repositioned if care is not taken. When repositioning a patient, obtain the assistance of at least one other person and use a sheet to lift the patient. Do not pull on the patient to reposition him or her.

- Use pillows, foam wedges, and heel protectors to minimize friction over common pressure points.
- Use mattress overlays, special mattresses, or specialty beds as needed.
- Keep bed linen wrinkle free.
- Provide well-balanced diet. Request nutritional evaluation if needed.

It is also important to have a systematic plan for implementing the above-mentioned interventions. Communication is important as well. Miscommunication may result in the omission of critical intervention and may result in actual skin breakdown. Each member of the treatment team should have clearly defined roles. There should be no question of who will provide skin care, when the patient will be turned, or who will ensure that the patient eats required meals and snacks.

In all instances, care should be provided in such a way that the patient's dignity is maintained. The nurse should also monitor the patient for signs of depression, feelings of hopelessness, and low self-esteem. Family members should be made aware of signs of these conditions and should be taught how to assist with meeting the patient's psychosocial needs. Additionally, the nurse should monitor ineffective family coping and should be on the lookout for caregiver role strain. If there is evidence of ineffective family coping or caregiver role strain, the nurse should identify community resources such as respite care for the family.

Interventions for Impaired Skin Integrity

Interventions and the level of care required for patients with altered skin integrity range from minor first aid and comfort measures to wound debridement, dressing changes (sterile and nonsterile), and wound irrigations. In more complex situations when there is an underlying disease or a disorder contributing to the impaired skin integrity, nursing care should be expanded to include interventions aimed at correcting the underlying cause.

Evaluation

The effectiveness of the plan of care for a patient experiencing impaired skin integrity is gauged by the goals and outcomes that were collaboratively established with the patient. Some goals may be fairly easy to achieve. For example, the discomfort associated with a first-degree burn on one finger may be resolved in a matter of a few minutes with cool running water and a topical pain reliever.

However, addressing the impact of a stasis ulcer on a patient who has diabetes is much more complex and requires more time to achieve. Goal achievement may be further compounded by coexisting psychosocial issues (depression, isolation, poor self-concept). It is always important to remember that the patient is the driver of care and that your perception of success or goal achievement may be completely different than the patient's perception. Ultimately, the success or lack thereof is significantly influenced by the nurse's ability to establish and maintain effective communication and a therapeutic relationship with the patient.

Conclusion

The discussion of impaired skin integrity, including influencing factors, assessment, and intervention, has by no means been exhausted in this text. Instead, the intent has been to facilitate your basic understanding of alterations in skin integrity. More specifically, you should be able to (1) describe the structure and function of the skin, (2) discuss factors influence normal skin function, (3) discuss key components that should be included when performing a skin assessment, (4) identify common nursing diagnoses that may be relevant for the patient experiencing alterations in skin integrity, and (5) discuss interventions for promoting healthy skin, preventing skin breakdown, and correcting impaired skin integrity.

REVIEW QUESTIONS

1. **While assessing a patient, the nurse observes a lesion on the skin that is raised, solid, and 0.25 cm in size. The nurse would be correct to document this lesion as a:**

   A. Bulla
   B. Macule
   C. Nodule
   D. Papule
   E. Vesicle

2. **A patient is brought to the emergent care facility with second-degree burns on the abdomen. The patient has large, water-filled lesions scattered throughout the burn. The nurse would be correct to identify the lesions as:**

   A. Bullae
   B. Macules

    C. Nodules

    D. Papules

    E. Vesicles

3. **When teaching a patient about proper skin care, the nurse should include all of the following EXCEPT:**

    A. Consume a well-balanced meal.

    B. Avoid excessive scrubbing and bathing.

    C. Use a tanning booth instead of sun bathing if a tan is desired.

    D. Exercise to promote healthy blood circulation.

4. **The nurse should include which of the following lesion characteristics when teaching a patient about warning signs to look for when observing the skin?**

    A. Asymmetrical shape

    B. Irregular borders

    C. Color variation within the same lesion

    D. A and B

    E. All of the above

5. **Which of the following body surfaces is more prone to skin breakdown when an immobilized patient is placed in the sidelying position?**

    A. Ears

    B. Shoulder blades

    C. Inner surface of the ankles and knees

    D. A and C

    E. All of the above

6. **A nurse is assessing a client's risk for pressure ulcer development. Which factor should be most concerning to the nurse?**

    A. The patient is only able to ambulate with an assistive device.

    B. The patient is visually impaired.

    C. The patient is elderly.

    D. The patient is incontinent of urine.

7. **A nurse is planning care for an immobile patient. The priority nursing action in the prevention of development of pressure ulcers is to:**

    A. Turn or reposition the client every 2 hours.

    B. Massage any reddened areas twice a day.

    C. Assess the patient's intake and output every shift.

    D. Wear gloves with any client contact.

ANSWERS

Routine Checkup

1. Epidermis, dermis.
2. Protection
   Temperature regulation
   Sensory perception

Review Questions

1. C
2. A
3. C
4. E
5. D
6. D
7. A

References

Craven RF, Hirnle CJ: *Fundamentals of Nursing: Human Health and Function*, 5th ed. Philadelphia, PA: Lippincott, 2006.

Daniels R: *Nursing Fundamentals: Caring & Clinical Decision Making.* New York, NY: Delmar Thomson Learning, 2004.

Potter PA, Perry AG: *Fundamentals of Nursing*, 6th ed. St. Louis, MO: Mosby Elsevier, 2005.

Ramutkowski B, Barrie A, Keller C, Dazarow L, Abel C: *Medical Assisting: A Patient-Centered Approach to Administrative and Clinical Competencies.* New York, NY: Glenco McGraw-Hill, 1999.

Additional Resources

American Geriatric Society: *Pressure Ulcers (Bed Sores).* Available at http://www.healthinaging.org/agingintheknow/chapters_ch_trial.asp?ch=30.

Medline Plus: *Skin Conditions.* Available at http://www.nlm.nih.gov/medlineplus/skinconditions.html.

Medline Plus: *Stasis Dematitis and Ulcers.* Available at http://www.nlm.nih.gov/medlineplus/ency/article/000834.htm.

Zeller JL, Lynm C, Glass RM: *Pressure Ulcers.* Available at http://jama.ama-assn.org/cgi/reprint/296/8/1020.pdf.

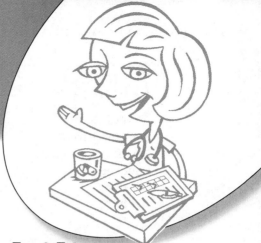

Chapter 9

Activity and Mobility

LEARNING OBJECTIVES

At the end of the chapter, the reader will be able to:

1. Describe the role that bones, muscles, joints, and central nervous system play in achieving movement.

2. Discuss factors that influence an individual's activity level and mobility.

3. Discuss the effects of immobility.

4. Describe the principles of proper body mechanics.

5. Discuss information that should be obtained when assessing an individual's activity or mobility level.

6. Discuss health promotion strategies that can be used to encourage an active lifestyle.

7. Describe restorative interventions that may be used to prevent complications of immobility and promote optimal function.

> ## KEY WORDS
>
> | | |
> |---|---|
> | Amphiarthrosis | Ligaments |
> | Body mechanics | Muscle |
> | Bones | Synarthrosis |
> | Dangling | Synovial |
> | Diarthrosis | Tendons |
> | Joints | |

Overview

The ability to move about freely is something that most people take for granted until presented with a situation in which their mobility is limited or altogether absent. Consequences of immobility extend beyond the lack of freedom to move about independently. It also minimizes or completely removes an individual's ability to perform self-care activities of daily living and alters the functional capacity of all body systems. Additionally, in today's world of technology-produced conveniences, we are faced with a growing sedentary population. Numerous studies have been published that reiterate the consequences of such a lifestyle and the need to integrate some form of physical activity into our daily routines on a consistent basis.

Physiology of Mobility

Movement is achieved through the combined actions of the musculoskeletal system and the nervous system. Movement is not limited to physical movement that we can see happening. It also involves critical life-sustaining activities unseen to the naked eye (ie, breathing, digestion, circulation). Key components of movement include bones, muscles, joints, and nerves:

- **Bones** (skeleton) provide the framework for movement. Weak bones yield a weak framework that may collapse at any time and thus prevent mobility. Weak bones can be compared to the structures that were built by the first little pig and the second little pig, both of which were easily blown down by the big bad wolf. On the other hand, the house that was built with bricks sustained the test.

- **Joints** are the points where bones meet. There are three different types of joints: **synarthrosis** or fibrous joints that do not allow movement (skull sutures); **amphiarthrosis** or cartilaginous joints that allow slight movement (vertebrae); and **diarthrosis** or **synovial** joints that allow for maximum movement. Synovial joints contribute the most to mobility. **Ligaments** are flexible bands of fibrous tissue that connect bones to one another. A torn ligament alters the stability of a joint and may impair movement.

- **Muscle** contraction and relaxation in conjunction with tendons (strong tube-shaped structures that attach muscles to bones) produce movement. The action produced mimics the action that occurs during the game of "tug of war." The rope represents the tendon that attaches one bone to another. The pulling action of the team member represents the muscle relaxation and contraction, and the actual movement of the team represents the bone movement.

- Just as bones cannot move without muscles and tendons, muscles cannot move without the assistance of the central nervous system (CNS). The CNS controls muscle contraction and relaxation, which in turn causes flexion (bending) and extension (straightening), which ultimately results in well-coordinated movements.

Factors Influencing Mobility

A multitude of variables may affect a person's activity level, including his or her personal preferences, values, beliefs, availability of resources, and health status (Box 9–1).

Some variables that influence mobility can be controlled or modified, but others cannot. For example, a person can make a choice of whether he or she wishes to lead a sedentary lifestyle or an active lifestyle within the person's physical

Box 9–1
Mobility-Influencing Factors

- Developmental stage
- Type of work
- Home environment
- Overall health status (nutrition, exercise, mental status)
- Therapeutic interventions (requiring immobility)
- Traumatic injuries
- Diseases or disorders (musculoskeletal, neurologic, cardiovascular, respiratory)

limitations. A person can choose to take the stairs or the elevator or to walk or drive a car; but he or she cannot decide whether or not to have a congenital defect of the skeletal system that impairs mobility. This example provides an oversimplified contrast between controllable and uncontrollable influencing factors. Differentiating between the two categories is not always that cut and dry. Unfortunately, we live in a society where resources are not always distributed equitably. Thus, what would usually be considered a controllable variable may well be uncontrollable for a particular individual. For instance, a homeless family may not have the resources to provide a well-balanced diet, which could result in iron-deficiency anemia, which could in turn alter a person's activity level. It is for this reason that the nurse uses the nursing process as a framework for meeting patients' needs. Doing so allows the nurse to accurately assess the individual patient's situation and collaboratively develop an effective plan of care.

Effects of Immobility

The effects of immobility are far reaching. Immobility can affect a person's physical well-being and his or her psychosocial well-being. The consequences range from an inability to perform simple activities of daily living (eg, feeding oneself, putting on clothes, putting on make-up) to more major limitations such as respiratory distress, circulatory problems, social isolation, depression, and bankruptcy. Table 9–1 provides a list of the most common physical and psychosocial effects of immobility.

> **NURSING ALERT**
>
> **Encourage Mobility**
> Patients should be self-reliant and responsible for their own care. The patient should care for themselves (ie, ADLS) unless the patient is unable to do so. Encouraging patients to perform self-care helps maintain mobility and self-esteem.

✔ # ROUTINE CHECKUP 1

1. _____, _____, _____, and _____ are key structures required for movement.

Answer:

2. Therapeutic interventions that require immobility may place a patient at risk for developing complications such as pneumonia and emboli. True/false?

Answer:

TABLE 9–1 Effects of Immobility	
Integumentary	• Skin breakdown, decubitus formation
Musculoskeletal	• Muscle atrophy: Weakness and contractures
	• Weakness
	• Contractures
	• Decreased joint mobility
	• Falls
	• Bone demineralization
Nervous	• Sensory deprivation
Endocrine	• Altered hormone function
	• Decreased metabolism
	• Activity intolerance
Cardiovascular	• Increased cardiac workload
	• Thrombi
	• Emboli
	• Stroke
	• Heart attack
	• Respiratory arrest
	• Orthostatic hypotension
Respiratory	• Pneumonia
	• Impaired gas exchange
Digestive	• Anorexia
	• Constipation
Urinary	• Urinary tract infections
	• Urinary incontinence (overstretched bladder)
	• Renal calculi (kidney stones)
Psychosocial	• Stress
	• Sleep interruption
	• Depression
	• Social isolation
	• Alteration in roles and relationships
	• Altered body image and self-esteem
	• Altered sexuality

The Nursing Process and Mobility

The nursing process ensures that a systematic approach is used to meet the patient's mobility-related needs. The expected outcome is that the patient will perform at his or her optimal level and remain injury free. When mobility is compromised, the goal is to prevent complications and restore as much mobility as possible.

Assessment

During assessment, the nurse collects information about the patient's functional capacity for mobility, his or her perception of what is an acceptable level of activity, and the impact that immobility may have on the patient. To obtain a complete and accurate database, the nurse should observe the patient while he or she is standing, sitting, and lying down and during ambulation (as tolerated by the patient). Specific observations that should be made include:

- Body alignment (scoliosis, kyphosis, lordosis)
- Gait, balance, and coordination
- Range of motion (ROM; active and passive)
- Joint deformities and musculoskeletal deviations (arthritic changes, muscle tone)
- Neurologic deviations
- Signs of discomfort and activity intolerance (nonverbal cues as well as verbal reports)
- Risk for falls
- Diagnostic test results (x-ray, magnetic resonance imaging, laboratory studies)
- Current therapeutic interventions and medications that may impact mobility
- Signs of complications (eg, skin breakdown, pneumonia, depression, social isolation)

NURSING ALERT

Difference Between Can Do and Won't Do
Some patients don't move because they are afraid of injury. The nurse should determine the extent of the patient's inability to move compared with the patient's lack of desire to move. For example, a patient recovering from a fractured leg may continue to use a wheelchair or crutches long after the leg has healed fearing that they will fall and reinjure the leg.

Nursing Diagnoses

The information collected during assessment drives nursing diagnoses identification. The nurse, with input from the patient, identifies and prioritizes
patient-specific nursing diagnoses. Chapter 2 provides specific guidelines for
how to successfully identify pertinent nursing diagnoses. It is important for the
nurse to remember that nursing diagnoses do not always mean that there is a
problem. Nursing diagnoses can also target maintenance and improvement of
current functional patterns. Some nursing diagnoses that may be appropriate
for addressing a patient's mobility needs include:

- Impaired physical mobility
- Activity intolerance
- Risk for falls
- Self-care deficit
- Impaired skin integrity
- Impaired social interaction

Planning

Planning involves the identification of expected outcomes and the means or
interventions for ensuring that the outcomes are achieved. At this point, the
nurse should also consider how he or she can implement the plan of care in a
safe manner. Achieving mobility in a safe manner rests partly on the use of
good body mechanics. **Body mechanics** can be described as the way an individual uses bones, muscles, and joints to create movement. Use of proper body
mechanics prevents injuries to the musculoskeletal system. To achieve proper
body mechanics, an individual must maintain proper alignment and balance
during movement (Box 9–2).

Implementation

Interventions for mobility fall into two broad categories: health promotion
interventions and restorative interventions. Health promotion interventions
keep individuals at their optimal level of functioning and target individuals
who are at risk for experiencing the consequences of being physically inactive.
Restorative interventions target individuals who are currently experiencing
some level of immobility and are implemented to minimize the negative
impact of immobility and to restore the individual to his or her optimal level
of functioning.

Box 9–2
Tips for Proper Body Mechanics

- Plan the task (eg, lifting, transfer) first.
- Allow the patient to assist as much as possible.
- Seek assistance as needed.
- Use mechanical devices as needed.
- Use smooth, coordinated movements instead of jerky movements.
- Tighten the gluteal and abdominal muscles for lifting.
- Push, slide, or pull instead of lifting or carrying when possible.
- Pivot the entire body, *do not twist the body*!
- Establish a wide base of support.
  - Feet planted firmly on floor
  - One foot slightly in front of the other foot
  - Knees slightly bent
- Use large leg muscles; *do not use back muscles*!
- Carry objects close to your body.
- Avoid stretching and reaching for objects.
- Adjust bed to waist height if possible.
- Teach family members and patients to use the same principles in the home setting.

Health Promotion

It is very important to encourage all individuals (from infancy through old age) to be active. This does not mean that every person should aim to be a marathon runner; instead, each individual should identify personal goals for activity and work toward reaching a level of optimal function. According to the Surgeon General's report on physical activity and health, "regular physical activity that is performed on most days of the week reduces the risk of developing or dying from some of the leading causes of illness and death in the United States." There are two key components to the success of a program to promote physical activity: (1) identifying enjoyable activities that the individual is capable of doing and (2) consistency in performing the activities. Thus, the nurse must work closely with the individual patient to tailor a program that meets the above criteria.

Restorative Interventions

As stated previously, the goal of restorative interventions is to prevent complications associated with immobility and assist the patient to achieve his or her optimal level of functioning. Specific interventions required depend on the nature of the patient's immobility as well as the phase of recovery. For example, during the immediate postoperative period for a patient who has had a total hip replacement, the goal may be to prevent acute complications of immobility through interventions such as positioning the patient, breathing exercises, and so on. After a couple of days, interventions to promote increased movement may be added. When the patient is ready to be discharged home, instructions on independent exercises to be used at home may be the focus. The following discussion highlights nursing interventions that may be used for the patient who is experiencing altered mobility.

Positioning and Transferring

Patients who are immobile may require the nurse's assistance to change positions or move from one location to another (eg, bed to chair, bed to stretcher). Positioning and transfer may be a matter of personal comfort or may be a part of the prescribed interventions to prevent complications and promote optimal function. When positioning or transferring a patient, the nurse should:

- Plan how activity will be performed before beginning.
- Use good body mechanics.
- Allow the patient to assist as much as possible.
- Use assistive devices (draw sheets, transfer belt, mechanical lifts, another person).
- Ensure proper body alignment (may require pillows, splints, footboard).
- Avoid pressure, especially over bony prominences (elbows, heels, sacrum).
- Develop a schedule (usually at least every 2 hours).

Range of Motion Exercise

Joint mobility is maintained by performing ROM exercises. ROM exercises can be performed actively or passively. In active ROM exercises, the patient performs the movement independently. Passive ROM exercises require the assistance of a nurse or a mechanical device. Before the initiation of ROM exercises, the degree of movement that can be achieved without causing injury should be established.

NURSING ALERT

Range of Motion Caution
When performing passive ROM exercises, never extend the joint beyond the point of resistance. Stop ROM exercises immediately if the patient complains of pain.

> ## NURSING ALERT
>
> **Medicate Before ROM Activities**
> Always medication an hour before performing ROM activities if the patient might be in pain as a result of the activities.

Ambulation

To promote safety and prevent injury to the patient and the nurse, the patient's readiness for walking must be assessed. Actual ambulation should not be attempted until the patient has the necessary strength and coordination to perform this task. It may be necessary to progress in steps, starting with sitting in the bed and then progressing to **dangling** (sitting on the bedside with the legs in a dependent position). Walking should be postponed if the patient complains of dizziness or if there is evidence that he or she is experiencing orthostatic hypotension. Assistive devices such as a transfer belt, cane, crutches, or walker should be used as needed (Figure 9–1).

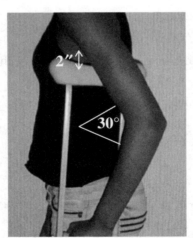

- The top of the crutch should be 2 inches below the armpit.
- The patient should bear body weight on the arms, **not** the shoulders and armpits.
- The handgrip should be adjusted to allow the elbow to be flexed 15 to 30 degrees (allows the elbow to fully extend when a step is taken).
- Rubber tips should be dry and should be replaced when worn.
- Crutches should be positioned 6 inches in front of each foot and 6 inches to the side of each foot.

FIGURE 9–1 · Proper use of crutches.

Evaluation

Consistency is critical to a successful plan for promoting an active lifestyle. Building in opportunities for evaluating the plan then becomes imperative to ensuring that the plan is appropriate and more importantly that the plan has not been abandoned. Additionally, the consequences of immobility often progress rapidly (eg, skin breakdown, pneumonia). Thus, evaluation of interventions and outcome achievement related to immobility must be conducted on a regular basis to minimize negative outcomes.

Conclusion

The benefits of physical activity have been well documented just as the consequences of inactivity have been. Nurses are challenged with convincing patients of the benefits of physical activity. One way of achieving this is by serving as a role model for the patient. The nurse should also work collaboratively with the patient to develop attainable individualized goals for physical activity. When the patient actually experiences immobility, the nurse must assist with preventing complications of immobility and help the client to achieve his or her optimal level of functioning. Doing so requires provisions for meeting psychosocial needs as well as physical needs.

REVIEW QUESTIONS

1. _____ connect bones to bones.
   A. Joints
   B. Ligaments
   C. Muscles
   D. Tendons

2. **Which of the following joints allow for the greatest amount of movement?**
   A. Amphiarthrosis
   B. Diarthrosis
   C. Metarthrosis
   D. Synarthrosis

3. **All of the following are proper principles of body mechanics EXCEPT:**
   A. Carry objects close to your body.
   B. Avoid stretching and reaching for objects.

    C. Lock your knees when lifting an object.

    D. Pivot your entire body; do not twist your body.

4. **Which of the following represents a consequence of immobility?**

    A. Altered sexuality

    B. Anorexia

    C. Constipation

    D. All of the above

5. **When teaching a patient how to crutch walk, the nurse should ensure that:**

    A. Each crutch is positioned 6 inches to the side of each foot and 6 inches in front of each foot.

    B. The hand grip is positioned to allow the arm to be fully extended before taking a step.

    C. The top of the crutch fits snuggly in the armpit.

    D. B and C

    E. All of the above

6. **When developing a plan for the integration of activity into a person's life, the nurse should:**

    A. Ask the patient to identify activities that he or she enjoys.

    B. Encourage the patient to enroll in a structured exercise program.

    C. Emphasize the benefit of engaging in some type of activity most days of the week.

    D. A and C

    E. All of the above

ANSWERS

Routine Checkup

    1. Bones, muscles, joints, and nerves.

    2. True.

Review Questions

    1. B

    2. B

    3. C

    4. D

    5. A

    6. D

References

Craven RF, Hirnle CJ: *Fundamentals of Nursing: Human Health and Function*, 5th ed. Philadelphia, PA: Lippincott, 2006.

Daniels R: *Nursing Fundamentals: Caring & Clinical Decision Making*. New York, NY: Delmar Thomson Learning, 2004.

Potter PA, Perry AG: *Fundamentals of Nursing*, 6th ed. St. Louis, MO: Mosby Elsevier, 2005.

Additional Resources

American College of Foot and Ankle Surgeons: *Instructions for Using Crutches.* Available at http://www.footphysicians.com/footankleinfo/crutches.htm.

Centers for Disease Control and Prevention: *The Link Between Physical Activity and Morbidity and Mortality.* Available at http://www.cdc.gov/nccdphp/sgr/mm.htm.

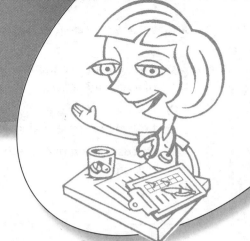

Chapter 10

Sensory and Cognition

LEARNING OBJECTIVES

At the end of the chapter, the reader will be able to:

1. Identify the eight mechanisms of external and internal sensory reception.
2. Describe how environmental stimuli reach the brain for cognitive processing.
3. Identify and describe four components of cognition.
4. Differentiate between immediate, remote, and long-term memory.
5. Discuss factors that influence sensory and cognitive function.
6. Explain the difference between a sensory deficit and sensory deprivation.
7. Differentiate between delirium, dementia, delusions, and hallucinations.
8. Describe the four forms of aphasia.
9. Identify information that should be collected during the mental status assessment.
10. List the five accepted NANDA nursing diagnoses for patients experiencing sensory and cognitive alterations.
11. Discuss health promotion interventions aimed at preventing sensory and cognitive dysfunction.

⑫ Describe interventions that may assist with minimizing the negative impact of a sensory deficit.

⑬ Discuss ways to prevent or minimize sensory deprivation and sensory overload both in the home setting and the acute care setting.

⑭ Discuss interventions appropriate for patients experiencing cognitive dysfunction.

KEY WORDS

Affect	Expressive language
Aphasia	Glaucoma
Cerumen	Hallucination
Congenital	Memory
Delirium	Ototoxicity
Delusion	Proprioception
Dementia	Receptive language
Equilibrium	

Overview

A person's ability to interact with his or her environment is contingent upon the presence of intact sensory and cognitive function. The senses serve as receptor sites for environmental stimuli. The absence of the ability to see, hear, smell, taste, or feel (sense of touch) impacts the quality of environmental interactions. The simultaneous absence of all sensory functions is equivalent to complete loss of the ability to interact with the environment. This not only interferes with pleasurable or desirable interactions but also presents safety issues. Likewise, to process stimuli that are encountered through the senses, the brain must be intact. Cognition is how meaning is given to the stimuli received via the senses. This chapter presents an overview of sensory reception, perception, and cognition. A discussion of influencing factors, common alterations, and nursing care of patients with altered sensory and cognitive function are also included.

Physiology of Sensory and Cognitive Function

Right now at this very moment you are receiving stimuli; receptors (ie, rental, touch sensors) translate stimuli into nerve impulses that travel to the brain where impulses are analyzed and, if necessary, new impulses are sent to respond to the stimuli. This is happening in seconds. In the absence of sensory and cognitive processing, you would not be able to read and understand what is printed on this page, and you would not be able to stop reading what is on this page when you need a break! The process of sensory reception, perception, and response is a fluid process. As demonstrated above, it occurs rapidly and ironically without the need for you to give it much thought. For the next couple of paragraphs, each component of the process will be discussed in "slow motion" to provide a basic understanding of the relationship between sensory and cognitive function and stimuli processing.

Sensory Reception

There are millions of stimuli in a person's external and internal environments. Stimuli from the external environment are received via the sensory organs. The sensory organs include:

- Eyes: sense of sight (vision)
- Ears: sense of hearing
- Nose: sense of smell
- Tongue: sense of taste via taste buds on tongue
- Nerve endings in skin: sense of touch

Stimuli that are mediated by the internal environment are responsible for a person's awareness of:

- Position and movement (also called **proprioception**)
- The size, shape, and texture of objects
- Large organs located inside the body (eg, stomach, liver, heart)

Cognitive Processing of Stimuli

The nerves, spinal cord, and brain make up the nervous system. The nervous system is the means by which an individual is able to interpret and respond to stimuli. Impulses created by sensory stimuli (external and internal) travel to the brain via the peripheral nerves or the cranial nerves. Stimuli received via the peripheral nerves travel to the brain by way of the spinal cord. Cranial nerves, on the other hand, originate from the brain. Impulses from stimuli travel through the brain stem or the "relay station" where they are screened to determine which ones will be processed immediately, which will be transmitted to a storage location (memory), and which will be discarded (Figure 10–1). Multiple cognitive processes influence the final fate of stimuli received by the brain.

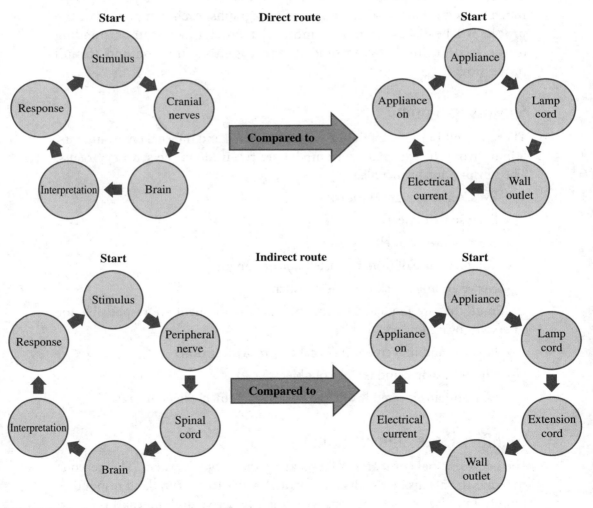

FIGURE 10–1 · Stimuli processing versus electrical current.

Cognitive Components

Consciousness

The reticular activating system (RAS), which is located in the brain stem, regulates a person's level of consciousness. A conscious state of mind is required to process sensory stimuli. In fact, one of the ways nurses assess a person's level of consciousness is by how the individual responds to certain types of stimuli (eg, whether the patient answers verbal commands or responds to painful stimuli).

Thinking and Judgment

When a conscious individual is presented with stimuli, he or she gives thought to what has been presented and subsequently makes a judgment about how to respond. The person's state of mind influences the soundness of his or her judgment. Whereas persons who are not in touch with reality or are disoriented may make poor judgment calls, those who are in touch with reality and oriented to person, place, and time are capable of making sound judgment calls.

Memory

Memory is simply storing information for later use. As discussed, an individual is presented with millions of stimuli simultaneously, and some of the stimuli are stored in a person's memory. Information stored in memory is recalled as needed to interpret stimuli that require an immediate response. For example, a person who has had an adverse drug reaction to a medicine in the past stores that information, and if that medication is recommended for use in the future, the person recalls from memory the fact that he or she previously had an adverse reaction to that medication. This information is then used in making a judgment about what course of action to take (eg, notifying the doctor that the medication caused a previous adverse reaction and requesting an alternate medication). There are three levels of memory:

- **Immediate memory (short term):** The ability to recall information for a very brief period of time (eg, viewing a safe combination number on a sheet of paper and holding it in memory long enough to go to the safe and open it)

- **Intermediate or recent memory:** Recall of stimuli stored within the past 24 hours (eg, recalling what you ate for breakfast yesterday)

- **Long-term or remote memory:** Recall of events that occurred earlier in life (eg, an adult recalls learning to ride a bicycle as a child)

✔ ROUTINE CHECKUP 1

1. Stimuli are transmitted to the brain by way of the _____ nerves, the _____ nerves, and the spinal cord.

Answer:

2. The ability to understand spoken and written words is referred to as receptive language. True/false?

Answer:

Language

Language is a major means of receiving and responding to stimuli and includes the ability to speak words, write words in a meaningful manner on a writing medium (eg, paper, chalkboard), and comprehend or understand spoken and written words. The ability to speak and write words is called **expressive language**, and the ability to understand spoken and written words is referred to as **receptive language**.

Factors Influencing Sensory and Cognitive Function

Multiple variables influence individual interpretations of sensory stimuli. Some of the common influencing factors are age, environment, past experiences, lifestyle, culture, health deviations, and medications.

Age

Sensory perception varies depending on the age and developmental status of the individual. During infancy, the immaturity of sensory organs and the nervous system as well as limited life experiences cause infants to have more generalized responses to environmental stimuli. For example, whereas an infant responds to noises such as a loud hand clap with his or her whole body (startle reflex), an older child or adult may turn his or her head to locate the source of the noise. Sensory perception diminishes as the individual ages. Vision and hearing may be less keen, resulting in slower response times in older adults. Knowledge of the variations in functional ability related to the age or developmental stage of the individual should be taken into consideration when planning nursing care.

Characteristics of cognitive function also vary at different developmental stages in an individual's life. Cognition increases as the nervous system matures and active environmental interaction occurs. Age in and of itself cannot be used to predict cognitive function in older adults. Instead, it seems that the level of cognitive activity in which the individual engages him- or herself is more of a determining factor.

Environment

The amount and type of stimuli present in an individual's surroundings influence his or her sensory and cognitive function. A person who lives in an isolated environment for any length of time may become disoriented and unable to respond to stimuli when reintroduced into his or her usual environment. Likewise, an individual who is bombarded with too many stimuli may become confused and have difficulty determining which stimuli to respond to and which ones to screen out.

Lifestyle and Previous Experiences

Everyday practices such as eating patterns, fluid consumption, and sleep habits affect cognitive function. Skipping meals as well as omission of certain types of foods may deprive the brain of nutrients and electrolytes essential for proper cognitive function. The brain not only needs certain nutrients to function properly; it also needs periods of rest and relaxation to assimilate information and recover. Sleep deprivation interferes with a person's ability to concentrate and process environmental cues. When a person makes the comment: "I'm so tired I can't think straight," he or she may be speaking symbolically, but actually his or her cognitive function is literally less than optimal. Thus, advising a person to "get a good night of sleep before taking the test tomorrow" is quite prudent advice.

Persons who are accustomed to a quiet environment with minimal stimulation may have a hard time adjusting to a noisy environment and vice versa. Other lifestyle characteristics that may impact sensory and cognitive function include work environment and leisure activities. Working in an environment where loud noise is constantly present or listening to very loud music may lead to hearing impairment over time. Recommending the use of ear plugs and educating those who listen to loud music about possible consequences are important. It is just as important to encourage patients, particularly older adults, to "keep their minds active" (eg, reading, crossword puzzles, and social gatherings).

Stress is another variable that may alter a person's sensory and cognitive function. When a person experiences a high level of stress (eg, job, family, financial, relationships), he or she may have difficulty concentrating, may make rash decisions, and may be vulnerable to safety hazards because of poor judgment or missing environmental signals. Stress sharpens critical thinking and decision-making abilities for a short time period such as with the fight or flight response to a threatening situation. However, continues stress decreases critical thinking and decision-making abilities. Some people such as staff in an emergency department develop coping skills that help them manage stressful situation. As a result, they can maintain a leveling of critical thinking and decision-making abilities for longer time periods.

Life experiences also play a significant role in a person's level of sensory and cognitive function. The more life experiences a person has had, the more options he or she has for responding to the various stimuli encountered. For example, a person who has never stepped in an ant bed might step in one and experience ant bites. However, the next time the person sees an ant bed, he or she will be more inclined to avoid stepping in it.

Culture, Values, and Beliefs

A person's culture and value system influence interpretation of environmental stimuli as well as how the individual responds to stimuli. For example, language varies depending on an individual's culture and may interfere with sensory perception and cognition in certain settings (eg, a person who is receiving healthcare in a setting where his or her native language is not spoken). Additionally, how a person perceives her- or himself has the potential to limit or expand his or her cognitive abilities. For example, a child who shies away from a spelling bee competition because of a perceived limited vocabulary may in fact be missing an opportunity to expand his or her language capacity. On the other hand, a person who is very confident may take on challenges and unchartered territories (eg, advanced classes, foreign languages, the school debate team) and use these activities to expand his or her cognitive abilities.

> ### NURSING ALERT
>
> **Cultural Diversity**
> Each nurse must assess their viewpoint caring for a diverse patient population in order to ensure that all patients receive the same level of care. The nurse must also be aware of how patients from various cultural backgrounds view the nurse and other members of the healthcare team. Some patients tend to view members of their healthcare team from the patient's cultural background, which might differ from that of healthcare team members.

Health Deviations

Conditions that directly affect the senses, such as congenital or acquired deafness and blindness, interfere with sensory perception. Additionally, infections, dementia, strokes, metabolic disorders, hypertension, multiple sclerosis, and head trauma may indirectly lead to alterations in both sensory and cognitive function. Assessing patients for risk factors, encouraging the use of preventive health strategies, and including health teaching are strategies that can be used to assist with minimizing the occurrence of impairment that occurs secondary to the above-cited health deviations. When health deviations cannot be avoided, the healthcare team should work collaboratively with the patient to promote his or her optimal level of sensory and cognitive function.

Medications

Medications may have a negative effect on cognitive and sensory function. Central nervous system medications such as narcotic analgesics, sedatives, antidepressants, and antipsychotics can impair cognitive function by causing drowsiness, confusion, and slowed reflex responses. Other medications may cause changes in sensory perception. For example, the antibiotic gentamicin, when given in high doses, may cause damage to the hearing organs (**ototoxicity**) and subsequently cause hearing impairment. Spinal and epidural anesthesia may also alter sensory and cognitive function either temporarily or in some cases, such as with nerve damage, permanently.

NURSING ALERT

Gentamicin Ototoxicity
Gentamicin is an antibiotic that may cause ototoxicity. One way to limit this occurrence is by monitoring the therapeutic level of the medication. The physician may order gentamicin peak (upper limit) and trough (lower limit) levels when the patient is taking gentamicin. It is important to make sure that the laboratory studies are ordered and drawn at the correct time to ensure the accuracy of the laboratory values.

NURSING ALERT

Assess Medication First
Be sure to understand the side effects of medication that the patient may have taken before assessing the cognitive status of the patient. The patient's medication may directly influence the cognitive presentation of the patient.

Alteration in Sensory and Cognitive Function

We usually progress through the course of a day without giving much thought to the "behind the scenes" activities that are required for "normal" function. We give little, if any, thought to the delicate balance that is being maintained until something goes wrong. Sensory alterations may occur because of an actual deficit or may be related to environmental deprivation or overload. Significant cognitive impairment may be caused by attention deficits, memory loss, disorganized thinking, or language impairment. This section discusses the aforementioned sensory and cognitive alteration. However, it is important to keep in mind that this discussion does not exhaust the list of possible cognitive and sensory alterations.

> **NURSING ALERT**
>
> **Normal Cognitive Function**
> Normal cognitive function is difficult to define. It is important for the nurse to assess why a patient appears to have abnormal cognitive functions. What might appear abnormal might be normal for the patient based on the patient's culture, experience, education, and cognitive capabilities.

Sensory Alterations

Sensory Deficit

Sensory deficits are the direct result of sensory organ damage and involve an actual loss of sight, hearing, taste, smell, or sense of touch. In the case of a sensory deficit, the individual is unable to process stimuli via a particular sense. Sensory deficits may be temporary (eg, temporary loss of ability to perceive touch after epidural anesthesia) or permanent (eg, blindness secondary to glaucoma). The onset may be sudden or slow. A person is usually able to prepare him- or herself and thus adapt better when the onset is slow.

Sensory Deprivation

Sensory deprivation, although it sounds a lot like *sensory deficit*, is not the same. Sensory deprivation occurs because of limited exposure to or poor quality of sensory stimuli. Persons who have sensory deficits are also sensory deprived. However, a person who is sensory deprived may or may not have a sensory deficit. For example, a prisoner who is placed in solitary confinement in total darkness does not have a sensory deficit because his or her vision is intact. However, he or she is at high risk for experiencing sensory deprivation (visual) because of the total darkness, minimal sounds, and lack of interaction with others. Poor quality of sensory input may also lead to sensory deprivation. For example, a person who is listening to a song for the first time may respond by singing along or dancing. However, if the song is played multiple times back to back, he or she will eventually become unresponsive to the song because of the monotony (poor quality).

Sensory Overload

Sensory overload occurs when a person is exposed to more sensory stimuli than he or she can process. The excess may be related to the number of stimuli encountered at one time or to the quality of the stimuli (eg, loud noise may cause sensory overload). The end result is that the individual may exhibit racing thoughts, anxiety, inability to think clearly, disorientation, and sleep deprivation. Acutely ill patients admitted to intensive care units (ICUs) where there is constant activity going on (eg, equipment beeping, alarms sounding, frequent visits and assessments) are at high risk for sensory overload. The same is true for a patient who is newly diagnosed with a severe or terminal illness. If the patient is bombarded with enormous amounts of difficult-to-understand information all at once, he or she may be overwhelmed and be unable to process the information and subsequently experience sensory overload.

Cognitive Alterations

Some of the more common cognitive alterations that an individual may experience include altered attention, memory impairment, disorganized thinking, and impaired language. Cognitive alterations may occur secondary to sensory impairments or for other reasons.

Altered Attention

Persons who are easily distracted may have difficulty completing tasks that involve focusing for more than a short period of time. All individuals at some time or another have experienced a short attention span (eg, having to read the same passage multiple times before grasping its meaning because your mind keeps trailing off to something else). However, when an individual's distractibility persists over time, the ability to learn, engage in meaningful interpersonal interactions, and perform activities of daily living may be hindered.

Memory Impairment

Memory is the means by which we store information for future use. Almost every activity that we perform requires the use of memory. When you open a banana peel the first time, you have to figure out how it is done. Every subsequent time, you open the banana peel as if it was second nature. Memory loss may be short term, intermediate, or long term (refer to the previous discussion of memory) and may be temporary or permanent depending on the underlying cause. Memory loss may occur as a result of head trauma, as an adverse effect of certain medication, or secondary to certain disease processes (eg, stroke, alcoholism, brain infections, tumors). Imagine the implications of memory loss. Performing simple activities of daily living would become a monumental task because each time the task would be performed would be like the first time the task was performed. Imagine the implications for you as a nursing student having to perform each skill you learn in fundamentals lab like it is the first time you have ever performed the skill. It would take forever to provide nursing care!

Disorganized Thinking

All of us get confused at one time or another in our lives, and in most cases we blame our confusion on someone else (eg, "You are confusing me!" or "That's confusing!"). However, there are occasions when confusion becomes a more serious matter. Two common forms of confusion are delirium and dementia. **Delirium** is a state of confusion characterized by a sudden onset that, in most cases, is short term. The person's presentation may range from being anxious, agitated, and fearful to being apathetic with limited reaction. Person with illnesses that are accompanied by a high fever may experience periods of delirium. Also, certain medications may trigger delirium. **Dementia**, on the other hand, usually has a slow onset and is irreversible. Dementia is not a disease in and of itself; instead, it occurs secondary to diseases such as strokes and Alzheimer's disease. Person's experiencing dementia may lose their ability to do things that were second nature to them in the past such as dressing themselves, paying their own bills, or going places independently without getting lost. A person who was previously very pleasant to be around may become rude and even violent. Family and friends of persons experiencing dementia require support and assistance in understanding and coping with the changes in their loved ones.

NURSING ALERT

Sundowners Syndrome
Sundowners syndrome usually occurs during the transition between day and night (at sundown or sunrise). The patient may exhibit varying levels of confusion; is at risk of wandering; and may have delusions, hallucinations, or both. It is important to identify specific triggers and to provide for the safety of the patient.

Persons experiencing delirium or dementia may also have delusions, hallucinations, or both. When a person has a **delusion**, he or she believes, without exception, that something is true when it is not. For example, a patient may believe that the nursing staff is trying to poison him or her with the medications that are being given. In this instance, nothing anyone says will convince the patient otherwise. A **hallucination** is an abnormal perception involving one of the five senses. A person may report seeing, hearing, or feeling something that in reality does not exist (eg, bugs crawling on their bodies or hearing voices). A cornerstone to responding to individuals experiencing delusions and hallucinations is the establishment of a trusting relationship; doing so gives the care provider more leverage when attempting to reorient the patient to reality. It is also advisable to acknowledge the distress that the delusion or hallucination is causing the patient but to also state the "real" circumstance. For example, if the patient thinks that there are bugs crawling on the wall; it would be appropriate to say, "I know you are upset, but I do not see what you are describing." It would be incorrect to go along with the false perception.

Impaired Language

Impaired language, also referred to as **aphasia**, occurs in four forms: expressive, receptive, anomic, and global. The individual is intellectually intact, but his or her language is impaired because of injury (eg, stroke, brain infection) to the parts of the brain that control language. The types of aphasia are:

- **Expressive aphasia:** Difficulty with speaking or writing thoughts. The individual is often very frustrated because the problem is not with knowing what to say but rather with verbalizing the words. As a result, the individual speaks slowly, and his or her words may be choppy.

✔ ROUTINE CHECKUP 2

1. _____ occurs as a result of the loss of function of one of the senses, and _____ occurs because of the lack of or poor quality of environmental stimuli.

Answer:

2. Whereas delirium is a slow-onset, permanent state of confusion, dementia occurs more suddenly and is usually temporary. True/false?

Answer:

- **Receptive aphasia:** The individual cannot understand spoken language (both verbal and written), although he or she may be able to speak fluently.
- **Anomic aphasia:** The individual has difficulty recalling the correct word for objects, places, or events he or she wants to communicate (eg, the object is a ball, but the person has a very difficult time recalling the word ball).
- **Global aphasia:** Total loss of language; receptive and expressive. The individual has difficulty or is unable to speak, read, write, or understand spoken language.

Nursing Process and Sensory and Cognitive Function

Nursing care for a patient experiencing sensory or cognitive alterations varies depending on the nature of the alteration(s) as well as the level of impact on the individual's ability to meet his or her daily needs. To ensure that the patient's needs are adequately met, the nurse must accurately assess the patient's sensory function and mental status as well as the impact of any identified alterations. Doing so facilitates the development of a comprehensive individualized plan of care that includes accurate problem identification and prioritization, appropriate interventions, and an effective implementation strategy.

Assessment

Assessment of sensory function includes a determination of whether the patient has difficulty hearing, seeing, smelling, or tasting or has problems with touch or feeling. In addition to inquiring about the level of function for each, the nurse should perform an objective assessment of sensory function (Table 10–1). Furthermore, the nurse should inquire about the impact of the alterations on the individual's ability to perform activities of daily living as well as the impact on his or her psychosocial well-being. Information about the patient's environment and possible sources of sensory deprivation or overload should also be obtained. The mental status assessment includes the collection of information about the individuals:

- General appearance and presentation
- Level of consciousness and orientation to person, place, and time
- Thought processes (memory, judgment, and problem-solving ability)
- Communication and language (ability to read, write, and carry on a conversation)

TABLE 10–1	Sensory Assessment
Sense	**Assessment**

Sight	• Inquire about:
	  • Problems with vision
	  • Family history
	  • Use of assistive devices (eyeglasses, contact lenses, magnifying glass)
	  • Eye injuries
	• Observe for structural defects of the eye
	• Perform vision screening tests (Snellen, Ishihara, and glaucoma)
	• Observe for squinting, tearing of the eyes, and voluntary placement of reading materials (close to face or away from face)

Hearing	• Inquire about:
	  • Problems with hearing (difficulty hearing, ringing in ears)
	  • Noise level in the work environment
	  • Use of a hearing aid
	  • Medications
	• Perform hearing screening (Rinne, Weber, audiometer)

Taste	• Inquire about:
	  • Current medications
	  • Smoker or not
	  • Appetite problems
	  • Illnesses (respiratory infections, gingivitis, Bell's palsy)
	  • Problems with smelling
	• Test the patient's ability to differentiate between salty, sweet, sour, and bitter
	• Check laboratory studies ordered by the doctor for vitamin B12 or zinc deficiencies

Smell	• Inquire about:
	  • Recent illnesses (cold, chronic sinusitis, head injuries)
	  • Current medication
	  • Allergies
	  • Exposure to toxic chemicals
	• Inspect nostrils for polyps
	• Test the sense of common smells (food, fragrances)

(*Continued*)

TABLE 10−1 Sensory Assessment (*Continued*)	
Sense	**Assessment**

Touch	• Inquire about:
	  • Medications
	  • Brain injuries and surgeries
	  • Numbness and tingling
	• Test the ability to perceive:
	  • Light touch
	  • Firm pressure
	  • Sharp object
	  • Dull object
	  • Temperature (hot, cold)

- Emotional state, including mood and **affect** (eg, flat, euphoric, or wide variations) and appropriateness of affect (eg, an individual laughs [inappropriate] or cries [appropriate] about someone's death)
- Motor function (gait, posture, muscles strength and tone, as well as facial expressions)

Each of the contributing factors discussed earlier in this chapter (ie, age and development, drug and medications use, health deviations, and lifestyle) should also be considered during the assessment of the patient.

NURSING ALERT

Be Clear in Your Questioning
Some patients may understand the intent of your question even if you did not phrase your question properly while other patients will respond literally to your question. You might ask the patient if she is hearing voices. Although you mean hearing voices that others don't hear, the patient may not read that into the question and respond yes—the patient is hearing your voice.

Nursing Diagnosis

Accepted nursing diagnoses for patients experiencing sensory and cognitive impairment include:

- Disturbed sensory perception
- Acute confusion

- Chronic confusion
- Disturbed thought processes
- Impaired verbal communication

Although the above identified diagnoses are the only ones directly related to sensory and cognitive impairment, many others may exist depending on the specific circumstances surrounding the impairment. Examples of other possible nursing diagnoses include:

- Ineffective role performance
- Impaired adjustment
- Impaired memory
- Risk for injury
- Risk for powerlessness
- Self-care deficit (specify what type)
- Situational low self-esteem
- Social isolation
- Wandering

Planning and Implementation

The ultimate goal of care is to prevent the occurrence of sensory and cognitive impairments. To accomplish this goal, the nurse must approach patient care in a proactive manner. Additional goals for patients who are already experiencing sensory or cognitive impairments include safety, assisting the patient in achieving his or her optimal functional level, and preventing further deterioration or secondary complications.

Health Promotion

Health promotion related to sensory protection begins even before a person is born. Expectant mothers are taught to avoid exposure to communicable disease such as rubella that may lead to **congenital** (acquired before birth) blindness. During the childhood years, children are at risk for permanent hearing impairment if they experience repeated ear infections; therefore, it is important to teach parents ways to minimize the occurrence of ear infections. Vision and hearing screening are important for both children and adults. Adults, especially African Americans, may be at risk for the development of **glaucoma** (increased pressure in the eyes), which can cause blindness. Damage associated with glaucoma cannot be reversed but can be prevented with medications if caught before any actual damage occurs. Protecting the eyes and ears is also important. Protective eye wear should be worn whenever there is a danger of a foreign object hitting the eyes (eg, during lawn work, welding, certain sports activities). Constant exposure to loud noises (eg, loud music, factory noise) can cause hearing impairment. During certain developmental periods, children are inclined to put foreign objects in their ears or nose, which may result in sensory impairments secondary to injuries. Hearing impairments may also be caused by **cerumen** (earwax) build-up. Healthcare workers can safely perform ear irrigation to remove ear wax build-up. Patients should be taught that it is not safe to probe in the ear with Q-Tip and hair pins to remove earwax.

Healthy cognitive development requires healthy lifestyle choices, including proper nutrition and exercise, avoiding bad habits (eg, smoking, alcohol abuse, recreational drugs use), and avoiding traumatic injuries (eg, motor vehicle accidents, firearm injuries). Anticipatory guidance and education about the aforementioned health promotion strategies should be integrated into the plan of care for the patient regardless of the setting in which patient presents. Of course, the nurse must set priorities and ensure that the circumstances are appropriate for health teaching. For example, if a patient presents to the emergency department in critical condition after a motor vehicle accident, it would not be appropriate to talk about preventive health at that point. However, before the patient is discharged, it would be appropriate to discuss safe driving strategies. Nurses should take advantage of every opportunity that presents itself (eg, routine doctor visits, community health fairs, school screenings) to educate individuals about strategies to promote optimal sensory and cognitive function.

Interventions for Sensory Deficits

Vision Persons who wear eyeglasses should have regular eye examinations and have their eyeglasses changed as needed. Magnification and enlarged print may also be beneficial. Individuals who wear contact lenses should clean the lenses regularly and with the correct solutions. Failure to do so may lead to the development of infections and further visual impairment. Patients who are blind may benefit from having their environment arranged in a set manner so they become accustomed to maneuvering themselves around. Other environmental modifications that will assist with promoting independence and safety include lighting adjustments, removal of throw rugs, removal of uneven door thresholds, and installation of ramps or handrails when ramps cannot be installed.

Hearing In the past, many patients with hearing deficits refused to wear hearing aids because of being stigmatized by others. Now hearing aids are designed to be barely noticeable. Nurses and other healthcare workers interacting with hearing impaired patients need to educate their patient about the new types of hearing aids, assist patients with identifying resources for obtaining hearing aids, and encourage patients to wear their hearing aids regularly. Sound amplification on home devices, such as doorbells, televisions, and telephones, may also be helpful. It is important to allow extra time for people with hearing impairments to respond. Additionally, persons experiencing hearing impairments may require the services of an interpreter in certain situations. The ears also influence a person's balance. Thus, some of the same precautions taken to promote safety in visually impaired people may also be necessary for elderly patients experiencing **equilibrium** (balance) changes.

Taste and Smell Taste and smell work hand and hand. An inability to smell food aromas may affect a patient's appetite. Good oral hygiene, enhanced flavoring of foods, and texture variety as well as serving individual foods instead of mixing the foods may enhance a person's ability to taste food. Besides affecting taste, a diminished sense of smell can lead to safety hazards. A person uses his or her sense of smell to detect dangerous gases, smoke, spoiled foods, and other potentially unsafe things in the environment. Visual gas sensors, food container labels, and smoke detectors may be required to promote safety.

Touch Patients with an altered sense of touch are at risk for developing pressure ulcers. Frequent repositioning, use of wrinkle-free linens, and prevention of skin contact with irritants are a few of the ways to minimize this risk. The patient can also be taught to rely on thermometer temperature reading of water to avoid scalding burns as well as weather temperatures when deciding how to dress. At the opposite end of the spectrum are patients with hyperesthesia, or excessive skin sensitivity to touch (eg, patients with shingles or nerve pain). In this case, the objective is to limit contact to promote comfort. Teaching the patient about proper use of medications to manage nerve pain may also be required.

Interventions for Sensory Deprivation and Overload

Sensory deprivation may occur in the absence of sensory deficits (vision, hearing, smell, taste, touch deficits). Environmental modifications for the home setting as well as for acute and long-term care settings that may minimize sensory deprivation include:

- Music
- Wall hangings and personal pictures of family and friends
- Clocks
- Bright wall colors
- Opening window shades during daylight hours
- Encouraging social interaction when possible (with nurses, family, friends, other patients when appropriate, pet visits)
- Range of motion exercises and repositioning for bedridden patients

When a patient is unconscious, healthcare team members should not assume that the patient cannot hear what is going on in the environment. The patient should be treated with respect. The nurse should talk to the patient and should encourage family members to talk to the patient during visits. Touch is also thought to be beneficial.

Persons experiencing sensory overload will benefit from a calmer environment. In the acute care setting, especially in ICUs, the nurse should make every attempt to organize care to minimize the number of times the patient has to be awakened. Care should be provided in an unhurried manner. Dim lighting should be maintained unless treatments require otherwise. The noise level should be kept at a minimum as much as possible. Stress should also be kept to a minimum, and any pain that the patient experiences should be managed effectively and in a timely manner.

Interventions for Cognitive Impairment

Persons experiencing cognitive impairment, particularly when confusion is manifested, may require frequent reorientation (reality and environmental). The use of written schedules and checklists may be helpful. Simple directions focusing on one thing at a time should be provided. Assistance with performing activities of daily living may be required. The establishment of environmental boundaries may be necessary for safety reasons. In the acute care setting, under extreme circumstances in which there may be a danger that the individual will harm him- or herself or others, restraints may be required.

A doctor's order is always required for the use of restraints. Restraints should only be used for the time that they are absolutely necessary. Patients requiring restraints should be checked frequently.

NURSING ALERT

Use of Restraints

The use of restraints requires a doctor's order. Restraints should *never* be used to facilitate staff convenience. Patients who require restraints should be monitored frequently, and restraints should be discontinued as soon as possible. A restraint includes holding the patient to administer an injection. The treatment team must use the least restrictive measures when caring for a patient. An alternative to restraints must be used first before the practitioner can order the patient placed in restraints.

Communication may be impaired when a patient has a cognitive impairment. In such cases, alternative methods of communication should be used, and extra time should be allotted. When verbal communication is impaired, written communication may be an alternative. Sometimes the patient may need to draw pictures instead of using words or may need to use gestures. Social interaction should be encouraged as appropriate to the individual's level of function and readiness.

Evaluation

The evaluation of the effectiveness of nursing care for the patient experiencing sensory or cognitive impairment is based on the earlier state goals: (1) prevention, (2) safety, (3) achievement of optimal function, and (4) prevention of further deterioration. The plan of care must be evaluated on an ongoing basis and adjusted as warranted. For patients who are cared for in acute care settings, it is also important at the time of discharge that the plan of care is evaluated and modified to meet the needs of the patient and family in the home or community setting.

Conclusion

This chapter has presented key information about normal sensory and cognitive function as well as common deviations. A review of normal physiology and influencing factors was presented as a foundation for understanding the application of the nursing process to the care of patients with sensory and cognitive impairments. Key concepts included in the chapter are as follows:

- The senses (sight, hearing, smell, taste, touch) serve as receptor sites for environmental stimuli.
- Cognition is the means by which meaning is given to stimuli received via the senses.
- Major components of cognition include consciousness, judgment, memory, and language.
- Memory can be divided into three subcategories: immediate memory, recent memory (within 24 hours), and long-term memory (recall from earlier periods in life).
- The ability to speak and write is expressive language and the ability to understand spoken and written words is receptive language.
- Whereas a sensory deficit involves the impairment of one of the senses, sensory deprivation occurs because of a limited exposure to or poor quality of sensory stimuli.
- Patients admitted to ICUs are at risk for sensory overload.
- Whereas delirium is a state of confusion that occurs suddenly and that is usually temporary, dementia has a slow onset and is permanent.
- The mental status assessment should include an evaluation of the level of consciousness, thought processes, ability to communicate, motor function, and emotional status.
- Accepted nursing diagnoses for patients experiencing sensory and cognitive impairment include disturbed sensory perception, acute and chronic confusion, disturbed thought processes, and impaired verbal communication.
- Nursing care for patients experiencing sensory and cognitive impairment is centered on promoting safety, promoting the individual's optimal level of functioning, and preventing further deterioration of the patient.

REVIEW QUESTIONS

1. _____ memory is the patient's ability to recall events or information stored within the past 24 hours.
    A. Immediate
    B. Recent
    C. Remote
    D. Long-term

2. **Environmental stimuli are received by which of the following sensory organs?**

   A. Eyes
   B. Mouth
   C. Skin
   D. A and C
   E. All of the above

3. **Which of the following should the nurse consider to be a significant risk factor for sensory and cognitive function impairment?**

   A. Recent lack of sleep
   B. Employment as a rock musician
   C. History of hypertension
   D. All of the above

4. **Which of the following medications may cause sensory or cognitive impairment?**

   A. Certain antibiotics
   B. Epidural or spinal medications
   C. Narcotics
   D. B and C
   E. All of the above

5. **All of the following may be valuable information when assessing a patient who is suspected of having an altered sense of taste EXCEPT:**

   A. Rinne screening test result
   B. Sense of smell
   C. Smoking habit
   D. Vitamin B_{12} level
   E. Zinc level

6. **A patient tells you that there are bugs crawling on the wall. When you observe the same wall, there is no evidence of crawling bugs. Your BEST response to the patient would be:**

   A. Change the topic of conversation.
   B. Acknowledge the patient's concern while at the same time telling the patient that there are no bugs on the wall.
   C. Pretend to kill the bugs on the wall.
   D. Summon a third objective party to the room to tell the patient that there are no bugs on the wall.

7. **All of the following interventions may be used, without limitation, for a patient who presents with confusion EXCEPT:**

   A. Frequent reorientation
   B. Written instructions and checklists

C. Restraints

D. Simple one-step direction

8. **A family member is visiting an elderly client who has Alzheimer's disease. The client becomes agitated and does not recognize the visiting family member. Which of the following actions by the nurse would be MOST beneficial? The nurse should instruct the family member to:**

A. Accept the inevitable decline and continue to visit "as a friend."

B. Increase the frequency of visits to increase the client's recall.

C. Remind the client as often as needed that the visitor is the client's family member.

D. Place pictures of family members, labeled with their names, and reminisce during visits.

ANSWERS

Routine Checkup 1

1. Peripheral, cranial.

2. True.

Routine Checkup 2

1. Sensory deficit, sensory deprivation.

2. False.

Review Questions

1. B

2. D

3. E

4. E

5. A

6. B

7. C

8. D

References

Craven RF, Hirnle CJ: *Fundamentals of Nursing: Human Health and Function*, 5th ed. Philadelphia, PA: Lippincott, 2006.

Daniels R: *Nursing Fundamentals: Caring & Clinical Decision Making*. New York, NY: Delmar Thomson Learning, 2004.

Potter PA, Perry AG: *Fundamentals of Nursing*, 6th ed. St. Louis, MO: Mosby Elsevier, 2005.

Additional Resources

American Association of Neurological Surgeons: *Anatomy of the Brain*. Available at http://www.neurosurgerytoday.org/what/patient_e/anatomy1.asp.

American Geriatrics Society: *Delirium (Sudden Confusion)*. Available at http://www.healthinaging.org/agingintheknow/chapters_ch_trial.asp?ch=57.

A Place for Mom: *Sundowners Syndrome*. Available at http://alzheimers.aplaceformom.com/articles/sundowners-syndrome/.

Mayo Clinic: *Sundowning: Late-Day Confusion*. Available at http://www.mayoclinic.com/print/sundowning/HQ01463/METHOD=print.

MedlinePlus: *Aging Changes in the Senses*. Available at http://www.nlm.nih.gov/medlineplus/ency/article/004013.htm.

MedlinePlus: *Aphasia*. Available at http://www.nlm.nih.gov/medlineplus/aphasia.html.

MedlinePlus: *Memory Loss*. Available at http://www.nlm.nih.gov/medlineplus/ency/article/003257.htm.

MedlinePlus: *Taste—impaired*. Available at http://vsearch.nlm.nih.gov/vivisimo/cgi-bin/query-meta?v%3Aproject=medlineplus&query=Mental+Status+Evaluation.

Merck: *The Merck Manuals Online Medical Library*. Available at http://www.merck.com/mmhe/index.html.

NIH Senior Health: *Problems with Smell*. Available at http://nihseniorhealth.gov/problemswithsmell/aboutproblemswithsmell/01.html.

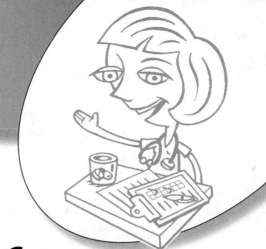

Chapter **11**

Sleep and Comfort

LEARNING OBJECTIVES

At the end of the chapter, the reader will be able to:

1. Differentiate between sleep and rest.

2. Discuss the characteristics of each phase of the sleep cycle.

3. Discuss factors that influence an individual's ability to obtain sleep and rest.

4. Discuss the effects and consequences of sleep disturbances.

5. Discuss information that should be obtained when assessing a person's sleep pattern and quality.

6. Discuss interventions that may be used to prevent, minimize, or resolve sleep disturbances.

7. Describe the pain transmission process.

8. Describe the difference between pain sensations mediated by A fibers and those mediated by C fibers.

9. Differentiate between acute pain and chronic pain.

10. Describe the various sources of pain.

11. Discuss variables that affect a person's pain experience.

12. Describe objective tools that can be used to assess an individual's level of pain.

⑬ List other information in addition to the quantity of pain that should be collected during the assessment phase of the nursing process.

⑭ Discuss nonpharmacologic interventions that can be included as a part of the pain management plan.

⑮ Describe the three categories of pharmacologic agents used for pain management.

KEY WORDS

Acute pain	Nociceptors
Adjuvant analgesics	Pain threshold
Allodynia	Pain tolerance
Chronic pain	Paresthesia
Circadian rhythm	Referred pain
Gate control theory	Rest
Idiopathic	Sleep
Modulate	Somatic pain
Neuron	Superficial or cutaneous pain
Neuropathic pain	Visceral pain
Neurotransmitters	

Overview

Imagine being actively involved in some form of activity 24 hours a day, 7 days a week, and 365 days a year. Just the thought of this idea is tiring. Thus, if for no other reason, we need sleep to gain energy to be able to engage in activity without experiencing excessive tiredness. By the same token, it is hard to imagine having to go through each and every day of your life in discomfort. This chapter presents basic information on the physiology of sleep and pain, influencing factors for each, the effects of sleep deprivation, the effects of acute and chronic pain, strategies for helping patients obtain adequate sleep and rest, and strategies to help patients prevent or control pain and its negative impact on daily living.

Sleep and Rest

Sleep is a reversible, altered state of consciousness characterized by minimal activity. Although it may be difficult to arouse some individuals from sleep, it is possible. Reversibility is the major factor that differentiates sleep from other undesirable states of altered consciousness such as a coma. **Rest**, on the other hand, is a conscious state of relaxation. It can involve relaxation of the entire body or may only involve resting a particular part of the body. For example, a person who is an avid reader may take a break from reading to rest his or her eyes. Rest is a more subjective experience because what is restful and relaxing to one person may be stressful to another person.

Physiology of Sleep

Sleep occurs in cycles alternating with periods of wakefulness. The sleep/wake cycle generally follows a **circadian rhythm** or a 24-hour day/night cycle. Most people are awake and busy during the day and sleep at night. Of course, there are exceptions to this rule, particularly for individuals who are employed in jobs that require working at night or rotating shifts. In addition to the sleep/wake cycle, sleep itself actually occurs in stages that progress in a cyclic manner. There are five stages of sleep (Table 11–1). Stages 1 through 4 are referred to as non-rapid eye movement (NREM) sleep and range from a very light state of sleep in stage 1 to very deep sleep in stages 3 and 4 (note: stages 3 and 4 are discussed as one stage, stage 3, by some sources). During NREM sleep, individuals usually experience a decrease in temperature, pulse, blood pressure, respirations, and muscle tone. The decreased demands on body function are thought to serve a restorative role, both physiologically and psychologically. Stage 5 is called rapid eye movement (REM) sleep. The REM stage of sleep is characterized by an increased level of activity compared with the NREM stages. The benefits of REM sleep seem to be related to an improvement in mental processes and emotional health.

Factors Influencing Sleep and Rest

Sleep requirements vary widely from individual to individual. Variables that influence the amount and quality of sleep include:

Age and Developmental Stage

Newborns spend most of their time sleeping (~16 hours in a 24-hour time period). Most of this time is spent in the REM stage. In general, as children progress through childhood, the number of hours spent sleeping decreases and the amount of time spent in the REM stage also decreases; the exception is adolescents and preteens, who may require more sleep during growth spurts.

TABLE 11–1 Sleep Stages and Sleep Cycle

	Non-Rapid Eye Movement Sleep (NREM)				Rapid Eye Movement
	Stage 1	Stage 2	Stage 3	Stage 4	Stage 5
Sleep level	Lightest sleep	Light sleep	Deeper sleep	Deepest sleep	—
EEG pattern	Brain waves become slow; theta waves are present	Brain waves become slower with burst of sleep spindles	Slow brain waves called delta waves	Same as stage 3 sleep with slow brain waves called delta waves	Beta waves, which are similar to those present when a person is awake
Description	• Lasts only a few minutes • Drowsiness; person may say he or she is not asleep; easily aroused • Vital signs, muscle tone, and metabolism begin to slow • May report a falling sensation accompanied by a muscle jerk as if to catch him- or herself.	• Lasts up to 20 minutes • Still fairly easy to arouse the person from sleep • Vital signs, muscle tone, and metabolism continue to slow	• Lasts 15–30 minutes • Person is difficult to arouse; may be disoriented for a while if awakened during this stage of sleep • Vital signs regular but slow; complete relaxation; little to no movement • Sleepwalking, sleep talking, enuresis, and nightmares may occur, especially in children	• Same as for stage 3 sleep	• Lasts an average of 20 minutes • Amount of REM increases as the night progresses; first period of REM begins approximately 110 minutes into the sleep cycle • Vital signs erratic • Rapid eye movements can be seen through closed eyelids • Vivid, colorful dreams • Feeling of being paralyzed is sometimes reported

Sleep cycle

Stage 1 → Stage 2 → Stage 3 → Stage 4 → Stage 3 → Stage 2 → Stage 3 → REM → Stage 2

The quality of sleep during the childhood years may be influenced by fears, nightmares, and the child's activity level immediately preceding bedtime. The amount of sleep and the intervals of sleep change as adults age. Older adults tend to awaken more during the night and may do more daytime napping, especially after retirement.

Psychosocial Influences

Psychosocial variables that impact a person ability to sleep as well the quality of sleep include:

- **Roles and relationships:** Persons who are married sometimes have difficulty falling asleep without their partners. The death of a spouse may have the same impact. In contrast, one spouse's sleep problems (eg, snoring, sleep apnea) may interfere with his or her partner's quality of sleep. Parents of young or sick children may have frequent sleep interruptions as well.

- **Work patterns:** The time of day a person works as well as the stability of his or her work hours may make it difficult to establish a sleep pattern. Daytime light and environmental noises may also make it difficult for the individual to fall and stay asleep.

- **Stress/depression:** Any type of stress, whether it is stress from one's job or stress generated from personal issues, can cause problems with falling asleep or staying asleep. Depression may have the same affect. Sleep problems may be further complicated because a person often tries to sleep to avoid depression; thus, he or she becomes frustrated on top of being depressed because of the lack of sleep.

Lifestyle

- **Activity and exercise patterns:** Although increased activity and exercise have an overall benefit, the timing is very important to promote optimal sleep. Engaging in increased activity and exercise close to bedtime may interfere with a person's ability to fall asleep. It is best to exercise early enough to allow the body to cool down and relax.

- **Eating habits:** The amount of food and types of food a person eats can affect the amount and quality of sleep obtained. Eating large amounts as well as eating high-fat or spicy foods immediately before going to bed may cause abdominal discomfort as well as indigestion and subsequently lead to problems with falling asleep and staying asleep. Consuming foods or beverages with caffeine and alcohol can also prevent restful sleep. On the other hand, attempting to go to bed hungry can also interfere with sleep. The discomfort and noise of a "growling" stomach may be distracting enough to prevent a person from falling asleep.

Environmental Conditions

The environmental temperature, noise level, and amount of lighting all affect a person's ability to sleep comfortably and without interruption. People require different environmental conditions for falling asleep and staying asleep. Some people sleep better in a cool environment, but others prefer a warm, toasty environment. Some people require some level of noise (eg, television, music) to fall asleep, but others must have a perfectly quiet environment to sleep. Likewise, some individuals can sleep through sirens, bad storms, loud music, and laughter without any knowledge of the events, but others awaken at the drop of a pin.

The amount of light in the environment may also influence a person's ability to fall and stay asleep. Some people require a night light to fall asleep, and others prefer to have complete darkness. Persons who work at night and sleep during the day may have difficulty falling asleep because of the sunlight. An interior room with no window or a room with window shades that completely block the light are options to facilitate sleep for persons falling into this category.

Health Deviations

Persons experiencing any type of acute illness are susceptible to sleep problems. Difficulty in breathing, pain, elevated temperature, and itching are examples of specific culprits that may interfere with sleep during an acute illness. Chronic health problems such as arthritis, emphysema, heart disease, and obesity may also disrupt sleep. Normal changes in the body that occur in such instances as pregnancy or menopause can also make it difficult to get the proper amount of rest and sleep.

Medical Interventions

The change of environment and individual bedtime routines associated with hospitalization often lead to sleep difficulties. Medications (both prescribed and over the counter) may also cause sleep problems. In some instances, the problem is related to the intended effect of the medication; in other instances, the problem may be the result of an adverse (unintended) effect. For example, a person taking a laxative may be awakened by the urge to evacuate (intended effect). On the other hand, a person may be taking an antibiotic for an infection and break out in an itchy rash (unintended effect) that interferes with his or her ability to sleep.

> **NURSING ALERT**
>
> **Coordinate Medication with Sleep**
> Some medications cause sleepiness as a side effect. It is important to remind the prescriber that such medications may disrupt the patient's normal sleep cycle if the medication is administered during awaken hours.

Effects of Sleep Disturbances

There are various forms of sleep disturbances (Table 11–2). Disorders are characterized by an inability to fall asleep, an interruption of sleep, the presence of unusual behaviors during sleep, or inappropriate timing of sleep episodes. The effect of sleep disturbances is far reaching and even dangerous in some situations. An inadequate amount of quality sleep has been associated with the occurrence of:

- Impaired memory or confusion
- Depression
- Altered coping abilities or mood swings
- Diminished motor performance
- Increased occurrence of automobile, home, and work-related accidents
- Impaired immune responses
- Cardiovascular disease
- Diabetes
- Obesity
- Depression

> **NURSING ALERT**
>
> **Sleeping Dangers**
> Nurses should teach patients who are at risk for daytime sleepiness secondary to sleeping disorders to use caution when driving and operating dangerous machinery.

TABLE 11–2 Sleep Disorders

Disorder	Description
Insomnia	Difficulty falling asleep or staying asleep. Causes include • Situational stress • Jet lag • Illnesses • Excessive use of hypnotics • Poor sleep habits Insomnia can evolve into a vicious cycle with the individual experiencing more difficulty with falling and staying asleep because of his or her anticipation of a sleep problem.
Sleep deprivation	Prolonged periods of inadequate sleep (amount and/or quality). Contributing factors include • Illness or hospitalization • Drug use (therapeutic or recreational) • Work pattern • Stress • Sleep environment
Narcolepsy	Excessive daytime sleepiness. Episodes usually last 10–15 minutes: • Rapid onset of REM (15–20 minutes) • Sleep paralysis may occur • Vivid dreams may occur • Cataplexy (sudden muscle weakness) may cause to individual to fall
Parasomnias	Activities occur during sleep that normally occur when a person is awake: • Sleepwalking • Sleep talking • Enuresis Other activities that fall into this category include • Nightmares • Teeth grinding
Sleep apnea	Periods of apnea lasting 10 or more seconds while an individual is asleep. Factors that contribute to sleep apnea include • Alcohol use • Obesity • Smoking • Sleeping position (sleeping on back) • Soft tissue obstructions • Jaw bone deformities Snoring and daytime sleepiness are two common manifestations that accompany sleep apnea. CPAP devices and surgery as well as lifestyle modifications may benefit patients who have sleep apnea.

CPAP = continuous positive airway pressure.

✔ ROUTINE CHECKUP 1

1. Stages 1 through 4 of the sleep cycle are referred to as _____ sleep, and stage 5 of the sleep cycle is called _____ sleep.

Answer:

2. Exercise just before going to sleep is thought to improve the individual's ability to fall asleep. True/false?

Answer:

3. Exercise just before going to sleep is thought to improve the individual's ability to fall asleep. True/false?

Answer:

_____

_____

_____

_____

_____

The Nursing Process and Sleep/Rest Disturbances

In the acute care setting, nursing, which is usually a helping profession, may actually contribute to sleep disturbance problems. The nurse uses the nursing process to minimize the occurrence of sleep disturbances resulting from nursing and other medical interventions. Nurses can also promote healthy sleeping behaviors for individuals in the community as well as assist patients who are recovering from illnesses to restore optimal levels of rest and sleep.

Assessment

Traditionally, the foundation of an effective assessment is built upon a well-round database of both subjective and objective data. However, when assessing a person's sleep pattern, the individual's perception of the quality and adequacy of his or her current pattern of sleep is the most powerful factor for determining whether there is a problem. Thus, the nurse should ensure that information about the patient's perception of the adequacy and quality of sleep is included when collecting data. Additionally, each of the variables previously mentioned during the discussion of factors influencing sleep should be considered during the assessment of an individual's sleep pattern (ie, age, developmental stage, marital status, diet, activity level, physical environment, work setting). It may also be helpful to have the patient keep a sleep diary to record information about his or her sleep patterns.

Nursing Diagnoses

As stated previously, sleep needs are highly individualized. The same is true of nursing diagnoses that may be applicable for a patient who is having difficulty sleeping. The two North American Nursing Diagnosis Association (NANDA) nursing diagnoses directly related to sleep are disturbed sleep pattern and sleep deprivation. There are numerous other nursing diagnoses that may be pertinent depending on the particular circumstances surrounding the individual's sleep difficulties. Examples of some diagnoses that may be appropriate include:

- Activity intolerance
- Ineffective coping
- Fatigue
- Ineffective breathing pattern
- Pain (chronic or acute)
- Impaired memory
- Risk for injury

Planning

Planning care for a patient who is experiencing an alteration in sleep pattern should revolve around what the patient perceives his or her needs to be. Realistic goals and measurable outcomes should be developed carefully and in collaboration with the patient. It is important to remember that the patient controls his or her sleep behaviors and that additional time may be required to change previously learned behaviors. When planning interventions the nurse must take into consideration the patient's available resources as well as the individual's willingness to make the suggested changes. If the patient does not buy in to the plan of care, compliance with required actions is likely to be low and goals/expected outcomes will not be achieved.

NURSING ALERT

Sleep Cycle Inpatient
Patients who are in a healthcare facility may experience disruption in their normal sleep cycle because they are bed-bound during their awake hours. The patient tends to sleep when in bed. Compounding the situation, the patient may be bored due to lack of activity. It is important for the nurse to identify the patient's normal sleep patterns and to maintain that pattern during the inpatient stay

Implementation

Nursing interventions that promote rest and sleep are mostly aimed at controlling the specific influencing variables (eg, sleep environment, stress, diet) that are causing the problem. In some instances, the fix may be very simple and easy to achieve, but in other situations, the fix may be complex and may only control the problem instead of completely eliminating it. For example, a simple fix for a child having difficulty sleeping because he or she is afraid of the dark may be to place a night light in the child's room. On the other hand, interventions to resolve sleep issues for a patient with sleep apnea may be more complex. The testing that is required to diagnose the problem, obtaining the equipment needed to control the problem, the willingness of the patient to use the prescribed equipment, and the impact of the patient's sleep disturbance problems on the spouse or significant other all have to be addressed. In some instances, the physician may prescribe medications to control the sleep disturbance. When this is the case, the nurse must educate the patient on the appropriate use of the medication and possible adverse effects. For a patient who is hospitalized or who resides in a long-term residential setting, sleep disturbances may be related to the interventions required as a part of the plan of care. Nurses should make every effort to coordinate care to minimize sleep interruptions. Environmental noise should be controlled as much as possible but not at the expense of safe care (eg, intensive care units where alarms serve life-preserving functions). An additional strategy to facilitate an effective sleep pattern for hospitalized and long-term care residential patients is to integrate measures the patients use at home to promote optimal sleep into the plan of care whenever possible. Box 11–1 includes a listing of interventions that may be used to promote sleep.

NURSING ALERT

Noisy Hospitals
An inpatient setting tends to be noisy 24/7 and not conducive to sleeping. Staff must make a conscious effort to reduce noise on the unit especially during the evening and night shifts.

NURSING ALERT

Dangers of Hypnotic Use
Patients who have respiratory disorders and who are also prescribed a hypnotic should be monitored closely for signs of respiratory depression. Outpatients who use hypnotics should also be cautioned about the potential for respiratory depression and instructed on what actions to take.

BOX 11–1
Sleep Interventions

- **Environmental modifications (according to individual preferences)**
  - Adjust lighting
  - Adjust room temperature
  - Adjust noise level
  - Use bedroom for sleeping only
- **Promote relaxation**
  - Increased activity and exercise during the day
  - Avoid vigorous activity and exercise just before bedtime
  - Back rub
  - Warm bath
- **Establish a sleep ritual**
  - Regular bedtime
  - Light activity (eg, reading, soft music, watching low-key television programs)
  - Bedtime snack (especially foods containing L-tryptophan such as milk)
- **Resolve stress and anxiety**
  - Avoid problem solving (eg, work or family issues) at bedtime
- **Pharmacologic interventions**
  - Hypnotics and sedatives (for short-term use only; long-term use may make sleep problems worse)
  - Benzodiazepines (safer than hypnotics and sedatives)
  - Herbal products (consult a physician first)
- **Additional strategies for hospitalized and long-term residential patients**
  - Organize or cluster care
  - Mimic the home environment and bedtime rituals
  - Control environmental noises unique to the healthcare setting

NURSING ALERT

Patient with Brittle Diabetes

A patient diagnosed with brittle diabetes usually requires blood glucose checks during their sleeping hours. There is a natural tendency not to disrupt the patient's sleep to check the patient's blood glucose. However, blood glucose must be checked and an appropriate intervention performed based on blood glucose levels.

✔ ROUTINE CHECKUP 2

1. During hospitalization, nursing interventions may interfere with a patient's ability to sleep. True/false?

Answer:

2. List two NANDA nursing diagnoses directly related to sleep.

Answer:

_____

_____

3. _____ should be used cautiously in patients who have breathing problems.

Answer:

Evaluation

Even though measurable outcomes are included in the plan of care to evaluate whether the goals are met, the true measure of success is whether the patient perceives that he or she is obtaining adequate sleep and rest. The amount of time that the patient reports he or she is sleeping may on the surface appear to be sufficient, but the patient's perception may be different. Reaching the goal of patient satisfaction may be challenging, but through continuous collaboration with the patient, reaching the goal is achievable and will be quite rewarding.

Pain and Comfort

According to one definition provided in *Merriam-Webster Dictionary*, pain is "a basic bodily sensation induced by a noxious stimulus, received by naked nerve endings, characterized by physical discomfort (as pricking, throbbing, or aching), and typically leading to evasive action," What a mind-boggling description. Everything included in this definition is true; however, the bottom line is that pain is a unique and personal experience that is based on the individual's perception of various stimuli. For instance, what is noxious for one individual may not be noxious for another. Also, physiological variations from person to person may alter the processing of potentially painful stimuli. Ultimately, this means that what is considered uncomfortable or painful to one individual may be completely acceptable to another. Healthcare providers (nurses included) must be cognizant of the requirement to accurately assess patients for pain and develop individualized plans of care for pain management. The following discussion of pain will focus on a basic understanding of the physiology of pain, factors influencing a person's pain experience, and utilization of the nursing process to address patient's needs for comfort and pain control or elimination.

Physiology of Pain

When a person is exposed to a painful stimulus, he or she usually reacts immediately. This being the case, one might incorrectly conclude that pain is a simple process. To the contrary, pain is quite complex (Figure 11–1). Pain receptors, also called **nociceptors**, are located in various parts of the body (the skin, muscles, blood vessels, organs). When a stimulus capable of producing pain (thermal, chemical or pressure) comes into contact with the nociceptors, chemicals called **neurotransmitters** are released. Neurotransmitters attach to receptors on the receiving nerve cell propagating the impulse. These chemicals (prostaglandin, endorphins) may also act to enhance or inhibit transmission of the pain signal and thus influence the individual's overall perception of pain. Once in the environment of the neurotransmitters, the impulse is transmitted to the spinal cord by way of two different types of nerve fibers, fast A fibers and slower C fibers. The A fibers are responsible for the transmission of an immediate, sharp, and localized sensation to the original injury site, whereas the C fibers produce a more generalized, long-lasting pain sensation. While still in

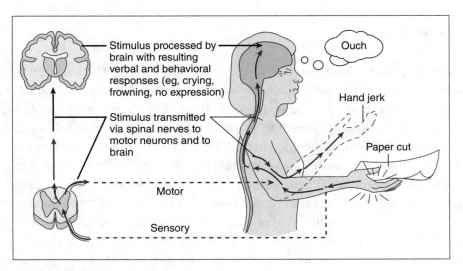

FIGURE 11–1 • Transmission of pain stimuli.

the spinal cord, the pain impulse may travel to a motor **neuron** (nerve cell). The motor impulse then travels back to muscles near the original injury site and causes movement at the site (eg, the jerk seen when a finger is pricked or touches a hot iron). The original impulse still eventually reaches the brain. Once in the brain, the pain impulse is processed within the context of the patient's past experiences with pain as well as cultural expectations and other psychosocial variables. The pain impulse then starts its descending journey away from the brain via the spinal cord and back to the original site of injury. During this journey, neurotransmitters are again released and may influence pain in the same manner as mentioned previously. The interpretive activity that occurs in the brain also dictates generalized responses to the pain stimulus (eg, crying, verbal responses).

Several theories have been developed in an attempt to explain how neurotransmitters, spinal nerves, and the brain work together to **modulate** (influence or alter) the pain experience. The most popular of these is the **gate control theory**, which suggests that "gates" along the nerve tracts as well as in the brain open and close under the influence of physiological, cognitive, sensory, emotional, and behavioral influences. When the gates are opened, pain impulses are permitted to continue to travel along the nerves and into the brain. When the gates are closed, the pain impulse is blocked. Massage, opiates, stimulation (eg, transcutaneous electrical nerve stimulation [TENS]), acupuncture, and acupressure are some of the therapies known to close the gate and inhibit pain transmission.

To bring this all together, think about when you get a paper cut on your finger. Initially, you might feel a stinging sensation at the exact site of the cut (under the influence of fast A fibers). At the same time, you may jerk your finger away from the paper (under the influence of the impulse partially crossing over to a motor neuron). However, over the next couple of days, the sensation becomes more generalized, and the area around the cut may feel "sore" (under the influence of the slower, longer lasting C fibers). Additionally, just how painful the experience is will depend on neurotransmitter release (inhibit or enhance stimuli), what the previous paper cut experience was like, and how you are expected to handle pain. This helps to explain why one person may score his or her pain level as a 1 (minimal pain) but another person with the same type injury may score the experience as an 8 (severe pain).

Types of Pain

There are several different ways to characterize or classify pain. Pain can be described by its onset and duration as well as by its origin or source.

Onset of Pain

Acute pain usually has a rapid onset and short duration. It is associated with tissue injury or disease and usually resolves itself with or without treatment when healing occurs. Additionally, acute pain is thought to serve a protective role by alerting us to the damage and causing us to take action to prevent further damage. This does not mean that acute pain is not serious. To the contrary, acute pain can be severe and can actually interfere with the healing process. For example, when a person who has pneumonia experiences severe chest pain, he or she tends to limit his or her movement and may refrain from coughing to minimize the pain. This in turn may actually worsen the condition by allowing secretions to continue to pool in the lungs. Thus, it becomes very important for the healthcare team to intervene to minimize the pain (eg, teaching the patient to splint when coughing, administering prescribed medications). Acute pain can also interfere with an individual's ability to perform activities of daily living that were once considered to be second nature. Fortunately, in most cases of acute pain, the negative effects are short lived, and the person can eventually return to a "normal" lifestyle."

Chronic pain persists beyond the healing phase, usually 6 months or more. It does not serve a protective function and is the source of useless suffering to the point that the individual's overall quality of life is negatively impacted. Cancer and arthritis are two conditions frequently associated with chronic pain. One of the most difficult characteristics of chronic pain is that sometimes it is not possible to determine just what is causing the pain (**idiopathic**). The person's life may be turned upside down, and the individual may find him- or herself incapable of working, socializing, or even performing basic activities of daily living. Persons who experience chronic pain may become frustrated or agitated, experience feelings of hopelessness, and may become depressed to the point of even considering suicide as an option. They are also sometimes mislabeled as "drug seekers" because of their constant request for pain medications or their frequent changes from one doctor to another. To the contrary, a person experiencing chronic pain who exhibits these behaviors may simply be trying to find relief from constant suffering.

NURSING ALERT

Suicide Precaution
Chronic pain is a risk factor for suicide attempts. The nurse should question patients who have chronic pain about suicidal thoughts and assess for other signs that the individual may be at risk. A safety plan should be implemented if the patient is at risk for suicide.

Sources of Pain

There are two main sources of pain. Nociceptive pain is pain that results from some type of injury or disease. **Neuropathic pain** is pain that results from actual nerve dysfunction. Nociceptive pain can be further broken down by its specific origins:

- **Superficial or cutaneous** pain originates from nerve endings located in the skin. As stated previously, noxious stimuli (chemical, thermal, or mechanical) trigger the nerve endings (in this case, located in the skin) to start the pain response. The initial response is localized to the area of the injury but may become more generalized.

- **Somatic pain** is nonlocalized and most often originates from muscles, tendons, and ligaments.

- **Visceral pain** originates in the various organs of the body, is nonlocalized, and is more slowly transmitted. A patient may identify the pain in an area remote to the actual organ from which the pain originates. This type pain is called **referred pain**.

Neuropathic pain occurs because of some type of damage to the actual nerves that are involved in the transmission of painful stimuli. Neuropathic pain, also called *nerve pain*, is often described as a burning or tingling sensation (**paresthesia**). Some individuals also compare it to an electrical shock. Patients experiencing nerve pain also often describe what are usually considered to be nonpainful stimuli, such as light touch, as being painful (**allodynia**). For example, a patient who has shingles may complain that the touch of a sheet against the affected area produces severe pain.

✔ ROUTINE CHECKUP 3

1. _____ are responsible for the transmission of immediate localized pain sensations.
Answer:

2. Acute pain serves a protective function. True/false?
Answer:

3. List the three categories of stimuli capable of producing pain.
Answer:

_____

_____

_____

Factors Influencing Comfort and Pain

Pain is a highly individualized experience. Many variables influence how a person perceives and responds to pain. A brief discussion of some of the more common influencing variables follows.

Age

Persons of all ages experience pain. However, the particulars of the experience vary depending on the age of the individual. The misconception that newborns do not experience "real pain" because their nerves are immature has long been dismissed. Newborns do indeed experience pain. However, their responses to pain are more generalized (ie, total body movement and crying) than localized. Additionally, newborns depend on their caretakers to recognize pain signals and control exposure to painful stimuli, thereby protecting them from harm. As a child becomes older, he or she will demonstrate a more localized response to pain and can eventually verbalize the location, intensity, and quality of the pain. Teenagers may avoid expressing pain to meet the expectations of their peers.

Growing old is not an automatic sentencing to pain. Elderly patients must be taught this fact. Otherwise, they may accept pain as a "normal" part of the aging process and miss an opportunity for pain relief. Even though pain does not come automatically with aging, older adults are at greater risk of experiencing disorders that are accompanied by pain. Thus, healthcare providers as well as other healthcare team members, including nurses, should include assessments of pain when interacting with older adults. Healthcare team members should also keep in mind that in the presence of disorders that affect mental status, elderly patients may have difficulty communicating their pain experiences.

Psychological State

Pain is usually heightened when a person is fatigued, agitated, depressed, or experiencing a high level of stress. This creates a vicious cycle because increased pain subsequently increases the level of fatigue, stress, agitation, and depression. Without intervention, this vicious cycle will continue, and pain management will become increasingly more difficult.

> **NURSING ALERT**
>
> **Anticipation of Pain**
> Patients who experience chronic pain anticipate when pain medication is going to be no longer effective and will request pain medication before the patient actually experiences pain.

Heredity

A person's genetic make-up is thought to influence his or her pain experience by influencing both the **pain threshold**, the level at which a person perceives painful stimuli, as well as his or her **pain tolerance**, how much pain the person is willing to endure. For example, during Lamaze classes, the labor coach may be instructed to pinch the expectant mother to simulate labor pains. The coach starts out with a light pinch and progresses to a stronger pinch to simulate the growing intensity of the labor pain. One expectant mother may perceive the pinch earlier than another expectant mother (pain threshold). Additionally, one expectant mother may instruct the coach to stop sooner than another expectant mother because she is not willing to experience any further discomfort associated with the pinching (pain tolerance).

NURSING ALERT

Nerve Damage
Some patients who have a high pain threshold may have nerve damage that prevents the normal sensation of pain. It is important that the nurse performs a head-to-toe assessment regularly to detect conditions that normally cause pain but may be hidden because the nerve damage.

Past Experiences

A person's past experiences with pain may influence future experiences with pain in a negative or a positive way. If the individual's past experience resulted in a positive outcome and effective means of controlling the pain were identified, then the individual is more likely to be prepared to effectively handle future instances of similar pain. However, if the experience did not result in a positive outcome, then the person is likely to be apprehensive, fearful, and unprepared to handle similar experiences in the future.

Culture and Support System

Available resources for coping with pain, including the presence of a support system, play a significant role in how a person handles pain. In some cultures, free expression of pain (eg, crying, body movements, other verbal expressions) is completely acceptable. Other cultures strictly prohibit expressions of pain. In such cases, silence and the absence of any type nonverbal cues are expected. Cultural and family values may also dictate that males respond to pain differently than females or that adults respond to pain differently than children. Cultural and family beliefs not only influence how pain is expressed; they may also influence what interventions are acceptable. Some parent refuse narcotics as an option for pain control in children for fear of addiction. Some people may believe that counseling, group therapy, the use of imagery, and other such interventions are not legitimate forms of treatment.

The Nursing Process and Pain

Pain is one of the most frequent reasons people seek medical care. Pain, particularly chronic pain, although not considered to be a life-threatening condition in the traditional sense, can be just as incapacitating and deadly as a heart attack, stroke, seizure, or cancer. Accurate identification of pain and its impact on a person is a key factor for ensuring the formulation of an effective plan of care for patients experiencing pain.

Assessment

The most critical information obtained during assessment is the patient's perception of his or her painful experience. Various tools have been developed to objectively document the patient's perception of his or her level of pain. Patients who are mentally alert may be asked to rate their pain on a scale of 1 to 10 with 1 being the least amount of pain and 10 being the worst level of pain. Children 3 years of age and older and adults, particularly those who are illiterate, may be shown faces with corresponding numbers and asked to identify the face that best correlates with their level of pain. The faces range from a smiling face (no pain, which is scored as a 1) to a face with a frown and tears (worst pain, which is scored as a 10). Tools have also been developed for use with patients who cannot communicate. Beyond obtaining a pain score, the nurse should also collect information about the following:

- Location of the pain (anatomical location, localized, diffuse)
- Quality of the pain (burning, tingling, aching, throbbing)
- Aggravating factors (what makes it worse)
- Alleviating factors (what makes it better)
- Effects (effects on activities of daily living, work, school, social interaction)
- Current and previous treatments, including effectiveness

Additionally, the nurse should include information related to all of the influencing variables discussed previously (ie, age or developmental stage, past experiences with pain, sleep pattern, psychological status, culture, support system). The initial assessment should be followed up by frequent reassessment of the patient's pain.

> ## NURSING ALERT
>
> **Addiction**
> Patients can become addicted to pain medication and may report pain without showing outward signs of pain. Pain is defined by the patient therefore the nurse should administer pain per the practitioner's order even if the nurse suspects that the patient is addicted to pain medication. The nurse should notify the practitioner of those concerns but still must administer pain medication to the patient per the practitioner's order.

Nursing Diagnoses

The two primary nursing diagnoses for patients experiencing pain are acute pain and chronic pain. Other related diagnoses that may be applicable include but are not limited to:

- Deficient knowledge
- Disturbed sleep pattern
- Hopelessness
- Impaired socialization
- Impaired physical mobility
- Low self-esteem (chronic or situational)
- Noncompliance
- Powerlessness
- Risk for injury
- Self-care deficit

Planning

Setting goals, identifying expected outcomes, and planning care for the patient experiencing pain requires collaboration between healthcare team members and the patient. It also requires that the nurse consider other coexisting problems that the patient may be experiencing or at risk of experiencing (see preceding nursing diagnoses). Ideally, a patient would like to have his or her pain completely resolved. In some instances, this may be possible. However, in other instances, achieving complete pain relief is not possible. When complete pain relief is not an option, the nurse and other members of the healthcare team must work with the patient to identify an acceptable level of pain. The patient must be involved in identifying possible interventions. The pros and cons of various interventions as well as a discussion of possible barriers to successful implementation of interventions should also be included. Open and honest

BOX 11–2
Realistic Pain Relief—Be Honest!

Pain cannot be completely relieved in all instances. This is especially true for patients experiencing chronic pain. Nurses must be honest with their patients about the level of pain relief that can be expected!

discussions as well as active listening are mandatory. Failure to acknowledge the patient's preferences and concerns, false promises to the patient, and coercive strategies all set the stage for failure of the plan of care (Box 11–2).

Implementation

Effective management of pain should begin with the use of strategies to control exposure to painful stimuli. For example, the nurse can premedicate a patient who is about to undergo a painful procedure to either prevent or minimize the occurrence of pain. Patients can also use assistive devices such as modified beds and chairs to achieve positions that will assist to minimize pain. Anticipatory guidance is another strategy that can be used to diffuse the pain experience. When people do not know what to expect, they often expect the worse. This mindset makes patients vulnerable to experiencing a higher degree of pain than if they were informed of what to expect and taught strategies to deal with the situation. For example, a patient who is taught beforehand how to splint the abdomen when coughing after having abdominal surgery will most likely have more success at pain control than one who is not given the same instructions until after the surgery. For patients who experience chronic pain, it is important to teach them ways to modify their lifestyles (eg, diet modifications, exercise, stress management, body mechanics) to manage their pain.

Management of pain requires a combination of independent, dependent, and interdependent nursing intervention. Interventions can be divided into two broad categories: nonpharmacologic and pharmacologic. However, this does not mean that one category of interventions is implemented exclusive of the other. In fact, in most cases, effective management of a patient's pain will involve a combination of both nonpharmacologic and pharmacologic interventions.

Nonpharmacologic Interventions   Nonpharmacologic interventions (Figure 11–2) are categorized as cognitive, behavioral, or physical. Cognitive and behavioral interventions are designed to alter the patient's perception of pain as well as

Health Promotion Strategies

- Teach patient ways to anticipate and manage painful situations and procedures
- Know triggers (eg, foods, movements, psychological stressors)
- Always practice good body mechanics

Physical Interventions

- Check for constrictive clothing
- Reposition
- Remove wrinkles from bedsheets
- Keep free of irritants (eg, urine, feces, tube leakage)
- Massage and vibration therapy
- Acupressure or acupuncture
- Transcutaneous electrical nerve stimulation (TENS)
- Heat and cold applications
- Contralateral stimulation (stimulate area opposite affected area)

Nonpharmacologic Interventions

Cognitive Interventions

- Anticipatory guidance
- Distraction (ie, watching TV, reading a book, music)
- Guided imagery (eg, imagining watching the sunset on a beach while feeling a light breeze from the water)
- Hypnosis (blocking pain through suggestion or substitution of another feeling while the person is in an altered state of mind)

Behavioral Interventions

- Relaxation
- Meditation
- Biofeedback (patient motivation important)

FIGURE 11–2 · Nonpharmacologic interventions for pain.

assist the patient to achieve control over the pain. Examples cognitive and behavioral interventions include biofeedback, distraction, guided imagery, hypnosis, meditation, reframing, and relaxation. Physical interventions, on the other hand, actually provide some level of comfort. Physical interventions include cutaneous stimulation (eg, acupuncture, acupressure, massage, heat and cold application, and TENS stimulation), positioning, and hygiene.

NURSING ALERT

Physical Intervention Safety
- Do not use TENS on patients with a pacemaker
- Heat application cautions
  1. Wait 24 hours after an injury to apply heat!
  2. Avoid use of heat when impaired circulation exists!
  3. Know the cause of pain before applying heat!

Pharmacologic Interventions Some pharmacologic agents (eg, aspirin, acetaminophen, ibuprofen) can be purchased over the counter by the patient, but others require a physician's order. The responsibility for administering pain medications rests primarily with the nurse; the nurse determines when to administer the medications, the effectiveness, and whether there is a need to notify the physician for adjustments in the prescribed medications. Pharmacologic options include nonopioid analgesics, opioids (narcotics), and **adjuvant analgesics**. Adjuvant analgesics are medications that are primarily used to treat other disorders but that have also been found to be effective in treating pain. Examples of adjuvant analgesics include anticonvulsants, antidepressants, and corticosteroids. When administering opioids, the nurse should monitor the patient for respiratory depression. Medications may be administered topically, orally, intramuscularly, intravenously, epidurally, or intrathecally. The type of pain, type of medication, origin of pain, desired duration, and patient preference are some factors that are considered when determining the most appropriate administration route. Patient-controlled anesthesia is also used and significantly improves pain control satisfaction because the patient can tailor the timing to his or her unique needs. The patient must be monitored closely to ensure early intervention if problems arise. Also, patients must be taught that they cannot overdose themselves while using patient-controlled anesthesia. Figure 11–3 provides additional information about common pharmacologic options used for pain management.

> **NURSING ALERT**
>
> **Opioid Antagonists**
> Naloxone is a common opioid antagonist that should be kept on hand to reverse respiratory depression that may occur with an adverse reaction to an opioid or when there is an opioid overdose.

Evaluation

The patient is the most reliable source for evaluating whether pain has been resolved or reached an acceptable level. At first glance, evaluation seems to be a pretty simple task to complete. However, this is not always the case. In some instances, the nurse has to decipher whether the patient is compliant with the recommended pain management plan, whether he or she is drug seeking, and whether the patient is hiding pain for fear of becoming addicted to certain types of medications. Addressing barriers during the planning phase minimizes less than desirable outcomes during evaluation. The evaluation phase is

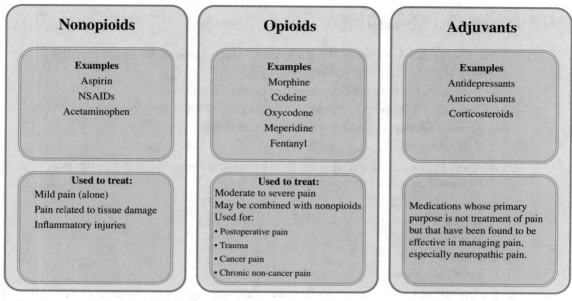

Nonopioids	Opioids	Adjuvants
Examples Aspirin NSAIDs Acetaminophen	**Examples** Morphine Codeine Oxycodone Meperidine Fentanyl	**Examples** Antidepressants Anticonvulsants Corticosteroids
Used to treat: Mild pain (alone) Pain related to tissue damage Inflammatory injuries	**Used to treat:** Moderate to severe pain May be combined with nonopioids Used for: • Postoperative pain • Trauma • Cancer pain • Chronic non-cancer pain	Medications whose primary purpose is not treatment of pain but that have been found to be effective in managing pain, especially neuropathic pain.

FIGURE 11–3 • Pharmacologic interventions for pain.

also the time when the nurse must be supportive of the patient and provide encouragement because when the plan does not effectively address the patient's pain issue, he or she may feel hopeless and may even show signs of depression.

Conclusion

Although sleep and pain are two different patient care issues, both share the commonality that the adequacy of each (ie, adequacy of sleep and pain relief) primarily depend on the patient's perception. Thus, meeting the patient's need for each can be quite a challenge. No matter how challenging, the nurse as well as other members of the healthcare team must take seriously the sleep and pain relief needs of the patient. Failure to do so can be costly or even deadly. To effectively address sleep and pain relief needs, nurses as well as other healthcare team members must have a clear understanding of the underlying physiology of both pain and sleep, be knowledgeable of treatment options, be open minded, and actively engage the patient in all phases of care planning (assessment through evaluation).

REVIEW QUESTIONS

1. **The most reliable indicator of the adequacy of the amount of sleep and of the quality of sleep for an individual is:**

   A. The number of hours of sleep reported by the patient
   B. The patient's stated perception of the adequacy of his or her sleep pattern
   C. Amount of sleep recorded in the patient's sleep diary
   D. Sleep study results

2. **Which of the following variables should be included when collecting information about a person's sleep pattern?**

   A. Diet
   B. Work schedule
   C. Marital status
   D. A and B
   E. All of the above

3. **During NREM sleep individuals usually experience which of the following?**

   A. Decreased temperature, pulse, and respirations
   B. Increased muscle tone
   C. Increased brain activity
   D. Numerous vivid dreams
   E. All of the above

4. **A patient, admitted to a busy intensive care unit, is having difficulty sleeping. Which intervention will best promote sleep for this critically ill client?**

   A. Administering a sleeping medication
   B. Keeping the television on to block the noise of other alarms
   C. Allowing the family to remain at the bedside to talk with the patient
   D. Clustering care and avoiding nonessential tasks

5. **A client is admitted to the Emergency Department having overdosed on an opioid. Which medication should be administered to the client to reverse the effects of the opioid?**

   A. Flumazenil (Romazicon)
   B. Dimercaprol (BAL in Oil)
   C. Naloxone (Narcan)
   D. Atropine sulfate (Atropine)

6. **A nurse administers pain medication to a client one hour before the client's scheduled physical therapy. One hour later, a physical therapist assists the client to ambulate in the hallway. Which type of intervention is this nursing action?**

   A. A nurse-initiated intervention
   B. A physician-initiated intervention

    C. A collaborative intervention

    D. An indirect care intervention

7. **A female client complains of severe pain following a bilateral mastectomy. Her husband explains to the nurse that he does not want his wife to receive analgesics because she might become addicted. Which action by the nurse is most appropriate?**

    A. Report the husband's request to the physician and medicate the client.

    B. Respect the beliefs of the husband and stop medicating the client.

    C. Ask the husband to leave the room and administer the pain medication.

    D. Educate the husband on postoperative pain and the action of analgesics.

8. **In the "gate control" theory of pain, gating mechanisms can be found in which structures?**

    A. Substantia gelatinosa cells within the dorsal horn of the spinal cord and the thalamus

    B. Spinal cord and central nervous system

    C. Peripheral nerves, cardiac muscles, and respiratory muscles

    D. Brain, motor nerves, and respiratory system

9. **The point at which a person becomes aware of pain is:**

    A. Behavioral response

    B. Physiological response

    C. Perception

    D. Pain threshold

10. **A behavioral theory that involves giving persons information about physiological responses and ways to exercise voluntary control over those responses to obtain nonpharmacologic pain relief is:**

    A. Relaxation

    B. Biofeedback

    C. Guided imagery

    D. Massage

ANSWERS

Routine Checkup 1

1. Non-rapid eye movement, rapid eye movement.
2. False.
3. Any of the following are the consequences associated with inadequate amounts of sleep:
   Impaired memory or confusion
   Depression

Altered coping abilities or mood swings

Diminished motor performance

Increased occurrence of automobile, home, and work- related accidents

Impaired immune responses

Cardiovascular disease

Diabetes

Routine Checkup 2

1. True.
2. Disturbed sleep pattern

    Sleep deprivation
3. Hypnotics.

Routine Checkup 3

1. A fibers.
2. True.
3. Chemical

    Thermal

    Mechanical

Review Questions

1. B
2. E
3. A
4. D
5. C
6. C
7. D
8. B
9. D
10. B

References

Craven RF, Hirnle CJ: *Fundamentals of Nursing: Human Health and Function*, 5th ed. Philadelphia, PA: Lippincott, 2006.

Daniels R: *Nursing Fundamentals: Caring & Clinical Decision Making*. New York, NY: Delmar Thomson Learning, 2004.

Potter PA, Perry AG: *Fundamentals of Nursing*, 6th ed. St. Louis, MO: Mosby Elsevier, 2005.

Additional Resources

Healthy Roads Media: *About Your Pain*. Available at http://www.healthyroadsmedia.org/english/Files/flv/engpain.htm.

How Stuff Works: *How Pain Works*. Available at http://health.howstuffworks.com/pain5.htm.

Institute for Clinical Systems Improvement: *Assessment and Management of Acute Pain Treatment Algorithm*. Available at http://www.guideline.gov/algorithm/ 6371/ NGC-6371_2.html.

Institute for Clinical Systems Improvement: *Assessment and Management of Chronic Pain Treatment Algorithm*, part 1. Available at http://www.guideline.gov/algorithm/6693/NGC-6693_1.html.

Institute for Clinical Systems Improvement: *Assessment and Management of Chronic Pain Treatment Algorithm*, part 2. Available at http://www.guideline.gov/algorithm/6693/NGC-6693_2.html.

MedlinePlus: *Pain*. Available at http://www.nlm.nih.gov/medlineplus/pain.html.

MedlinePlus: *Pain: Treatment*. Available at http://www.nlm.nih.gov/medlineplus/pain.html#cat3.

National Pain Foundation: *Chronic Pain and Suicide Risk*. Available at http://www.nationalpainfoundation.org/articles/290/chronic-pain-and-suicide-risk.

National Sleep Foundation: Available at http://www.sleepfoundation.org/atf/cf/%7BF6BF2668-A1B4-4FE8-8D1A-A5D39340D9CB%7D/Sleep-Wake_Cycle.pdf.

National Sleep Foundation: *Diet, Exercise and Sleep*. Available at http://www.sleepfoundation.org/article/sleep-topics/diet-exercise-and-sleep.

National Sleep Foundation: Available at http://www.sleepfoundation.org/site/c.huIXKjM0IxF/b.4809783/k.5FBD/Diet_Exercise_and_Sleep.htm.

NIH Pain Consortium: *Pain Intensity Scales*. Available at http://painconsortium.nih.gov/pain_scales/index.html.

Nursing Times: *Anatomy and Physiology of Pain*. Available at http://www.nursingtimes.net/ntclinical/2008/09/anatomy_and_physiology_of_pain.html.

Pain. In *Merriam-Webster Dictionary*. Available at http://www.merriam-webster.com/dictionary/pain.

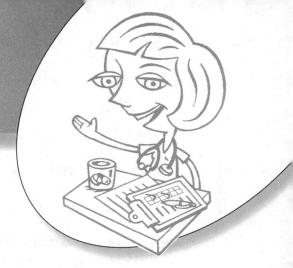

Chapter 12

Oxygenation

At the end of the chapter, the reader will be able to:

1. Briefly describe the process of oxygenation.

2. Identify age and developmental factors that influence the oxygenation process.

3. Discuss how diet may influence oxygenation.

4. Discuss how lifestyle choices may influence oxygenation.

5. Identify health deviations that may contribute to impaired oxygenation.

6. Describe manifestations of impaired oxygenation.

7. Identify subjective and objective data that should be collected during the assessment of the patient who has a potential or actual alteration in oxygenation.

8. Identify nursing diagnoses appropriate for the patient experiencing an alteration in oxygenation.

9. Discuss interventions that may be used to prevent or resolve altered oxygenation.

10. Describe actions that can be taken to prevent complications during the care and suctioning of a tracheostomy.

11. Discuss why evaluation is critical for a patient who is experiencing impaired oxygenation.

KEY WORDS

Alveoli	Capillaries
Atherosclerosis	Septicemia

Overview

Oxygen is a life-sustaining gas that is transported to cells in the body by way of the respiratory system and the cardiovascular system. Under normal circumstances, the process of oxygenation occurs without any real thought about what is happening. However, when the body is deprived of oxygen, an individual immediately recognizes the effects. In other words, "you don't miss your oxygen until your well runs dry." This chapter presents an overview of the process of oxygenation, factors that influence oxygenation, alterations in oxygenation, and use of the nursing process to address alterations in oxygenation.

Physiology of Oxygenation

Oxygen enters the respiratory tract through the nose and mouth. It is then transported through the respiratory airways (pharynx, trachea, and bronchi) to the **alveoli**, which are air sacs surrounded by capillaries. The **capillaries** are small blood vessels with thin walls that allow for easy gas exchange. Gas exchange begins when oxygen that is inhaled passes across the capillary walls surrounding the alveoli and is picked up by the blood cells that are circulating inside of the capillaries. Oxygen picked up by the blood cells in the capillaries is transported to the heart and then it is pumped throughout the body by way of the aorta. The aorta branches into smaller arteries and even smaller arterioles, which eventually become capillaries. The very thin walls of the capillaries allow diffusion of the oxygen into cells in the various body tissues (Figure 12–1).

Factors Influencing Oxygenation

Physiological Factors

Several systems work together to make possible normal oxygenation. We have already described the role that the lungs and heart play in

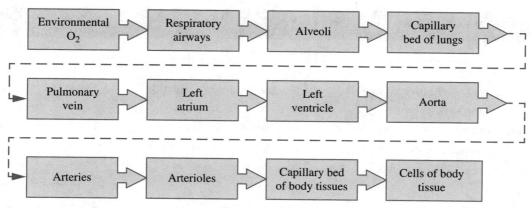

FIGURE 12–1 · Physiology of oxygenation.

oxygenation, but it is also important to recognize that other processes also directly impact the proper functioning of the lungs and heart. The diaphragm, a large muscle located just below the lungs, assists with inhalation and exhalation of gases in the lungs. The contraction and relaxation of cardiac muscles make it possible for the heart to pump blood efficiently. Contraction and relaxation of both the diaphragm and cardiac muscles depend on proper signaling from the neurologic system. Blood vessels are also made of smooth muscles that assist with the circulation of oxygen-rich blood to target tissue.

Age and Developmental Stage

An immature respiratory system and immune system coupled with a smaller heart place younger children at a greater risk for impaired oxygenation. Older adults are also at risk for impaired oxygenation because the functional capacity of the lungs and heart diminish as the individual ages (Table 12–1).

Environmental Factors

Several variables in the environment impact an individual's ability to meet his or her oxygen needs. Pollutants and allergens in the air (eg, pollen, smog, toxic chemicals) as well as secondhand smoke may damage lung tissue and lead to long-term consequences such as lung cancer and chronic obstructive pulmonary/lung disease (COPD or COLD). High altitudes also impair oxygenation because there is a decreased amount of oxygen in inspired air.

TABLE 12–1	Age and Developmental Influencing Factors
Characteristic	**Effect**
Young Children	
• Short, narrow respiratory airways • Immature immune system	↑ Risk for respiratory infections
• Smaller number of airways and alveoli	↑ Respiratory rate
• Immature respiratory muscles	Abdominal breathing
• Immature heart	↑ Heart rate
Older Adults	
• ↓ Elasticity of lungs	Less effective air exchange
• ↓ Cilia in respiratory tract • ↓ Strength of cough	Ineffective airway clearance, which causes ↑ risk for infection
• ↓ Elasticity in blood vessels	Less effective delivery of oxygen to tissues

Diet

The consequences of a poor diet are well documented. Food content as well as the amount of food ingested may cause problems that directly impact oxygenation.

Food Content

High-fat, high-cholesterol foods are associated with plaque build-up in the blood vessels, also known as **atherosclerosis**. The build-up of plaque can occur in any blood vessel. If it occurs in the coronary arteries of the heart, the individual will be at risk for a heart attack. If the arteries leading to the brain are blocked, the person may experience a stroke. If vessels in the extremities are blocked, then the person will experience peripheral artery disease, which can cause pain, tingling, and ulcers. High-fat, high-cholesterol, and high-sodium diets can also predispose an individual to hypertension. Consumption of large amounts of caffeine may increase the heart rate and the blood pressure. Poor nutrition also increases the risk for infection and may lead to anemia, both of which increase cardiac workload.

Food Amount

Obesity increases the workload of heart, which can diminish the heart's effectiveness as a pump and eventually results in heart failure. Obesity can also limit chest movement, which in turn decreases the room for lung expansion and limits inhalation of oxygen. Persons who are obese are usually less active. Inactivity can interfere with muscle strength, including muscles that assist with breathing and cardiac muscles ("if you don't use it, you lose it").

Lifestyle

How an individual chooses to live his or her life may also contribute to impaired oxygenation. A few examples of lifestyles choices and associated consequence include:

- A sedentary lifestyle increases cardiac workload because it promotes obesity and decreases muscles strength (eg, diaphragm and heart).
- Smoking is associated with chronic respiratory disorders and cancer. Additionally, nicotine causes constriction of the coronary arteries and increases blood pressure (increasing the workload on the heart). At the same time, nicotine increases the amount of carbon monoxide in the blood, which causes a decrease in the amount of oxygen available for circulation to body tissues.
- Drug and alcohol abuse are associated with the following risks:
  - Narcotics and large amounts of alcohol may cause respiratory depression.
  - Aspiration may occur secondary to alcohol intoxication.
  - IV drug users have an increased risk of **septicemia** (blood infections) and damaged blood vessels from repeated needlesticks.
  - Cardiac arrest is known to occur in some persons who abuse cocaine.

Health Alterations

Health alterations directly related to respiratory and cardiovascular function as well as those related to other body functions have the potential to influence oxygenation. Many of the deviations that are mentioned occur secondary to unhealthy life choices (eg, diet, smoking, sedentary lifestyle). Thus, one key intervention is health teaching to prevent, control, or reverse the adverse impact of such choices. Examples of respiratory system deviations include:

- Pneumonia
- COPD and COLD
- Hypoventilation (collapsed lung, COPD, COLD)
- Hyperventilation (anxiety, infections, drugs, acid–base imbalances, fever)

Examples of cardiovascular health deviations include:

- Dysrhythmia
- Coronary artery disease (related to plaque build-up)
- Hypertension
- Heart attack
- Impaired heart valve function
- Anemia
- Hypovolemia (massive bleeding, severe dehydration)
- Peripheral vascular disease
- Congenital (birth) defects

Other health deviations that may alter oxygenation include

- Pain (eg, abdominal surgery, fractured ribs), which causes shallow breathing
- Infections or wound healing (increase demand for oxygen)
- Neurologic disorders (eg, spinal cord injuries, Guillain-Barré syndrome)
- Muscle disorders (may affect muscles used for breathing and cardiac muscles)
- Ingestion of foreign object (eg, foods, toys)
- Pregnancy (enlarged uterus decreases room for lung expansion and causes shortness of breath)

✔ ROUTINE CHECKUP

1. _____, which is found in cigarettes, decreases the amount of oxygen available for delivery to body tissues.

Answer:

2. _____ are small blood vessels with thin walls that allow for easy gas exchange.

Answer:

3. Name four environmental factors that impact a person's ability to meet his or her oxygen needs.

Answer:

_____

_____

_____

Alterations in Oxygenation

Alterations in oxygenation have the potential to affect all body systems. Why? Because body systems consist of organs, organs consist of tissue, and tissues are made of cells that depend on oxygen to carry out their work. For example, a lack of oxygen to the brain may cause altered mental status. If the brain is slowly deprived of oxygen, the patient exhibits confusion and agitation. If the brain is deprived of oxygen for a long time, the damage will be more severe and may be permanent (eg, stroke, paralysis, coma). If you were to look at each body system, you could identify an example of how oxygen deprivation can alter the function of each one. Even more significant is the fact that the changes that occur in body function as a result of impaired oxygenation ultimately impact the functional capacity of an individual. Activities once taken for granted (eg, bathing, eating, independent toileting) now become very challenging. A person may not even be able to speak or take a few steps without becoming short of breath.

Certain cues may be present that signal that a patient is having problems with oxygenation, including:

- Anxiety, confusion, disorientation
- Changes in vital signs (temperature, pulse respirations, blood pressure)
- Shortness of breath
- Cyanosis (late sign)
- Chest wall retractions
- Abnormal breath sounds
- Cough
- Fluid in the lungs and increased sputum production
- Chest pain (respiratory or cardiac in nature)
- Heart murmur
- Clubbing of fingers and toes (with chronic lack of oxygen)
- Capillary refill <3 seconds
- Edema
- Dark discoloration of the skin and ulcers (peripheral tissue oxygen deprivation)
- Muscle cramps

The Nursing Process and Oxygenation

Remember that the focus of the nursing process is to identify the patient's response to human or life processes and to develop a plan of care in collaboration with the patient to promote health as well as restore optimal function when there is a health alteration.

Assessment

Data collected during assessment help the nurse determine potential and actual patient responses to alterations in oxygenation. In some instances, the patient may present in acute distress. When this is the case, the nurse should focus on collecting critical information to address the immediate crisis. A more detailed assessment is conducted for patients who are stable and not experiencing acute distress. Data should be collected from the patient, the physical assessment, and diagnostic laboratory studies and procedures. Refer to Table 12–2 for a more comprehensive listing of data that should be collected.

Nursing Diagnoses

Nursing diagnoses for a client experiencing alterations in oxygenation include those related to respiratory function and cardiovascular function.

TABLE 12–2 Assessment Data for Potential and Actual Impaired Oxygenation

Patient Data (Subjective)	Physical Assessment (Objective)	Labs and Diagnostic Test (Objective)
Habits (eating and exercise habits, smoking, drugs, and alcohol use) Ability to perform activities of daily living	Respiratory status (eg, cough, abnormal breath sounds, retractions, cyanosis, sputum amount, and content)	Laboratory results (eg, CBC, blood gases, cardiac enzymes, cholesterol levels, triglycerides)
Past and present illnesses	Mental status changes (eg, anxiety, confusion)	Chest radiographs CT scans
Medications and allergies	Vital signs and weight	Pulmonary function test
Family history	Heart murmur	TB skin test
Sleep pattern	Clubbing of fingers and toes	EKG, echocardiogram
Environment (home and work)	Capillary refill <3 seconds	Stress test
Chest pain (respiratory or cardiac in nature)	Edema	Heart catheterization
Shortness of breath	Skin (color, moisture, temperature)	

CBC = complete blood count; CT = computed tomography; EKG = electrocardiography; TB = tuberculosis.

TABLE 12–3 Nursing Diagnoses for Potential and Actual Impaired Oxygenation		
Respiratory	**Cardiovascular**	**Related**
• Ineffective airway clearance • Ineffective breathing pattern • Impaired gas exchange • Impaired spontaneous ventilation	• Decreased cardiac output • Ineffective tissue perfusion (specific type: cerebral, peripheral, renal, and so on)	• Anxiety • Activity intolerance • Self-care deficit • Chronic low self-esteem • Ineffective coping • Ineffective family coping • Excess fluid volume • Risk for infection • Imbalanced nutrition • Disturbed sleep pattern • Impaired home maintenance • Deficient knowledge

Related diagnoses should also be included if the data support the presence of such diagnoses. Table 12–3 identifies examples of diagnoses for patients with altered oxygenation.

Planning

Goals and outcomes for patients with potential or actual altered oxygenation are highly individualized and are driven by the data collected during assessment. The goals and outcomes should be realistic in terms of expectations and time frames for the particular patient and should be consistent with the patient's desires. Noncompliance is more likely to occur if the patient does not buy in to the goals and established outcomes. Refer to Box 12–1 for an example of a goal and outcome for the patient experiencing altered oxygenation.

BOX 12–1
Goals and Expected Outcomes

Goal

Patient will demonstrate effective gas exchange

Expected Outcome

- Oxygen saturation (SaO_2) will be between 90% and 100%.
- Hemoglobin will be 12–14 g/dL for women and 14–18 g/dL for men.
- Refill will be <3 seconds.
- Mucous membranes will be pink in color.

> ## NURSING ALERT
>
> **Normal Levels of Oxygen Saturation**
> A patient with normal respiratory function should have an oxygen saturation level between 95% and 100%. A patient who receives supplemental oxygen is expected to have a 100% oxygen saturation level, if the patient has normal respiratory function. However, a patient experiences chronic respiratory function (ie, COPD) will have a normal oxygen saturation lower than expected normal for a patient who has normal respiratory function. It is not unusual for such a patient to have a normal oxygen saturation level of 88–90% because of impaired gas exchanged related to the patient's disease.

Implementation

Just as goals and outcomes are driven by the data, nursing interventions are driven by the goals and expected outcomes. Teaching is a primary intervention for both the patient who is at risk for altered oxygenation and the patient who is experiencing an actual alteration in oxygenation. It is important that the nurse tailor the instructions at a level the patient or caregiver will understand. Validation may be achieved by having the patient or caregiver restate the instructions or perform demonstrations. Examples of interventions include:

- Preventing respiratory infections through vaccinations (eg, pneumococcal and influenza)
- Reducing or eliminating allergic responses (eg, skin testing, desensitization, rescue medications)
- Offering smoking cessation programs (Box 12–2)

> ## NURSING ALERT
>
> **Oxygen Therapy**
> It is very important for the nurse to emphasize to the patient that it is very dangerous to smoke during oxygen therapy.

> ## NURSING ALERT
>
> **Oxygen Therapy for COPD**
> Supplemental oxygen therapy should be set at PaO_2 to between 60 and 65 mm Hg or the saturations from 90% to 92% for patients diagnosed with COPD. Higher values decrease the level of carbon dioxide in the blood. A relatively high level of carbon dioxide in the blood drives the patient's desire to breath. Reducing the level of carbon dioxide decreases the patient's desire to breath.

BOX 12–2
Safety Tip

Caution!
- Secondhand smoke causes heart disease and lung cancer in nonsmokers.
- Smokeless tobacco (chewing tobacco and snuff) also causes cancer.

- Managing dyspnea with independent and collaborative interventions (eg, positioning, medications)
- Maintaining an open airway with independent and collaborative interventions (eg, coughing, fluid, humidifier, nebulizer, chest physiotherapy, postural drainage, suctioning, positioning, incentive spirometry, artificial airway care) (Box 12–3)
- Performing cardiopulmonary resuscitation

Evaluation

Respiratory and cardiac arrest can ensue rapidly in a patient who is experiencing impaired oxygenation. Evaluation of the patient's status and the effectiveness of interventions must be ongoing. To prevent the occurrence of life-threatening situations, the nurse must read cues accurately and respond quickly.

NURSING ALERT

Cyanosis Significance
Cyanosis of the mucous membranes inside the mouth is most likely a sign of central cyanosis, a very serious condition. Bluish discoloration of the nail beds is more likely attributable to cold extremities. In dark skin patients, cyanosis is better detected in lips, gums, and around the eyes.

Evaluation of goals, expected outcomes, and the effectiveness of interventions is also important for a patient who is not experiencing an acute episode of altered oxygenation. If goals and expected outcomes are not being met, the nurse must determine whether it is because the interventions are not effective, the goals or expected outcomes are inappropriate, or the patient is noncompliant. In any of the above-cited situations, the nurse and the patient must collaboratively revise the plan to better meet the patient's needs. Continuous monitoring and revisions are particularly important for a patient who is at risk for or who actually has altered oxygenation.

BOX 12–3
Procedure Tip: Artificial Airway Care and Suctioning

The danger of compromising oxygenation during the care of an artificial airway is very real and scary, especially for students and novice nurses. The following tips are presented to highlight steps that will minimize the risk of compromising oxygenation.

Tip	Rationale
• When changing the ties on a tracheostomy, have a second person available to hold the tracheostomy tube in place.	• If the patient coughs, the tracheostomy tube may be dislodged, thereby cutting off the patient's oxygen source.
• Before suctioning the tracheostomy, hyperinflate or hyperoxygenate (or both) the patient with an Ambu bag connected to the oxygen source.	• Hyperinflation or hyperoxygenation decreases the risk of hypoxia and atelectasis that may occur during tracheostomy suctioning.
• Only handle the suction catheter with your sterile-gloved, dominant hand.	• This controls the risk of respiratory infections secondary to introduction of potentially infectious microorganisms into the trachea via the suctioning catheter.
• Insert the catheter into the trachea (preferably during inhalation) *without* applying suctioning until you feel resistance. Then pull back about 0.5 inch before applying suctioning.	• This prevents damage to the tissue inside the trachea that may occur if catheter is resting on the inner wall of the trachea and decreases the risk of hypoxia.
• While withdrawing the catheter from the trachea in a rotating motion, intermittently apply suctioning.	• Intermittent suctioning and catheter rotation removes secretions from trachea without damaging the inner wall of the trachea.
• Achieve suctioning, both insertion and withdrawal, over a time span of no more than 5–10 seconds.	• This prevents hypoxia.
• Hyperinflate and hyperoxygenate before each cycle of suctioning.	• This prevents hypoxia.
• If at any time during suctioning the patient shows signs of respiratory distress, discontinue and administer oxygen.	• This prevents respiratory arrest.

Conclusion

The impact of insufficient tissue oxygenation can be massive. To intervene effectively, the nurse must have knowledge of the oxygenation process, the impact of impaired oxygenation, and the manifestations of impaired oxygenation. This chapter has provided an overview of each of the above as well as interventions to promote oxygenation. Key concepts presented include:

- The respiratory system and cardiovascular system play a central role in oxygenation.

- Age, developmental stage, exercise, environmental conditions, lifestyle choices, and health status all influence the oxygenation process.

- Impaired oxygenation affects the function of all body systems.

- Both behavioral and physiological findings provide cues about whether a patient is experiencing impaired oxygenation.

- Impaired oxygenation, if not corrected, will result in a rapid deterioration of the patient's health status even to the point of respiratory and cardiac arrest.

- Health teaching is a major component of the plan of care for patients who have a potential or actual alteration in oxygenation.

- Vaccinations and smoking cessation programs are two preventive interventions for patients who are at risk for impaired oxygenation.

- Interventions that may be included in the plan of care for patients experiencing impaired oxygenation include nebulizer treatments, oxygen therapy, medications, chest physiotherapy, suctioning, cardiopulmonary resuscitation, and artificial airway management.

- Quick and accurate evaluation of patients experiencing impaired oxygenation is pivotal to preventing life-threatening situations.

REVIEW QUESTIONS

1. Which one of the following is a late sign of impaired oxygenation?

A. Anxiety

B. Cough

C. Cyanosis

D. Capillary refill <3 seconds

2. **Which of the following may occur as a result of plaque build-up in blood vessels?**
   A. Stroke
   B. Heart attack
   C. Peripheral artery disease
   D. All of the above

3. **Which of the following patients is at risk for experiencing alterations in oxygenation?**
   A. A patient who has an acute infection.
   B. A toddler who is choking on a toy.
   C. A postoperative patient after abdominal pain.
   D. B and C
   E. All of the above

4. **Which of the following should be included when teaching patients about modifications that can be made to promote oxygenation?**
   A. It is just as important to avoid secondary smoke as it is not to personally smoke.
   B. Even an occasional alcoholic beverage can increase the risk for aspiration.
   C. Chewing tobacco and dipping snuff are acceptable alternatives to smoking.
   D. A and B
   E. All of the above

5. **To safely suction a tracheostomy, the nurse should:**
   A. Insert the suctioning catheter while applying suction.
   B. Discontinue suctioning if the patient shows any sign of respiratory distress.
   C. Complete suctioning cycle within 10–20 seconds.
   D. All of the above

ANSWERS

Routine Checkup

1. Nicotine.
2. Capillaries.
3. Allergens
   Pollutants
   Secondhand smoke
   High altitude

Review Questions

1. C
2. D
3. E
4. A
5. B

References

Craven RF, Hirnle CJ: *Fundamentals of Nursing: Human Health and Function*, 5th ed. Philadelphia, PA: Lippincott, 2006.

Daniels R: *Nursing Fundamentals: Caring & Clinical Decision Making*. New York, NY: Delmar Thomson Learning, 2004.

Potter PA, Perry AG: *Fundamentals of Nursing*, 6th ed. St. Louis, MO: Mosby Elsevier, 2005.

Additional Resources

National Heart, Lung, and Blood Institute: *What is Atherosclerosis?* Available at http://www.nhlbi.nih.gov/health/dci/Diseases/Atherosclerosis/Atherosclerosis_WhatIs.html.

National Heart, Lung, and Blood Institute: *Your Guide to Living Well with Heart Disease*. Available at http://www.nhlbi.nih.gov/health/public/heart/other/your_guide/living_well.pdf.

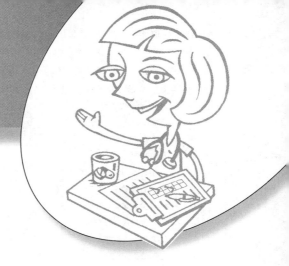

Chapter **13**

Nutrition

LEARNING OBJECTIVES

At the end of the chapter, the reader will be able to:

1. Differentiate between macronutrients and micronutrients.

2. Describe the major function of each of the macronutrients.

3. Briefly describe the four processes of food breakdown.

4. Briefly discuss factors that influence nutrition.

5. Identify subjective and objective data that should be collected for a patient who has a potential or actual alteration in nutrition.

6. Discuss health promotion interventions that are appropriate for an individual with a potential or actual alteration in nutrition.

7. Describe basic actions that can be taken to assist patients who are experiencing altered nutrition to achieve adequate nutrient intake.

8. Briefly describe the various special diets that may be prescribed for patients with certain medical conditions.

9. Briefly describe the various types of enteral tube feedings, including any necessary precautions.

10. Discuss the nursing care of patients who are receiving total parenteral nutrition (TPN) or lipids.

KEY WORDS

Absorption
Anabolism
Anorexia
Anthropometric
Bariatric surgery
Calorie or kilocalorie
Carbohydrates
Catabolism
Celiac disease
Digestion
Enteral nutrition
Fats
Fiber
Gastrostomy

Hypervitaminosis
Jejunostomy
Macronutrients
Metabolism
Micronutrients
Minerals
Nasogastric
Orogastric
Parenteral nutrition
Pica
Pneumothorax
Proteins
Villi
Vitamins

Overview

Nutrients are a primary source of essential substances needed to sustain life. Health is promoted when an individual consumes the right combination of nutrients in the right amounts. A major concern facing healthcare providers (eg, physicians, nurse practitioners) today is the overconsumption of nutrients, both those good for you and those that are not good for you. Obesity has been linked to many chronic illnesses, including heart disease, diabetes, cancer, and arthritis. Each of these diseases impacts the quality of life, and some are even life threatening. Nutritional deficiencies can also contribute to less than optimal health. Traditionally, we think of a malnourished patient as being one who is underweight. However, an individual may be overweight and at the same time be malnourished if he or she is not consuming the right nutrients. Malnourishment may lead to stunted growth, impaired oxygenation, or arrhythmias, to name a few. Thus, it is critical that healthcare providers, particularly nurses, intervene to promote healthy nutritional patterns and correct nutritional deviations.

Physiology of Nutrition

Nutrients

Nutrients are obtained through the consumption of food substances. There are two broad categories of nutrients, and both are further broken down into subcomponents.

Macronutrients

Macronutrients include carbohydrates, fats, and proteins (Table 13–1). Each macronutrient provides a source of calories. A **calorie** or **kilocalorie** is the basic unit of energy available in a particular food substance. For example, if you eat a piece of bread that has 70 calories, then you have that much energy available for use. Engaging in activity equivalent to the amount of calories consumed results in neither a gain nor a loss of weight. However, if the caloric intake is more than what is required for the level energy exerted, then there will be a weight gain. On the other hand, if the caloric intake is less than the amount of energy expended, then there will be a weight loss (provided there is not an excess amount of calories stored in the body). A brief description of each macronutrient follows.

- **Carbohydrates:** Also referred to as sugars, these are our main source of energy. Some carbohydrates cannot be completely digested and absorbed by the body. The undigested carbohydrates are called **fiber**. Even though

TABLE 13–1 Macronutrients

	Carbohydrates	Proteins	Fats
Calories	4 kcal/g	4 kcal/g	9 kcal/g
Function	Provide energy source	Tissue building	Concentrated energy and energy storage
Recommended intake	45–65% of calories	10–35% of calories	20–35% of calories
Sources	Fruits and vegetables Breads, cereals, and other grains Milk and milk products Foods with added sugar	Meats, poultry, and fish Dry beans and peas Tofu Eggs Nuts and seeds Milk and milk products	Nuts Vegetable oils Fish

fiber is not absorbed by the body, it serves many beneficial functions (Box 13–1).

- **Proteins:** These are composed of amino acids. Proteins are important for growth and development, tissue building and repair, immune processes, and the transport of other nutrients and some medications. In the absence of carbohydrates, proteins provide a source of energy. However, this situation should be avoided because of the key role that protein plays in other body functions.

- **Fats:** Certain types of fats are important to include in the diet, but others can lead to health problems. Good fats (unsaturated) in the right amount are important because they provide a source of energy as well as a means to store energy. Fats also transport other nutrients (eg, vitamins), insulate the body, and protect certain organs.

Dietary guidelines published jointly by U.S. Department of Health and Human Services (HHS) and U.S. Department of Agriculture (USDA) suggest that you encourage patients to develop healthy eating patterns by eating

- a variety of vegetables
- whole fruits, grains at least half of which are whole grains
- fat-free or low fat dairy
- a variety of protein foods including seafood, lean meats, beans, peas, nuts, seeds, and soy products

Patient should also

- Limit saturated fats, trans fats, added sugars, and sodium
- Consume less than 10% of calories per day from added sugars
- Consume less than 10% of calories per day from saturated fats

BOX 13–1
Benefits of Fiber

Fiber is found primarily in fruits and vegetables and is good for you because it:
- Prevents constipation
- Lowers cholesterol
- Prevents hemorrhoids and diverticuli
- Helps with weight loss
- Controls blood sugar levels

- Consume less than 2300 mg per day of sodium
- Alcohol should be consumed in moderation—one drink per day for women and two drink per day for men

> ### NURSING ALERT
>
> **Proteins as a Source of Energy**
> Nurses should warn patients about the dangers associated with using proteins as a source of energy because doing so may interfere with tissue building, growth and development, and immune processes.

Micronutrients

Micronutrients include vitamins, minerals, and water. They are required in small amounts by the body. Micronutrients do not provide a source of energy for the body, but they do serve the important role of regulating body processes. In fact, in some instances, a lack of certain micronutrients may alter the body's ability to use certain macronutrients.

- **Vitamins** aid in the regulation of metabolic activities at the cellular level. There are two broad categories of vitamins: fat-soluble vitamins and water-soluble vitamins. The fat-soluble vitamins include vitamins A, D, E, and K. Fat is required for the body to absorb fat-soluble vitamins. The B-complex vitamins and vitamin C are water soluble. The body can store fat-soluble vitamins, but the majority of unused water-soluble vitamins are excreted from the body via the kidneys. Because some vitamins can be stored by the body, particularly fat-soluble vitamins, patients must be warned against overconsumption to prevent the adverse effects of **hypervitaminosis** (an excessive amount of a particular vitamin).

- **Minerals** are inorganic substances that are used by the body to regulate various body processes. For example, potassium is a mineral that plays a role in regulating heart rhythm. There are two categories of minerals: macrominerals, which are required in larger amounts, and trace minerals. Numerous minerals are found in the body. Some of the more common minerals are calcium, iron, sodium, chloride, potassium, iodine, fluoride, zinc, phosphorous, and magnesium.

- **Water** is just as important for proper body functioning as are the other nutrients. Water is needed to carry out cellular processes. An individual usually obtains water by drinking fluids and by eating foods high in water content (eg, fruits and vegetables). Fluid balance is discussed in more detail in Chapter 14.

Digestive Process

The digestive or gastrointestinal system consists of the mouth, pharynx (throat), esophagus, stomach, small intestines, and large intestines. Accessory organs are also required to complete the digestive process and include the salivary glands (located in the mouth), the liver, the gallbladder, and the pancreas (Figure 13–1).

Four processes occur during the breakdown of food: digestion, absorption, metabolism, and elimination.

- **Digestion** is the process whereby food is broken down into a form that can be absorbed by the body for use. It begins in the mouth and involves both the mechanical breakdown of foods that occurs with chewing and the chemical breakdown of nutrients that is aided by various enzymes. The partially digested food is transported to the stomach by way of the esophagus. When it is in the stomach, the food continues to be mechanically

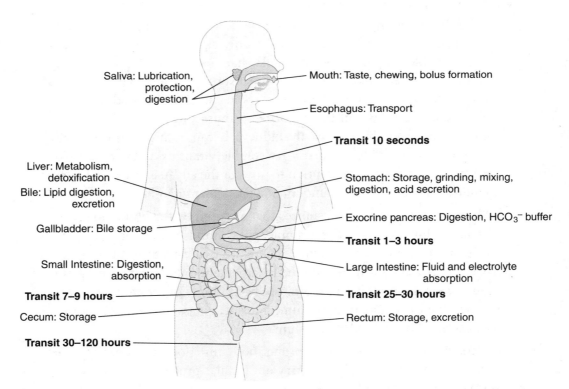

FIGURE 13–1 · The digestive process breaks down food as the food passes through the GI tract via digestion, absorption, metabolism, and elimination. (Reproduced with permission from Kibble JD, Halsey CR: *The Big Picture: Medical Physiology*. New York, NY: McGraw-Hill; 2009, Fig 7-1.)

and chemically broken down. Food content leaves the stomach in a liquid form and enters the first segment of the small intestines, the duodenum. Additional enzymes are secreted from the liver and gallbladder by way of the bile duct as well as from the pancreas. These enzymes further aid nutrient breakdown.

- **Absorption:** After nutrients are broken down, they must have a means for entering the bloodstream, lymphatic system, and ultimately the cells. Absorption takes place in the **villi** (small finger-like projections) in the small intestines.

- **Metabolism:** At the cellular level, chemical reactions occur to release energy from nutrients for use by the various tissues, organs, and organ systems. Metabolism is the combined action of **anabolism**, building complex substances from simple substance, and **catabolism**, breaking down complex substances into simple substances. Nutrients not needed immediately are stored for later use, primarily in the form of fat.

- **Elimination:** Substances left over after absorption in the small intestines enter the large intestines, where most of the water content is absorbed, leaving behind formed stool, which is eventually excreted from the body via the anus.

✔ ROUTINE CHECKUP 1

1. Whereas _____ provide calories, _____ serve a role in regulating body processes.

Answer:

2. List the four processes involved in food breakdown.

Answer:

_____

_____

_____

_____

Factors Influencing Nutrition

Factors that influence an individual's nutritional intake and status include those related to the person's age or developmental stage, lifestyle and culture, health alterations, and adverse effects of certain medical interventions. Although some variables are not controllable, many are. Nurses play a key role in assisting patients and their families and significant others to modify the variables that can be changed to benefit the patient.

Age and Developmental Stage

Periods of time in an individual's life when growth is rapid require higher levels of energy expenditures and a greater intake of nutrients. Two such times are at the beginning of life and during the adolescent years, when there is a growth spurt. An infant's ability to meet energy needs is compounded by the fact that he or she has an immature digestive tract. Thus, the forms of food used to meet the infant's needs must be modified to match the level of functioning of his or her digestive tract. During the adolescent years, the challenge is to ensure that the proper nutrients are consumed. Adolescents are very active and on the go. They have a higher level of independence and are more likely to select fast foods that are high in calories and fat and that are easy to eat on the go. Adolescents, particularly young women, are very concerned about their body image and may become victims of eating disorders such as anorexia nervosa and bulimia (Box 13–2).

Older adults also have challenges related to their developmental stage. Although energy and caloric needs decrease with aging, the need for certain nutrients does not. Remember that an individual can be overweight and malnourished at the same time. Thus, an elderly patient may need to monitor his

---

BOX 13–2
Eating Disorders

Types
- Anorexia nervosa: Very thin but refuses to eat because of the perception of being fat
- Bulimia: Overeating followed by purging by self-induced vomiting or laxative use
- Binge eating: Overeating even when not hungry or uncomfortably full

Prevalence
Affects females more than males

Treatment
Treatment usually involves a combination of psychotherapy, nutrition education, family counseling, medications, and hospitalization

or her caloric intake while at the same time ensuring the intake of required nutrients such as calcium and iron. Certain changes that occur during this time period make it more difficult for elderly patients to achieve this goal. Examples of such changes include:

- Loss of teeth or poorly fitting dentures (affects the ability to chew foods)
- Decreased ability to smell and taste food
- Appetite changes secondary to prescribed medications
- Decreased vision (affects the ability to read food labels)
- Presence of multiple chronic illnesses

Additionally, older adults may have a limited income and may be socially isolated, making it difficult to obtain groceries or prepare meals.

Lifestyle and Culture

The lifestyle of an individual or family also has a bearing on eating behaviors. Examples of lifestyle variables that may influence eating behaviors include:

- Whether or not both parents work outside of the home may influence the types of meals eaten (eg, fast foods, boxed meals, balanced meals including selections from each of the food groups)
- Income (eating out at restaurants, ability to purchase variety of foods)
- When and where meals are eaten (eg, at the dinner table, as a family, individually, in front of the television, at distinct mealtimes, eating throughout the day)
- Beliefs (eg, religious beliefs, the belief that eating everything on your plate will make you healthy, intolerance of "wasting food," using food as a reward, what and how much men vs. women should eat, pica [eating non-food items])
- Activity level (affects amount of calories needed)
- Consumption of alcohol and drugs

Health Alterations and Therapeutic Interventions

Certain illnesses may alter an individual's nutritional status. Nausea, vomiting, mouth ulcers, toothaches, swallowing impairment, or an inflamed esophagus can affect a person's ability to mechanically process food as well as alter the desire for food. Certain disorders (eg, infections, hyperthyroidism) increase the metabolic rate, which subsequently leads to an increased demand for nutrients. Patients with inflammatory disorders or malabsorption disorders such as gastric ulcers and **celiac disease** (an intolerance of foods containing gluten, including wheat, rye, oats, and barley) will also experience altered nutrition. Other familiar diseases associated with altered nutrition include diabetes mellitus and the "wasting syndrome" associated with HIV.

Some therapeutic interventions, although effective for their intended purpose, have an adverse effect on nutritional status. Chemotherapy and radiation may cause nausea, vomiting, **anorexia** (loss of appetite), and mouth sores. Gastric resections and **bariatric surgery** (surgery to cause weight loss) both have an associated risk of malabsorption of nutrients. Surgical patients, particularly those who have had oral or gastrointestinal procedures, may experience nutritional issues ranging from an inability to ingest nutrients to malabsorption of nutrients. Certain medications, both prescribed and over the counter, have associated side effects that may alter taste; produce nausea, vomiting, or diarrhea; or interfere with one or more of the digestive processes. There is also a risk for adverse effects associated with drug-to-drug interactions as well as drug-to-food interactions.

✔ ROUTINE CHECKUP 2

1. The two periods of life during which growth is more rapid and energy requirements are higher are _____ and _____.

Answer:

2. Surgical patients as well as those who are receiving chemotherapy and certain types of medications may experience alterations in nutrition secondary to these therapies. True/false?

Answer:

The Nursing Process and Nutrition

The nurse is a key player in bringing the pieces of the puzzle together for proper diagnosis and treatment of patients experiencing altered human function related to nutritional imbalances. Achieving an optimal outcome partially depends on the nurse's ability to establish a trusting relationship with the client. Doing so is more likely to yield accurate information, correct diagnoses, and an effective plan of care with buy-in from the patient.

Assessment

During the assessment phase of the nursing process, the nurse should collect data about the client's perception of his or her diet patterns and nutritional status as well as obtain objective evidence of the patient's nutritional status (Box 13–3). Subjective data should include:

- Types of foods eaten, including food likes and dislikes
- Food allergies
- Food preparation
- Timing and frequency of meals, including any rituals

How the above information is obtained may vary from situation to situation. Some options include the 24-hour recall format or a diet diary.

NURSING ALERT

Stay Positive
Patients may be sensitive about their weight. Expect apprehension when the patient is asked to step on a scale or when their waist is measured. Make small talk when taking measurements to distract the patient and lower anxiety. Document the results without making any comment. Encourage the patient to be honest when providing dietary information. You and the patient together will help the patient lose weight.

BOX 13–3
Signs of Altered Nutrition

- Weight (underweight, overweight, significant changes)
- Complaints of tiredness or weakness
- Flaccid or wasted appearance
- Loss of appetite
- Constipation or diarrhea
- Fragile skin or slow healing
- Pale conjunctiva
- Hair loss
- Brittle nails or nail shape changes
- Tooth decay or gum disease
- Skeletal deviations (bowed legs, knock-knees, fractures)
- Altered mental status (irritability, listlessness, confusion)
- Tachycardia or irregular heart beat
- High or low blood pressure

The nurse obtains objective data during the physical assessment as well as from a review of laboratory results. Key data to obtain include:

- **Anthropometric** (human body) measurements: Height, weight, skin fold measurements, upper arm measurements, abdominal circumference
- Appearance: Hair, nails, skin, gums, muscle mass, posture
- Mental status
- Laboratory data: Prealbumin, albumin, transferrin, hemoglobin, cholesterol, creatinine, lymphocyte count

> **NURSING ALERT**
>
> **Relationship Between Body Shape and Health Risk**
> People who have a larger waist and abdomen compared with their hips and thighs are at a greater risk for weight-related health problems.

Nursing Diagnoses

It is not possible to derive a standard list of nursing diagnoses for a patient experiencing alterations in nutrition because each individual brings a unique set of circumstances to the healthcare encounter. Therefore, what may be appropriate or applicable for one patient may not be pertinent for another. Imbalanced nutrition, more than body requirements and imbalanced nutrition, less than body requirements are the two nursing diagnoses directly related to patients with altered nutrition. Other nursing diagnoses that may be applicable include:

- Impaired swallowing
- Deficient knowledge (nutrition-related)
- Activity intolerance
- Altered body image
- Self-care deficit, feeding
- Ineffective therapeutic regimen management
- Impaired skin integrity
- Diarrhea
- Constipation
- Risk for infection
- Self-esteem disturbance

Planning and Implementation

During the planning phase of the nursing process, the nurse and patient jointly decide on the goals and establish outcomes. This can be a major task because in many instances it requires the patient to make significant changes in practices that have been a part of their life for many years. The implementation phase involves not only the identification of interventions but also the dynamics of effective deployment of the interventions. Patients who are obese realize excessive weight is a health risk. They likely tried countless diets to curb their weight gain but failed. Consistent failure brings hopelessness and the resolve that barring surgical intervention that losing weight is unrealistic. The nurse must be able to instill hope that the patient can reduce weight by following a plan devised by the nurse and the patient. Therefore, the initial intervention is to change a negative attitude to a positive attitude.

Health Promotion Interventions

Health promotion is the mainstay of interventions for all potential health deviations, the premise being that "an ounce of prevention is worth a pound of cure." This is especially true in the case of the prevention of health deviations associated with altered nutrition. The nurse should include interventions aimed at promoting healthy nutrition practices at every afforded opportunity. This includes teaching about good food choices (Figure 13–2), proper portion sizes, and safe handling and preparation of food.

NURSING ALERT

Cut Portions in Half
Some patients are looking for a quick fix to losing weight and shy away from calorie counting. A good intervention is for the patient to cut current portions in half. Instead of drinking an 8-oz glass of soda, drink a 4-oz glass, for example. This reduces caloric intake without the patient having to count calories or drastically disrupting their dietary routine.

Altered Nutrition Interventions

Patients experiencing acute illnesses often lose their appetite or have difficulty ingesting nutrients. Basic actions that may assist the patient to achieve an adequate intake of nutrients include:

- Provision of a pleasant environment for eating (free of odors and unpleasant sights)
- Allowing the patient to provide input into food selection

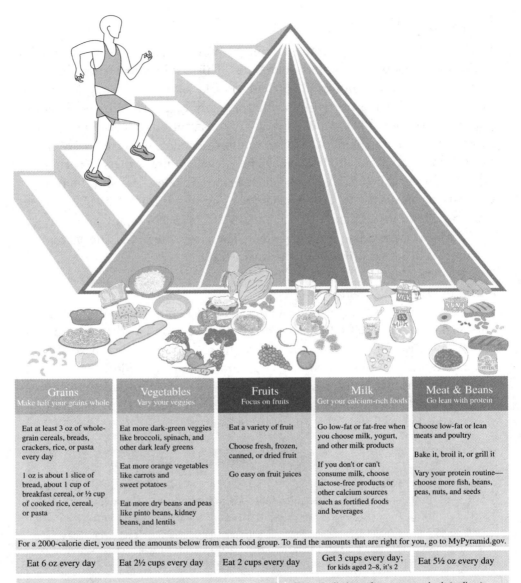

Grains Make half your grains whole	Vegetables Vary your veggies	Fruits Focus on fruits	Milk Get your calcium-rich foods	Meat & Beans Go lean with protein
Eat at least 3 oz of whole-grain cereals, breads, crackers, rice, or pasta every day 1 oz is about 1 slice of bread, about 1 cup of breakfast cereal, or ½ cup of cooked rice, cereal, or pasta	Eat more dark-green veggies like broccoli, spinach, and other dark leafy greens Eat more orange vegetables like carrots and sweet potatoes Eat more dry beans and peas like pinto beans, kidney beans, and lentils	Eat a variety of fruit Choose fresh, frozen, canned, or dried fruit Go easy on fruit juices	Go low-fat or fat-free when you choose milk, yogurt, and other milk products If you don't or can't consume milk, choose lactose-free products or other calcium sources such as fortified foods and beverages	Choose low-fat or lean meats and poultry Bake it, broil it, or grill it Vary your protein routine—choose more fish, beans, peas, nuts, and seeds

For a 2000-calorie diet, you need the amounts below from each food group. To find the amounts that are right for you, go to MyPyramid.gov.

Eat 6 oz every day	Eat 2½ cups every day	Eat 2 cups every day	Get 3 cups every day; for kids aged 2–8, it's 2	Eat 5½ oz every day

Find your balance between food and physical activity

- Be sure to stay within your daily calorie needs.
- Be physically active for at least 30 minutes most days of the week.
- About 60 minutes a day of physical activity may be needed to prevent weight gain.
- For sustaining weight loss, at least 60–90 minutes a day of physical activity may be required.
- Children and teenagers should be physically active for 60 minutes every day, or most days.

Know the limits on fats, sugars, and salt (sodium)

- Make most of your fat sources from fish, nuts, and vegetable oils.
- Limit solid fats like butter, margarine, shortening, and lard, as well as foods that contain these.
- Check the Nutrition Facts label to keep saturated fats, *trans* fats, and sodium low.
- Choose food and beverages low in added sugars. Added sugars contribute calories with few, if any, nutrients.

FIGURE 13−2 · "Food pyramid" diagram showing sensible choices for planning meals.

- Serving foods in an appealing manner (hot foods hot, cold foods cold, appropriate condiments)
- Providing assistance during mealtimes as needed (positioning the patient, cutting foods, adding condiments)

The patient's medical condition may make it necessary for the healthcare provider to prescribe a special diet (Table 13–2). The nurse is responsible for ensuring that the patient receives the prescribed diet. To promote compliance, the nurse should teach the patient or significant others, as appropriate, about the required modifications.

NURSING ALERT

Be Proactive

Work with the patient and the patient's support group to devise a dietary plan immediately when the patient is diagnosed with an illness or before treatment begins if there is a tendency that the patient's appetite will decrease. The patient and the patient's support group can then expect the loss of appetite and will have a plan in place to respond to the change in appetite.

A healthcare provider may decide that a patient should not receive anything by mouth (NPO) or the patient may not be able to tolerate anything by mouth. When a patient is NPO for an extended period of time, an alternate route of nutrient intake is necessary. Alternate routes of intake can be divided into two broad categories: **enteral nutrition**, which refers to the provision of nutrients into the digestive tract by means other than ingestion through the mouth, and **parenteral nutrition**, which involves the infusion of nutrients intravenously (directly into the bloodstream).

Enteral Nutrition   Enteral tube feedings are ordered for various reasons. Patients who have an altered state of consciousness, those who are not able to ingest an adequate amount of nutrients to meet the body's needs, and those who have some type of digestive tract obstruction (eg, edema, tumor, or trauma) are all potential candidates for enteral tube feedings. There are multiple types of tube feedings. **Nasogastric** feedings are administered via a tube that is inserted into the stomach by way of the nose. When the nose cannot be used, the tube may be inserted via the mouth, in which case the feeding is called an **orogastric** feeding. If the feedings are to be administered over an extended period of time or permanently, the patient may require the placement of a **gastrostomy** tube (tube inserted directly into the stomach) or **jejunostomy** tube (tube inserted into the jejunum segment of the small intestines). The type of tube used for the

TABLE 13–2 Special Diets

Diet and Purpose	Description
Nothing by mouth (NPO) • Preoperatively • Procedure preparation • Immediate postoperative period • Rest the GI tract	Individual is not to ingest anything solid or liquid by way of the mouth.
Clear liquid • Postoperatively • Immediately after being NPO	Any liquid that does not contain pulp or solid components, including: • Plain water • Fruit juices • Broth • Gelatin • Popsicles • Tea or coffee without cream
Full liquid • After individual tolerates clear liquids	All fluids and foods that are liquid or semi-liquid at room temperature, including: • Milk • Puddings • Strained cream soups • Pureed vegetables • Cooked cereals
Soft or low residue • Difficulty chewing or swallowing • Impaired digestion or absorption (eg, irritable bowel diseases)	Persons on a low-residue diet should avoid fried foods, spicy foods, and seeded or raw fruits and vegetables. The following foods are generally allowed on both the soft and low-residue diets: • Enriched white bread • White rice • Plain pasta • Low-fiber cereals • Moist or tender meats, poultry, and fish • Eggs • Smooth peanut butter • Milk, yogurt, and cheese (limit amounts) • Desserts without nuts or coconut
High fiber • Constipation • Diverticulosis • To lower high cholesterol	Good food sources of fiber include: • Grains, especially whole-grain products • Fruits and vegetables • Legumes (beans, peas) • Nuts and seeds
Sodium restricted • Excess fluid (edema) • Hypertension • Congestive heart failure • Kidney disease	Level of restriction varies from "no added salt" to stringent restriction (no more than 500 mg/day). Individuals on a sodium-restricted diet should not only monitor the use of table salt but should also check food labels for the amount of sodium in foods purchased. Canned and prepackaged foods (eg, chips, boxed meals) may contain high levels of sodium.

GI = gastrointestinal

enteral feeding varies depending on the length of time the feeding will be continued, the placement of the tubing, and the method of delivery (eg, continuous vs. intermittent). There are also different types of formulas for enteral tube feedings depending upon the condition of the gastrointestinal tract and the intended purpose of the feeding. The healthcare provider is the individual responsible for making the decision about the type of feeding, tube, and formula. Professional nurses may insert enteral tubes via the nose or mouth. Tube placement should be confirmed before the initiation of feedings. The most reliable method of checking for correct tube placement is radiography (especially for initial placement confirmation). Assistive personnel may be delegated the responsibility of actually administering the enteral feedings. However, professional nurses are responsible for assessing the patient and must always verify tube placement before the feeding is administered. Furthermore, it is critical that the nurse monitor the patient for complications that may occur secondary to enteral tube feedings.

NURSING ALERT

Confirming Enteral Tube Placement
After initial placement of an enteral tube has been confirmed by radiography, subsequent checks can be confirmed by checking gastric aspirate color and pH. Radiographic confirmation of placement should be performed anytime there is doubt about tube placement.

NURSING ALERT

Replacement of Residual
When checking for residual, replace aspirated gastric contents back into the stomach to prevent fluid and electrolyte imbalances (unless otherwise instructed by the physician).

NURSING ALERT

Sit the Patient Upright
The head of the patient should be raised 30 degrees or be in an upright position during feeding and an hour after feeding unless contraindicated. Patients are at risk for aspiration.

Parenteral Nutrition Parenteral nutrition is required when the patient cannot adequately obtain nutrients by the enteral route or when doing so would result in adverse effects on the patient. Parenteral nutrition can be administered through peripheral veins or through central venous lines. The route chosen (peripheral or central) depends on the solution used and the length of time the parenteral nutrition will be required. Short-term administration of solutions that contain no more than 10% dextrose and 5% protein can safely be administered through a peripheral intravenous line. This form of parenteral nutrition is referred to as partial parenteral nutrition (PPN). Total parental nutrition (TPN), which is the administration of a solution containing more than 10% dextrose and 5% protein as well as the administration of lipids (fats), always requires the use of a central venous line (larger vessels that have rapid blood flow). TPN and lipids provide all of the essential nutrients required by a patient. The specific amount of nutrients and calories are tailored to meet the individual patient's needs. Specially trained nurses may insert peripherally inserted central catheters (PICCs). All other central lines (subclavian, jugular, tunneled catheters, implanted vascular access) must be inserted by a physician. In all instances, sterile technique must be used. Professional nurses are delegated the responsibility of caring for the central line insertion site, administering TPN, tubing and bag changes, and monitoring the patient for complications. Meticulous care should be given when carrying out these duties. Sterile technique should be maintained during dressing changes. Any sign of infection at the insertion site should be reported to the physician. Tubing and TPN bag changes should be performed according to policy (usually every 24 hours). The patient should be monitored for signs indicating a **pneumothorax** (collection of air in the pleural space), air embolism, infection, fluid overload, and metabolic imbalances. Refer to Box 13–4 for a more thorough discussion of nursing care of patients receiving TPN.

NURSING ALERT

Safe Infusion of Hyperosmolar Solutions
Infusing hyperosmolar solutions (dextrose >10% or protein >5%) into a peripheral intravenous site may cause irritation and hardening of the veins.

NURSING ALERT

Safe TPN Infusion Rate
Administer TPN at the rate prescribed by the physician. Speeding up or slowing down the infusion may cause complications such as electrolyte shifts, fluid overload, or hypoglycemia.

BOX 13–4
Procedure Tip: Total Parenteral Nutrition and Lipids

Life-threatening complication may occur in patients receiving TPN and lipids. The following tips will assist the nurse to minimize, if not prevent, such complications from occurring.

Tip	Rationale

• After the insertion of a central venous line, monitor the patient closely for
  • Difficulty in breathing
  • Sharp chest pain
  • Coughing
Report findings to the physician immediately!
	• There is a danger of puncturing the patient closely for lung with the insertion of the central venous line. The puncture will create pain a pneumothorax and may lead to lung collapse. Respiratory distress will occur if left untreated.

• During insertion of the central venous line as well as during tubing changes:
  • Have the patient assume the left sidelying position
  • Have the patient bear down and hold his or her breath (Valsalva maneuver)
	• Air can enter the tubing or catheter, increasing the likelihood of an air embolism. The left sidelying position and the Valsalva maneuver increase venous pressure and may prevent air from entering the bloodstream

• Monitor the patient for signs of an air embolism (tachypnea, tachycardia, hypotension, and anxiety) for at least 24 hours	• Signs of an air embolism may develop slowly

• Perform tubing and dressing changes using sterile techniques:
  • Wash hands thoroughly
  • Wear a sterile mask and gloves
	• This prevents infection

• Monitor the following:
  • Temperature
  • Blood sugars (per doctor orders)
  • Weight
  • Intake and output
  • Dressing
	• Early detection of possible complications (eg, infection, hyperglycemia, hypoglycemia, fluid overload)

• Do not use the TPN line for the administration of anything other than TPN and lipids	• Minimize breaks in the central line, thereby diminishing the risk of infection

• Inspect lipid solution closely before administering
  • Do not administer if separated into layers or if oil droplets are present
  • Do not mistake for tube feeding formulas (both are milky in appearance)
	• May cause fat embolisms if infused
	• May administer wrong solution by the wrong route

Evaluation

The success of the plan of care for the patient experiencing a potential or actual alteration in nutritional status relies heavily on whether mutually developed realistic goals were established during the planning phase, a task that in most cases is easier said than done. Therefore, it is even more important to begin the evaluation process early on and to continuously evaluate the appropriateness of goals, expected outcomes, and interventions. Modification should be made as the need arises, and the patient and/or significant other(s) should be actively involved as much as is possible.

Conclusion

Nutrition and its impact on health is a very hot topic currently. The literature supports, over and over again, the relationship between an individual's health status and his or her nutritional habits. Nurses, just as other healthcare professionals, are challenged to intervene to promote healthy eating patterns. Nurses also play an important role in caring for patients who experience alterations in health caused by nutritional problems or who experience nutritional problems secondary to other health problems. This chapter has presented key information about nutritional requirements, alterations in nutrition, and interventions to assist patients to maintain healthy diet habits and to deal with alterations in nutrition. Key concepts presented include:

- Macronutrients (carbohydrates, fats, and proteins) and micronutrients (vitamins, minerals, and water) in the right amounts are needed to perform life-sustaining processes.
- Carbohydrates are the preferred source of energy for the body.
- Proteins serve an important role in tissue building and repair, growth and development, and immune processes.
- Good fats in the right amounts are an important part of the diet.
- Vitamins are fat soluble (A, D, E, K) or water soluble (B complex and C). Overconsumption of vitamins, especially fat-soluble vitamins, can cause adverse effects on the body.
- Water is needed by the body to carry out important cellular processes.
- The four processes involved in food breakdown are digestion, absorption, metabolism, and excretion.
- Age, developmental stage, lifestyle, culture, disease, and certain medical interventions can all affect a person's nutritional status.

- Assessment should include the collection of data about a patient's eating patterns as well as body measurements, laboratory data, appearance, and mental status.

- Nursing diagnoses vary widely from patient to patient. The two primary North American Nursing Diagnosis Association (NANDA) diagnoses directly related to nutrition are imbalanced nutrition, more than body requirements and imbalanced nutrition, less than body requirements.

- Health teaching related to nutrition should include information about good food choices, proper portion sizes, and safe handling and preparation of food.

- Enteral (nasogastric, orogastric, gastrostomy, jejunostomy) and parenteral nutrition (TPN) may be required for patients who are unable to ingest nutrients orally.

- Patients receiving TPN are at risk for developing a pneumothorax, air embolism, and infections.

REVIEW QUESTIONS

1. **Which of the following nutrients plays a major role in tissue repair?**
   A. Carbohydrates
   B. Fats
   C. Proteins
   D. Vitamins

2. **Nutrients enter the bloodstream through the process of:**
   A. Absorption
   B. Digestion
   C. Metabolism
   D. Elimination

3. **When caring for an elderly patient who has a potential or actual alteration in nutrition, the nurse should:**
   A. Assess the patient's visual acuity.
   B. Determine whether the patient wears dentures.
   C. Assess the patient's financial resources.
   D. All of the above

4. **All of the following actions may improve nutrient intake for the patient with a poor appetite EXCEPT:**
   A. Providing a pleasant eating environment
   B. Providing condiments

C. Serving foods hot

D. Providing the patient with choices

5. **All of the following may be signs of poor nutrition EXCEPT:**

A. Slowly healing wound

B. Pink conjunctiva

C. Brittle nails

D. Bowed legs

6. **Which of the following foods is/are not recommended for a patient who is on a soft or low-residue diet?**

A. Raw fruits and vegetables

B. Milk

C. Eggs

D. All of the above

7. **Which of the following types of enteral tube feedings is preferred when long-term feedings are required?**

A. Gastrostomy

B. Nasogastric

C. TPN

D. A or C

8. **Which of the following methods of enteral tube placement verification is preferred when there is any uncertainty about tube placement?**

A. Aspiration of gastric content

B. Checking the pH of gastric content

C. A and B combined

D. Radiography

E. Both C and D are acceptable

9. **Which of the following nursing diagnoses would be generally appropriate for the patient who is receiving TPN?**

A. Constipation

B. Impaired nutrition, less than body requirements

C. Risk for infection

D. B and C

E. All of the above

10. **When providing care for a patient who is receiving TPN, the nurse should include all of the following EXCEPT:**

A. Have the patient bear down and hold his or her breath during tubing changes.

B. Place the patient in the left sidelying position if there are signs of an air embolism.

C. Clean the port thoroughly before administering IV push medications into the TPN line.

D. Monitor the patient's glucose levels.

E. Wear sterile gloves and a mask during dressing and tubing changes.

ANSWERS

Routine Checkup 1

1. Macronutrients, micronutrients.
2. Digestion
   Absorption
   Metabolism
   Elimination

Routine Checkup 2

1. Infancy, adolescence.
2. True.

Review Questions

1. C
2. A
3. D
4. C
5. B
6. A
7. A
8. D
9. D
10. C

References

Craven RF, Hirnle CJ: *Fundamentals of Nursing: Human Health and Function*, 5th ed. Philadelphia, PA: Lippincott, 2006.

Daniels R: *Nursing Fundamentals: Caring & Clinical Decision Making*. New York, NY: Delmar Thomson Learning, 2004.

Potter PA, Perry AG: *Fundamentals of Nursing*, 6th ed. St. Louis, MO: Mosby Elsevier, 2005.

Additional Resources

Centers for Disease Control and Prevention: *Dietary Fat.* Available at http://www
.cdc.gov/nccdphp/dnpa/nutrition/nutrition_for_everyone/basics/fat.htm#
polyunsaturated.

KidsHealth: *Digestive Health.* Available at http://kidshealth.org/parent/general/body_
basics/digestive.html.

Kimberley-Clark Medical Devices: *The MIC-KEY.* Available at http://www.mic-key
.com/animediaUSA08enduser.swf.

Mayo Clinic: *Dietary Fiber: Essential for a Healthy Diet.* Available at http://www
.mayoclinic.com/print/fiber/NU00033/METHOD=print.

Mayo Clinic: *Eating Disorders.* Available at http://www.mayoclinic.com/print/eating-
disorders/DS00294/DSECTION=all&METHOD=print.

Merck: *Disorders of Nutrition and Metabolism.* Available at http://www.merck.com/
mmhe/sec12.html.

Merck: *Minerals and Electrolytes.* Available at http://www.merck.com/mmhe/sec12/
ch155/ch155a.html.

U.S. Department of Agriculture: *Dietary Guidelines for Americans 2005.* Available at
http://www.cnpp.usda.gov/Publications/DietaryGuidelines/2005/2005DGPolicyDoc
ument.pdf.

U.S. Department of Agriculture: *MyPyramid.* Available at http://www.mypyramid
.gov/mypyramid/index.aspx.

U.S. Food and Drug Administration: Available at http://www.fda.gov/consumer/
updates/vitamins111907.html.

Chapter **14**

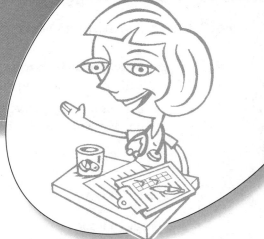

Fluid, Electrolyte, and Acid–Base Balance

LEARNING OBJECTIVES

At the end of the chapter, the reader will be able to:

1. Describe the distribution of fluids in the body.
2. Describe six ways fluid balance is maintained.
3. Differentiate between isotonic, hypotonic, and hypertonic fluids.
4. Compare and contrast passive transport and active transport.
5. Compare and contrast acids and bases.
6. Discuss the role of buffers in maintaining acid–base balance.
7. Compare and contrast how the lungs and the kidneys manage acid–base imbalances.
8. Discuss factors that influence fluid, electrolyte, and acid–base balance.
9. Discuss the major types of fluid, electrolyte, and acid–base imbalances, including signs, symptoms, and risk factors.

⑩ Identify actual and related nursing diagnoses that may be appropriate for patients experiencing fluid, electrolyte, and acid–base imbalances.

⑪ Discuss nursing interventions that may be appropriate for addressing the needs of patients experiencing fluid, electrolyte, and acid–base balance.

KEY WORDS

Active transport	Hypertonic
Buffer	Hypotonic
Diffusion	Isotonic
Electrolytes	Osmolality
Endocytosis	Osmolarity
Exocytosis	Osmosis
Facilitative diffusion	Passive transport
Filtration	Solutes
Homeostasis	Tonicity

Overview

Water is a critical medium in the human body. It accounts for 50–75% of a person's body weight and is the major element in blood plasma, which is used to transport nutrients, oxygen, and electrolytes throughout the body (Box 14–1). Water also gives shape and form to cells, regulates body temperature, lubricates the joints in the body, and cushions the body organs. Thus, it is easy to see that water plays an important role in maintaining health and normal body function. **Electrolytes**, which are electrically charged minerals suspended in the body, work in unison with the water to maintain **homeostasis**, or achieve the precise balance required to sustain life. Acid–base balance is also

---

Box 14–1
Body's Water Composition by Weight

- Infants: 75%
- Men: 60%
- Women: 50%

important for maintaining homeostasis. Slight deviations outside of the normal range can significantly affect the body in a negative way. This chapter discusses basic concepts related to the processes of fluid, electrolyte, and acid–base balance. Additionally, treatments and nursing care required to prevent, control, and resolve alterations are included.

Physiology of Fluid, Electrolyte, and Acid–Base Regulation

A basic understanding of the dynamics of fluid, electrolyte, and acid–base balance is required for the nurse to correctly assess patients for imbalances and to implement effective plans of care.

Fluids

If cells are to survive and function normally, the fluid medium in which they live must be in equilibrium. That means being in the right place at the right time in the right amount.

Fluid Distribution

Body fluids are contained in two primary compartments that are separated by a semipermeable membrane. The two compartments are referred to as the intracellular and extracellular compartments. About 65% of the body's fluids are contained inside the cells, or intracellular. The remaining 35% of body fluids is located outside of the cell, or extracellular. The extracellular compartment is further broken down into three subdivisions (Figure 14–1):

- **Interstitial:** Fluid between the cells and around the blood vessels (25%)
- **Intravascular:** Fluid inside the blood vessels; also called blood plasma (8%)
- **Transcellular:** Eye humors as well as spinal, synovial, peritoneal, pericardial, and pleural fluids (2%)

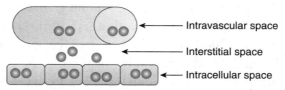

FIGURE 14–1 · Body fluid is located between cells (interstitial), inside blood vessels (intravascular), and inside cells (transcellular).

Fluid Balance

Extracellular fluid balance is maintained through close regulation of intake and output of fluids. Thirst is one mechanism used to achieve this end. When the body does not have an adequate amount of water, the sensation of thirst is triggered, which, under normal circumstances, will cause a person to drink liquids and eat fluid-containing foods.

Internal controls, besides thirst, also work to ensure that the right amount of fluid is located in the right place at the right time. Water constantly moves back and forth across the selectively permeable cell membrane through the process of **osmosis**, flowing from a lesser concentration of **solutes** (substances dissolved in the fluid) to a greater concentration of solutes, thereby facilitating equal distribution of both the water and solutes.

Fluid regulation also depends on the sensing of the **osmolality** (solute concentration in a given weight of fluid) or **osmolarity** (solute concentration in a given volume of fluid). Osmolality and osmolarity, although technically different, are often used interchangeably. The body responds to an increase in osmolality by stimulating the release of antidiuretic hormone (ADH), which causes the retention of fluid and lowers the osmolality of body fluids.

Fluid volume plays a part in regulation of fluid levels as well. Sensory receptors located in the blood vessels are able to sense when the volume of blood is low. This condition triggers a sympathetic nervous system response that results in constriction of the arterioles. Constricted arterioles slow the flow of blood to the kidneys and subsequently decrease urine output, thereby retaining body fluid. The opposite response occurs when the blood volume is high.

The renin–angiotensin–aldosterone mechanism is another means by which the body responds to changes in fluid volume. If the circulating blood volume is low, cells in the kidneys release renin. Renin triggers the production of angiotensin I, which is almost immediately converted to angiotensin II. Angiotensin II causes vasoconstriction and triggers the production of aldosterone. Aldosterone plays a key role in the reabsorption of sodium. Sodium, in turn, causes water reabsorption. The net result of these activities is increased circulating blood volume.

An additional mechanism for regulating sodium reabsorption and likewise fluid volume is the atrial natriuretic peptide (ANP) mechanism. When an increase in fluid volume is detected in the atrium of the heart, ANP is secreted. ANP directly influences renal function by decreasing sodium reabsorption, which subsequently results in sodium and water loss from the body in the form of urine.

Solutions introduced into the body can also affect the body's intracellular fluid balance. The ability of a solution to affect the flow of intracellular fluid is called **tonicity**. There are three types of solutions with regard to tonicity. Each is described below along with its effect on movement (Figure 14–2).

- **Isotonic** fluids have the same concentration of solutes as cells; thus, there is no fluid movement one way or the other. For example, normal saline is an isotonic intravenous fluid; therefore, when it is administered, it does not change the cell (ie, it does not make it swell or shrink).
- **Hypertonic** fluids have a higher concentration of solutes (hyperosmolality) than is found inside the cells, which causes fluid to flow out of cells and into the extracellular spaces. This causes cells to shrink.
- **Hypotonic** fluids have a lower concentration of solutes (hypo-osmolality) than is found inside the cells, which causes fluid to flow into cells and out of the extracellular spaces. This causes cells to swell and possibly burst.

Electrolytes

Electrolytes are electrically charged minerals that are found inside and outside the cells of the body (Table 14–1). They are ingested in fluids and foods and eliminated primarily through the kidneys. Electrolytes are also eliminated through the liver, skin, and lungs to a lesser degree. Electrolytes are most often measured in units called milli-equivalents (mEq) per liter rather than in milligram weights

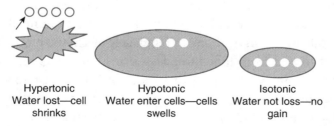

Hypertonic	Hypotonic	Isotonic
Water lost—cell	Water enter cells—cells	Water not loss—no
shrinks	swells	gain

FIGURE 14–2 • Tonicity is the ability of solution to affect the flow of intracellular fluids. These fluids are classified as isotonic solution, hypertonic solution, and hypotonic solution.

TABLE 14–1 Major Electrolytes

	Function	Location	
		Intracellular (mEq/L)	Extracellular (mEq/L)
Sodium (Na$^+$)	Neuromuscular function and fluid management (most abundant extracellular electrolyte)	12	145
Potassium (K$^+$)	Neuromuscular and cardiac function (most abundant intracellular electrolyte)	150	4
Calcium (Ca^{++})	Bone structure, neuromuscular function, and clotting	5	<1
Magnesium (Mg^{++})	Active transport of Na$^+$ and K$^+$ neuromuscular function	40	2
Chloride (Cl$^-$)	Osmolality, acid–base balance	103	4
Phosphate (HPO$_4^-$)	ATP formation, acid–base balance	4	75

Modified with permission from Johnson JY: *Fluids and Electrolytes Demystified*. New York: McGraw-Hill, 2008:12.

because of their chemical properties as ions. The milliequivalent measures the electrochemical activity in relation to 1 mg of hydrogen. Electrolytes may also be measured in millimoles (mmol), an atomic weight of an electrolyte that is often equal to the milliequivalent but on occasion may be a fraction of the milliequivalent measure.

> ### NURSING ALERT
>
> **Caution! Is it a Milliequivalent or a Millimole?**
> Care should be taken when interpreting the value of an electrolyte to ensure which measure, mmol or mEq, is being used and the normal range for the electrolyte in that measure.

Electrolyte levels in the body are regulated through absorption and elimination to maintain desired levels for optimal body function. In the case of calcium, parathyroid hormone and calcitonin are secreted to stimulate the storage or release of calcium from the bone to regulate levels in the blood. Other electrolytes are absorbed from foods to a lesser or higher degree or retained or excreted by the kidneys or bowels to a lesser or higher degree as needed to reduce or elevate the level of the electrolyte to the level needed for optimal body function (Figure 14–3). For this feedback mechanism to be effective, the organs or systems responsible for absorption and excretion (gastrointestinal) or reabsorption and excretion (renal) must function properly.

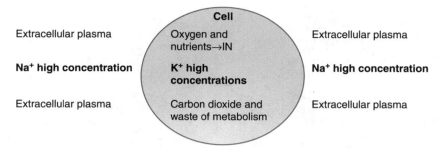

FIGURE 14–3 · The relationship between the cell and its extracellular environment regarding transport of electrolytes across the cell membrane. (Reproduced with permission from Johnson JY: *Fluids and Electrolytes Demystified*. New York: McGraw-Hill, 2008:6.)

The human body is composed of about 70 trillion cells. Cells make up tissues, tissues form organs, and organs form organ systems. Various processes take place at each of the aforementioned levels (cellular, organ, and system) to maintain a relatively constant internal state in the context of the ever changing surrounding environment. All cells are bound by a selectively permeable plasma membrane. Useful substances such as oxygen and nutrients enter through the membrane, and waste products such as carbon dioxide leave through it. Electrolytes travel into and out of the cell as needed to maintain an appropriate concentration gradient.

Electrolyte movement is achieved either passively or actively. **Passive transport** (movement without the requirement of energy expenditure) occurs in the following ways:

- **Diffusion** is movement of molecules from an area of high concentration to an area of low concentration.

- **Facilitative diffusion** is movement of molecules from an area of high concentration to an area of low concentration using a carrier cell to accelerate diffusion.

- **Filtration** is a selective allowance or blockage of substances across a membrane. Movement is influenced by a pressure gradient.

Active transport involves the movement of molecules against a concentration gradient and requires energy in contrast to passive transport, which does not require energy (visualize riding a bicycle uphill for active transport vs. downhill for passive transport). Methods of active transport include (Figure 14–4):

- **Endocytosis:** Plasma membrane surrounds substance being transported and takes substances into the cell with the assistance of adenosine triphosphate (ATP).

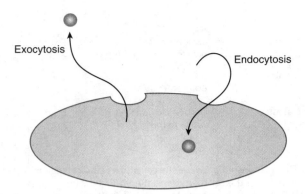

FIGURE 14–4 · A substance can be transported into the cell (endocytosis) with the assistance of ATP. Substances from inside the cell are released to outside the cells (exocytosis).

- **Exocytosis:** Manufactured substances are packaged in secretory vesicles that are fused with plasma membrane and then released outside of the cell.

The "sodium–potassium pump" is a specific example of active transport. To maintain the appropriate balance inside and outside of the cell, sodium and potassium move against the concentration gradient with the help of ATP, an energy source produced in the mitochondria of the cell (Figure 14–5).

Acid–Base Balance

Proper acid–base balance is critical to life. Too much of either can disrupt the delicate homeostatic environment required by the body to perform

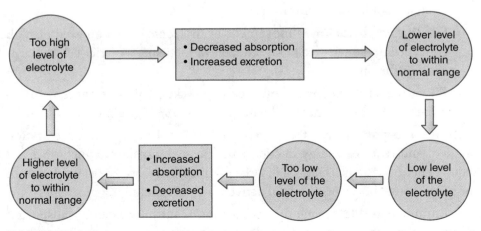

FIGURE 14–5 · Example of feedback mechanism for regulation of electrolyte levels. (Reproduced with permission from Johnson JY: *Fluids and Electrolytes Demystified*. New York: McGraw-Hill, 2008:14.)

life-sustaining functions. The margin for error (to either side) is very narrow. Fortunately, under normal circumstances, the body is able to maintain the required level of balance.

Acids

An acid is defined as any chemical that releases hydrogen ion (H^+) in solution. When acids are placed in water, they release hydrogen ions, which cause the water to become more acidic. Some acids are called strong acids (eg, hydrogen chloride [HCl]) because they dissociate (separate) completely when placed in water. Conversely, some acids are called weak acids (eg, carbonic acid [H_2CO_3]) because they only partially dissociate when placed in water.

Bases

A base is defined as any substance that can accept hydrogen ions. A base is also called an alkali. Similar to acids, bases can be either strong or weak. Whereas strong bases dissociate completely, weak bases dissociate only partially. Most, but not all, bases dissociate to produce hydroxide ions (OH^-). When a hydroxide ion (OH^-) is combined with or accepts hydrogen ions (H^+), water (H_2O) is formed. Therefore, hydroxide ions tend to neutralize substances.

pH

The amount of acid or base in a solution is represented by its pH value. The pH value can range from 1 to 14. Whereas a pH value of 1 represents a very strong acid, a pH value of 14 represents a very strong base. A pH of 7 is considered neutral. Weak acids and weak bases fall to either side of 7 (weak acids a little less than 7 and weak bases a little more than 7).

The pH scale functions just like a thermometer. Just as there is an optimal temperature range, there is an optimal pH range. The acceptable pH level varies depending on the solution. For example, the pH of a lemon is different than the pH of milk. In the human body, several different body fluids have their own acceptable pH ranges. Whereas stomach content and urine are more acidic, blood and intestinal content is more alkaline. Maintaining an appropriate pH level in the blood is very important. The normal pH level of blood should be between 7.35 and 7.45.

Acid–Base Regulation

Chemical buffers, the respiratory system, and the renal system are the key mechanisms for regulating acid–base balance in the human body.

A **buffer** is a substance that regulates the body's pH by attaching to or releasing H^+ ions. One of the most important buffers in the human body is bicarbonate.

- Carbon dioxide (CO_2) is released from body tissue and is picked up by the red blood cells (RBCs).
- The CO_2, once in the RBC, combines with water and under the influence of carbon anhydrase (an enzyme) is immediately converted to carbonic acid.
- The carbonic acid ionizes or separates into bicarbonate (HCO_3^-) and H^+.
- The bicarbonate leaves the RBC and travels in the plasma toward the lung.
- The free H^+ ion remaining in the RBC quickly interacts with oxyhemoglobin in the cell and causes the release of oxygen (O_2) from the RBC into the tissue for use in cellular respiration.

The reverse happens in the lungs:

- O_2 diffuses from the lungs into the RBC, where it is converted to oxyhemoglobin.
- This triggers a shift of the bicarbonate back into the RBC.
- Once in the RBC, the bicarbonate combines with the free H^+ (by-product of oxyhemoglobin formation) to form carbonic acid.
- Under the influence of carbon anhydrase, carbonic acid breaks down into water and CO_2.
- The CO_2 diffuses out of the RBC into the lung, where it is eliminated from the body during exhalation.

The aforementioned buffer system facilitates acid–base balance, the elimination of carbon dioxide from the body, and the transport of oxygen to various body tissues for use in cellular respiration.

The role of the lungs in maintaining acid–base balance under normal circumstances has already been described. When there is an excessive amount of acid in the body (acidosis), the lungs kick in to cause deeper and faster breathing to eliminate the excess. The opposite occurs when there is an excessive amount of base in the body (alkalosis). However, it is important to note that respiratory control of acid–base imbalance is a rapid regulatory measure occurring over minutes and cannot be maintained as a long-term strategy for correcting imbalances. The limitations include the fact that (1) retention or release of CO_2 does not address the underlying cause of the imbalance unless it is respiratory in nature, (2) extreme acid–base imbalances are not always fully corrected or compensated back to the normal level, (3) the energy needed for rapid

✔ ROUTINE CHECKUP 1

1. Extracellular fluid is distributed in the _____, _____, and
   _____.

   Answer:

2. Hypertonic fluids can cause cells to swell and possibly burst. True/false?

   Answer:

3. A _____ is a substance that regulates the body's pH by attaching to or releasing
   H^+ ions.

   Answer:

4. Active transport requires energy in contrast to passive transport, which does not require
   energy. True/false?

   Answer:

breathing places a high demand on the body, and (4) decreased respiratory rate
and depth can decrease oxygenation and compromise tissue.

The kidneys control acid–base balance by secreting or retaining H^+ or
HCO_3^- from the body to reverse acidosis or alkalosis. The kidneys respond to
acidosis by increasing the elimination of H^+ from the body via excretion of
urine and by retaining HCO_3^-. Bicarbonate retained by the kidneys is circu-
lated in the blood and is available to neutralize free H^+ ions circulating in the
blood. In the case of alkalosis, the opposite occurs. Hydrogen ions are retained,
and bicarbonate is eliminated via urine. Renal regulation of pH is a slow process, but it results in a long-term efficient correction of acid–base imbalances
and, unlike the respiratory system, can fully return the pH to a normal range.

Factors Influencing Fluid, Electrolyte, and Acid–Base Balance

Maintaining fluid, electrolyte, and acid–base balance affects metabolic processes
in the body. Imbalances may speed up processes, slow them down, prevent
proper use of nutrients, affect oxygen levels in the body, or cause our body to
retain toxic wastes.

Although the body is designed to keep everything in balance, we have to
help the body to achieve this end. Just as we help to regulate our body temperature by regulating environmental temperature, putting on or taking off clothes,

avoiding infectious organisms, and so on, we must do the same to regulate our fluid, electrolyte, and acid–base balance.

Food and Fluid Intake

The foods and fluids we eat and drink play a big role in fluid, electrolyte, and acid–base regulation. In addition to beverages, we consume foods, particularly fruits and vegetables, that provide us fluids. The type of fluids and foods we take in may alter electrolyte and acid–base balance.

Drugs

Drug (prescribed, over the counter, recreational) intake is another influencing factor. Certain medications may cause fluid retention, and others may increase urination. Drugs may also alter electrolyte levels or their functionality by competing with them for receptor sites at the chemical level. This same turn of events may affect acid–base balance.

> **NURSING ALERT**
>
> **Safe Use of Antacids and Laxatives**
> Patients should be educated regarding the danger of electrolyte and acid–base imbalances with excessive use of antacids and laxatives.

Health Alterations

Alterations in health, acute and chronic as well as physiological and psychological, may also impact the body's ability to maintain fluid, electrolyte, and acid–base balance. Acute alterations in output, as in the case with vomiting and diarrhea, can rapidly lead to fluid, electrolyte, and acid–base imbalances. Chronic illnesses such as heart failure, renal failure, and respiratory failure will ultimately alter fluid, electrolyte, and acid–base balance. A person experiencing stress, regardless of the source, is more likely to retain fluid.

Age

A person's age affects organ function. Very young individuals may have organs that have not developed to the point of maximum function, and very old individuals may start to have diminished organ function as a part of the aging process. In both cases, the ability of the organs (eg, heart, kidneys, lungs) to efficiently manage fluid, electrolyte, and acid–base balance is affected. Because age is an uncontrollable influencing factor, it becomes even more important to regulate the aforementioned controllable influencing factors for very young and very old individuals.

Alterations in Fluid, Electrolyte, and Acid–Base Balance

Alterations in fluid, electrolyte, or acid–base balance may impact all body systems. Frequently, an alteration in electrolyte balance can result in an acid–base imbalance and vice versa because electrolytes frequently involve ion exchange, and hydrogen ions are exchanged along with other ions, resulting in acid–base shifts and possible imbalances. The impact of an imbalance will depend on the degree of imbalance in fluid, electrolyte, acid, or base, as well as the role that the electrolyte plays in controlling body functions. Additionally, imbalances that occur over a short period may have a greater impact than those that occur gradually because of the body's ability to better adapt to gradual changes.

Fluid Imbalances

Hypovolemia

Hypovolemia is a deficiency of body fluids caused by inadequate intake or excessive losses. Multiple factors may contribute to an inadequate intake of fluids, including an inability to swallow or chew, an inability to self-feed along with the absence of assistance, the lack of access to clean water or food, anorexia, and nausea. On the other hand, excessive fluid losses may occur when there is vomiting, diarrhea, bleeding, overuse of diuretics, trauma to the kidneys or kidney disease, aldosterone deficits, and third spacing with burns and ascites. Third spacing occurs when fluids shift into the interstitial spaces instead of actually being lost from the body.

Hypervolemia

Hypervolemia is fluid overload caused by an excessive intake or decreased excretion of fluids. Excessive intake of oral fluids is a rare occurrence; instead, most cases of excessive intake of fluids are related to the infusion of excessive amounts of intravenous fluids. Conditions that lead to decreased excretion of fluids include cardiac failure, renal disease, endocrine disorders, and occasionally central nervous system and pulmonary disorders. Certain medications may also cause fluid retention.

> **NURSING ALERT**
>
> **Safe Infusion of Intravenous Fluids**
> Never attempt to catch up fluids that have fallen behind (eg, if patient was supposed to have received 1000 cc in 8 hours but only received 700 cc in 8 hours, do not try to make up for the 300 cc deficit). Instead, notify the physician for guidance.

Electrolyte and Acid–Base Imbalances

Electrolyte imbalances occur either because there is too little or too much of an electrolyte in the body. Electrolyte imbalances can be caused by ingesting too much or too little of the electrolyte in the diet, medication usage, or underlying disease processes. As previously stated, there is a relationship between electrolyte balance and acid–base balance because electrolytes are electrically charged ions. Thus, a person may experience electrolyte imbalances and acid–base imbalances simultaneously. Table 14–2 describes major fluid, electrolyte, and acid–base imbalances, including the signs, symptoms, risk factors, and interventions.

✔ ROUTINE CHECKUP 2

1. List four factors that influence fluid, electrolyte, and acid–base balance.
   Answer:
   _____
   _____
   _____
   _____

2. Excessive oral intake of fluids is the most common cause of hypervolemia. True/false?
   Answer:

3. A person may experience electrolyte imbalances and _____ at the same time.
   Answer:

TABLE 14–2 Imbalances: Risk Factors, Signs, Symptoms, and Interventions

Imbalance	Risk Factors	Signs and Symptoms	Interventions
Fluid Imbalances			
Fluid volume excess or water excess	• Excessive IV fluid intake • Excessive water intake (uncommon) • Excessive Na$^+$ intake • Renal disease • Neurologic disorders • Respiratory disorders • Heart failure • SIADH • Cirrhosis of the liver • ↑ Aldosterone or steroid levels	• Rapid weight gain • ↑ BP • Bounding pulses • Neck vein distention • Edema • Dyspnea* • Rales* • Ascaria* • Ascites* • Headache+ • Lethargy+ • Personality • changes+ • Irritability+ • Confusion+ • Seizure+ • Coma+	• Restrict Na$^+$ intake as ordered • Administer diuretics as ordered • Dialysis as ordered • Monitor I & O • Daily weights • Monitor for signs of overcorrection (see Hypovolemia) • Monitor for electrolyte imbalances • Hyponatremia • Hypophosphatemia • Hypercalcemia • Hypomagnesemia
Fluid volume deficit or water deficit	• Diarrhea • Vomiting • ↓ Oral fluid intake • Draining tubes • Burns • Hemorrhage • Excessive perspiration • Fever • Diuretics • Third space shifting	• Weight loss • ↑ Thirst • Poor skin turgor • Dry mucous membranes • ↓ BP with standing (orthostatic hypotension) • Slow vein filling • Weak rapid pulse • ↓ Urine output • ↑ Urine specific gravity • Neurologic changes (dizziness, confusion, seizures, coma, agitation)	• Oral and IV fluid replacement as ordered • Blood transfusion as ordered • Fall precautions

(*Continued*)

TABLE 14–2 Imbalances: Risk Factors, Signs, Symptoms, and Interventions (*Continued*)

Imbalance	Risk Factors	Signs and Symptoms	Interventions
		Fluid Imbalances	
Hyponatremia (<134 mEq/L)	• Renal disease • Adrenal insufficiency • ↑ Water intake • Excess D5W IV infusion • Diuretics • Anorexia • GI losses • Vomiting • Diarrhea • Tap water enemas • Burns • Heart failure • Cirrhosis • SIADH	• Headache • Tiredness • Dry mucous membranes • Nausea or vomiting • Abdominal cramping • Dry pale skin • Disoriented • Muscle cramps and muscle weakness • Tachycardia • Seizures	• Administer IV fluids as ordered • Restrict free water intake as ordered • Monitor for excessive fluid and Na^+ intake • Monitor I & O • Monitor weights • Monitor laboratory values (glucose, electrolytes) • Monitor for neurologic changes • Seizure precautions
Hypernatremia (>146 mEq/L)	• Diabetes insipidus • High Na^+ intake • Vomiting • Diarrhea • Excessive amounts of hypertonic IV solution • ↑ Water loss • Excessive sweating • Overcorrection of acidosis with sodium bicarbonate	• Thirst • Dry flushed skin • Sticky tongue or mucous membranes • Fever • Nausea or vomiting • Anorexia • Excessive urination (polyuria) • Tachycardia • Neurologic changes (restlessness, agitation, irritability, confusion, seizures)	• Verify fluid orders before initiating IV infusion. • Infuse fluids at prescribed rate (should be infused slowly) • Avoid overhydrating patient • Seizure precautions • Monitor for neurologic changes • Provide oral hygiene care

TABLE 14–2 Imbalances: Risk Factors, Signs, Symptoms, and Interventions (*Continued*)

Imbalance	Risk Factors	Signs and Symptoms	Interventions
		Fluid Imbalances	
Hypokalemia (<3.4 mEq/L)	• Diuretics • Excessive sweating • Diarrhea • Fasting or starvation • Crash diets • Anorexia nervosa • Magnesium deficiency • Alkalosis • Insulin therapy • Cirrhosis • Heart failure • Hyperaldosteronism • Alcoholism	• Disorientation or confusion • Tiredness • Abdomen distention • Paralytic Ileus • Nausea and vomiting • Constipation • Polyuria • Tachypnea • Tachycardia or dysrhythmia • EKG changes • Coma	• Oral potassium replacement as prescribed • Intravenous potassium as prescribed with serious deficits • Patient teaching— potassium-rich foods • Monitor pulse rhythm (apical also) • Monitor EKG changes • Monitor IV site for phlebitis and infiltration
		Electrolyte Imbalances	
Hyperkalemia (>5.0 mEq/L)	• Renal disease • K^+ sparing diuretic use • Addison disease • Excess K^+ supplement • Hemolysis • Burns • Crush injuries • Rapid IV infusion of K^+ • Chemotherapy • Acidosis • Infusion of old blood	• Dysrhythmia • EKG changes • Cardiac arrest with rapid IV infusion of K^+ • Diarrhea • Abdominal cramping • Irritability	• Caution patient against excessive salt substitute use • Check expiration date on blood products before giving • Restrict oral and IV K^+ intake • Monitor I & O • Monitor vital signs • Monitor EKG changes • IV calcium gluconate (severe cases) • Dialysis (severe cases) • Kayexalate (severe cases)

(*Continued*)

TABLE 14–2 Imbalances: Risk Factors, Signs, Symptoms, and Interventions (*Continued*)			
Imbalance	**Risk Factors**	**Signs and Symptoms**	**Interventions**
	Electrolyte Imbalances		
Hypocalcemia (<8.6 mg/dL or 4.5 mEq/L)	• Inadequate dietary intake • Malabsorption disorders • Vitamin D deficiency • Hyperphosphatemia secondary to chronic laxative use • Hypoparathyroidism • Alcoholism • Renal disease • Pancreatitis	• Respiratory distress or bronchospasms • Cardiac dysrhythmia or EKG changes • Tetany • Tingling or numbness • Seizures • Irritability • Pathologic fractures • Osteomalacia • Osteoporosis • Rickets (children)	• Patient teaching regarding adequate intake of calcium • Sunlight exposure • Monitor vital signs • IV calcium as ordered • Monitor IV site closely • Thiazide diuretic as ordered
Hypercalcemia (>10 mg/dL or 5.5 mEq/L)	• Hyperparathyroidism • Cancer • Excessive intake of Ca^{++} • Prolonged immobilization • Osteoporosis • Thiazide diuretics • Steroid therapy	• Anorexia • Nausea and vomiting • Thirst • Dry mucous membranes • Constipation • Abdominal pain • Kidney stones • Polyuria • Pathologic fractures • Dysrhythmia • Impaired memory • Mood swings • Coma	• Patient education (plenty of fluids, only medication cleared by doctor, no smoking, weight bearing and strength exercise after cleared by doctor) **Severe Cases** • Calcitonin or glucocorticoids as ordered • Loop diuretics as ordered • Monitor I & O • Possible hemodialysis • Prevent stress and strain on bones • Exercise after cleared by doctor • Parathyroid removal • Emotional support

TABLE 14–2 Imbalances: Risk Factors, Signs, Symptoms, and Interventions (*Continued*)			
Imbalance	Risk Factors	Signs and Symptoms	Interventions
Electrolyte Imbalances			
Hypomagnesemia (<1.3 mEq/L)	• Malnutrition • Alcoholism • Low K^+ levels • Malabsorption related to GI disorders (Crohn, gluten-sensitive enteropathy) • Antibiotics (gentamicin, amphotericin, cyclosporine) • Antineoplastics (cisplatin) • Vomiting • Diarrhea • Polyuria • NG drainage • Aldosterone excess	• Tremors • Cramps • Hyperactive reflexes • Seizures • Premature ventricular contractions • Ventricular fibrillation • Anorexia • Nausea and vomiting • Confusion • Memory loss • Fatigue	• Treat underlying causes as prescribed • Monitor IV infusions carefully to prevent cardiac or respiratory arrest • Oral supplements • Patient teaching regarding dietary intake
Hypermagnesemia (>2.5 mEq/L) (rare)	• Renal disease • Overtreatment of hypomagnesemia • Overuse of magnesium-based laxative • Antacids (Riopan, Milk of Magnesia, Epsom salt)	• Diarrhea • Flushing • Slurred speech • Profuse sweating • Vomiting • Weakness • Shallow breathing • Bradycardia • ↓ Deep tendon reflexes • Hallucinations (severe cases) • Coma (severe cases) • Cardiac/respiratory arrest (severe cases)	• Check vital signs and reflexes frequently • Monitor neurologic status • Educate patient against excessive use of laxatives and antacids

(Continued)

TABLE 14—2 Imbalances: Risk Factors, Signs, Symptoms, and Interventions *(Continued)*

Imbalance	Risk Factors	Signs and Symptoms	Interventions
Electrolyte Imbalances			
Hypophosphatemia (<2.5 mg/dL)	• Diabetic ketoacidosis • Respiratory alkalosis • Sepsis • Refeeding syndrome (secondary to malabsorption • Malabsorption disorders • Overuse of aluminum-based antacids • Hyperparathyroidism • Alcoholism • Loop diuretics • Vitamin D deficiency • Anorexia nervosa • Severe burns	• Muscle weakness • Respiratory distress • Hypotension • Pale skin secondary to hemolytic anemia • Altered mental status (ranging from irritability to coma) • Worsening infection (secondary to WBC destruction)	• Patient teaching (foods containing phosphorous and food preparation to minimize phosphorous loss) • Monitor for respiratory distress • Monitor for bleeding • Implement measures to protect against infection • Administer IV phosphate as ordered • Administer slowly • Dilute • Do not infuse with calcium
Hyperphosphatemia (>4.5 mg/dL)	• Renal disease • Hypoparathyroidism • Excess intake (foods, laxatives, enemas) • Prolonged exercise (rhabdomyolysis) • Chemotherapy • Respiratory acidosis • Calcium or magnesium deficiency • ↑ Vitamin D level	• Numbness • Tingling • Muscle spasms • Tetany • Seizures • Tachycardia • Anorexia • Nausea • Vomiting • Diarrhea • EKG changes	• Patient teaching (excessive intake, foods containing phosphorous, reading labels, laxative, and enema use) • Monitor vital signs • Check reflexes • Monitor urine output • Administer calcium as ordered

TABLE 14–2 Imbalances: Risk Factors, Signs, Symptoms, and Interventions (*Continued*)			
Imbalance	Risk Factors	Signs and Symptoms	Interventions
Acid–Base Imbalances			

Metabolic acidosis pH <7.35 HCO_3^- ≤20 mEq/L CO_2 ≤23 mEq/L BE <2 mEq/L	• Diabetic ketoacidosis
	• Lactic acidosis
	• Hypoxemia
	• Respiratory or heart failure (causing ↓ tissue perfusion)
	• Renal failure
	• Hyperaldosteronism
	• Diarrhea
	• Laxative overuse
	• Excessive intake of iron or aspirin
	• Acetazolamide
		Note: Signs and symptoms depend on the underlying cause of the acidosis and are nonspecific. Possible signs and symptoms include:
		• Blurred vision ⎫ Asprin
		• Tinnitus ⎭ overdose
		• Vertigo
		• Neurologic changes (headache, confusion, coma)
		• Dyspnea
		• Tachypnea
		• Hyperpnea
		• Hyperventilation
			• Monitor vital signs closely
			• Monitor respiratory status closely (especially if patient is on O_2 therapy)
			• Monitor blood gases and report any abnormal values
			• Correct underlying causes
			• Bicarbonate as ordered with severe cases
			• Monitor patient closely for complications if bicarbonate is given:
			  • Fluid overload
			  • Hypokalemia
			  • ↑ CO_2
			  • Tissue hypoxia
			  • Alkalosis

Respiratory acidosis pH <7.35 $PaCO_2$ >45 mm Hg HCO_3^- >28 mEq/L	• COLD • Neuromuscular disorders • Chest wall deformities • Obesity • OSA • CNS depression	• Kussmaul breathing • Chest pain or palpitations (severe academia) • Nausea and vomiting • Abdominal pain • Generalized muscle weakness • Bone malformations pain, or fractures (chronic metabolic acidosis)	• Bronchodilators, respiratory stimulants, and assisted ventilation may be ordered for patients with respiratory acidosis in whom case supportive nursing care would be provided as appropriate • Surgical interventions may be required with bone malformations, in which case supportive nursing care would be required

(*Continued*)

TABLE 14–2   Imbalances: Risk Factors, Signs, Symptoms, and Interventions (*Continued*)

Imbalance	Risk Factors	Signs and Symptoms	Interventions
Acid–Base Imbalances			
Metabolic alkalosis pH >7.45 HCO_3^- >28 mEq/L BE >2 mEq/L	• Vomiting • Nasogastric suctioning • Hypokalemia (diuretic induced) • Overtreatment with bicarbonate • Excess use of antacids • Steroids • Low chloride level	• Neurologic symptoms (lightheadedness, confusion, stupor) • Muscle twitching, hand tremors • Muscle spasms • Numbness or tingling in face or extremities • Nausea and vomiting • Dysrhythmia • Electrolyte alterations	• Monitor vital signs closely • Monitor neurologic status • Monitor I & O • Monitor blood gases • Patient teaching about antacid use
Respiratory alkalosis pH >7.45 $PaCO_2$ <35 mm Hg	• Extended periods of hyperventilation • Extreme anxiety • Hypoxemia (lung disease, high altitudes)		• Encourage patient to take slow, deep breaths • Have patient breathe into a paper bag • Approach patient in a calm manner • Implement interventions to decrease patient's anxiety • Monitor blood gases

*Secondary to pulmonary edema.
⁺Related to water excess.

BP = blood pressure; CNS = central nervous system; COLD = chronic obstructive lung disease; D5W = dextrose 5% in water; EKG = electrocardiography; I & O = input and output; IV = intravenous; NG = nasogastric; OSA = obstructive sleep apnea; SIADH = syndrome of inappropriate secretion of antidiuretic hormone; WBC = white blood cell.

The Nursing Process and Fluid, Electrolyte, and Acid–Base Balance

Fluid, electrolyte, and acid–base imbalances may be detected when symptoms are noted or may be discovered with routine laboratory testing (Table 14–3). Use of the nursing process facilitates prevention, early detection, and implementation of interventions to minimize the negative impact of imbalances.

TABLE 14–3 Common Laboratory Tests Related to Fluid, Electrolyte, and Acid–Base Balance

Test	Normal Values	Significance and Purpose
Urine specific gravity	1.015–1.025	• Monitor for fluid volume excess or deficit • Fluid volume excess causes urine dilution and decreased urine specific gravity • Fluid volume deficit cause urine concentration and increased urine specific gravity
Urine osmolality	Random urine sample: 50–1200 mOsm/kg H_2O	• Measures the concentration of particles dissolved in urine • Shows how well kidneys are able to clear metabolic waste and excess electrolytes
Serum osmolarity	285–295 mOsm/kg H_2O	• Measures the concentration of particles dissolved in blood • ↑ Serum osmolality levels with fluid volume deficit • ↓ Serum osmolality levels with fluid volume excess
Hematocrit	Men: 39–49% Women: 35–45%	• Measures the number of RBCs per volume of blood • ↑ Hematocrit with hypovolemia • ↓ Hematocrit with hypervolemia
Electrolytes	Potassium: 3.5–5.5 mEq/L Sodium: 135–145 mEq/L Chloride: 98–106 mEq/L Calcium: 8.5–10.5 mEq/L Magnesium: 1.3–2.1 mEq/L Phosphate: 3.0–4.5 mg/dL	• Measure concentration of electrolytes in the blood
pH	7.35–7.45	• Measures hydrogen ion concentration in the blood • ↑ pH reflects alkalosis • ↓ pH reflects acidosis
pCO_2	35–45 mm Hg	• Measures partial pressure of CO_2 • As CO_2 ↑ pH ↓ leading to acidosis • As CO_2 ↓ pH ↑ leading to alkalosis
Bicarbonate HCO_3^-	21–28 mEq/L	• As HCO_3^- ↑ pH ↑ leading to alkalosis • As HCO_3^- ↓ pH ↓ leading to acidosis
pO_2	80–100 mm Hg	• An indirect measure of the oxygen content in arterial blood • Measures effectiveness of ventilation with regard to providing oxygen for the tissue
Base excess	+ or −2 mEq/L	• Negative base excess (≤−3 mEq/L) indicates metabolic acidosis • Positive base excess (≥3 mEq/L) indicates metabolic alkalosis

Assessment

Awareness of the risk for or symptoms of fluid, electrolyte, or acid–base imbalance promotes early recognition of an imbalance and treatment to minimize a negative impact. Some symptoms may be caused by both electrolyte and acid–base imbalances, and treatment of both is needed to restore proper body function and the patient's well-being. Signs, symptoms, and risk factors associated with fluid, electrolyte, and acid–base balance are presented in Table 14–2. This information should be referenced when assessing a patient suspected of having a fluid, electrolyte, or acid–base disturbance.

Nursing Diagnosis

Nursing diagnoses for a patient experiencing alterations in fluid and electrolyte or acid–base balance vary and may reflect the resulting symptoms or the underlying cause. Frequently, the diagnosis may be related to any combination of altered renal, respiratory, gastrointestinal, or cardiovascular function. Related causes should be included as a part of the nursing diagnoses to ensure that the healthcare needs of the patient are fully addressed. Examples of diagnoses for a patient with altered fluid, electrolyte, or acid–base balance include:

- Actual or risk for deficient fluid volume
- Excess fluid volume
- Risk for imbalanced fluid volume

Additional related nursing diagnoses include:

- Impaired gas exchange
- Urinary elimination, impaired
- Cardiac output, decreased
- Self-care deficit
- Diarrhea
- Risk for injury

Planning

Goals and outcomes for a patient with potential or actual altered fluid, electrolyte, and acid–base balance are highly individualized and are driven by the data collected during assessment. The goals and outcomes should be realistic in terms of expectations and time frames for the particular patient and should be consistent with the patient's desires. Noncompliance is more likely to occur if the patient does not agree with the goals and established outcomes.

Nursing Interventions

Nursing interventions can be grouped into two major categories—health promotion interventions and interventions to address alterations in fluid, electrolyte, and acid–base balance.

Health Promotion

Many of the actions taken by an individual on a day-to-day basis have the potential to facilitate normal fluid, electrolyte, and acid–base balance or contribute to imbalances. The amount of fluid intake, the types of foods eaten, stress level, medications, and how we take care of our body are all examples of how individuals can influence whether imbalances will occur. Nurses are in a key role to help patients achieve fluid, electrolyte, and acid–base balance. Nutritional counseling helps patients make wise food choices. Teaching patients about how to properly take medications and cautioning them about possible adverse effects of self-medicating may also help patients avoid imbalances. Encouraging patients to live a healthy lifestyle includes but is not limited to:

- Exercising (proper hydration)
- Developing effective coping strategies to handle stress
- Avoiding the use of recreational drugs and smoking

It is also important to teach the patient about the early signs of fluid, electrolyte, and acid–base imbalances (eg, thirst, dry mouth, weight loss or gain) and risk factors.

Nursing Interventions for Alterations in Fluid, Electrolyte, and Acid–Base Balance

The following interventions may be required when providing care for a patient experiencing an actual alteration in fluid, electrolyte, or acid–base balance:

- Daily weights
- Vital sign assessment
- Skin and mucous membrane assessment
- Monitoring for jugular vein distension
- Monitoring and reporting laboratory values
  - Urine specific gravity
  - Serum electrolytes
  - Serum osmolarity
  - Urine osmolarity
  - Arterial blood gases

- Intake and output measurement
- Skin care
- Oral fluid replacement
- Fluid restriction
- Intravenous fluid therapy (Box 14–2)
- Blood transfusion (Box 14–3)

BOX 14–2
Procedure Tip: Administering Intravenous Fluids

Life-threatening complications can occur during the administration of intravenous (IV) fluids. The following tips are presented to highlight actions that will minimize the risk of adverse outcomes during fluid administration.

Tip	Rationale
• Always check the physician's orders and correctly identify the patient to ensure that you have the correct fluids for the correct patient.	• Serious adverse outcomes may occur if the patient is given the wrong fluids.
• Vigilantly monitor the patient for signs of fluid overload (eg, neck vein distention, edema, rales) and if discovered, reduce the IV fluid rate and notify the doctor.	• Fluid overload can result in serious complications just like fluid deficits. Also, electrolyte imbalances may occur with fluid overload.
• Before starting an infusion, trace the tubing back to its point of insertion, especially when the patient has multiple tubes.	• Misconnections (eg, central venous catheters, peripheral lines, epidural catheters) have resulted in serious adverse events, especially when the connection tip was a Luer lock tip (Luer lock tips are found on many types of tubing, including blood pressure cuffs as well as the tubing listed above).
• Caution patients and nonclinical staff not to disconnect or reconnect tubing; instead, instruct them to notify the nurse.	• Same as above.
• Monitor the IV site for signs of infiltration (especially when administering calcium gluconate).	• Serious tissue damage may occur as a result of IV fluid infiltration even to the point of requiring plastic surgery.
• Do not use markers to label IV fluid bags.	• Ink may diffuse into the bag and contaminate the fluids.

BOX 14–3
Procedure Tip: Administering a Blood Transfusion

Life-threatening complications can occur during the administration of blood transfusions. The following tips are presented to highlight actions that will minimize the risk of adverse outcomes during a transfusion.

Tip	Rationale
• Before administering blood, perform a baseline assessment that includes assessment of the following: 1. Vital signs 2. Skin rashes 3. Signs of respiratory distress (listen to lungs) 4. Itching 5. Pain Repeat assessment for signs of transfusion reaction at a minimum of 15 minutes after initiation of the transfusion and at the conclusion of the transfusion	• Transfusion reactions may be life threatening. Collecting baseline information will make it easier for the nurse to recognized signs of a transfusion reaction.
• Check the size of the catheter that the patient has in place. A larger bore catheter (18-gauge preferably) is used because of the thickness of the blood.	• An incorrect catheter size may result in interruption of the transfusion or may result in the blood not infusing within the prescribed time frame.
• Check blood for compatibility and integrity (with a second person) before initiation of the transfusion.	• This is done to ensure that the correct person receives the correct blood as well as to prevent a hemolytic reaction.
• Hang only normal saline with blood products.	• Using other types of fluids may cause clumping of the red blood cells.

Evaluation

Evaluation of the patient's status and the effectiveness of interventions must be ongoing. To prevent the occurrence of life-threatening situations, the nurse must evaluate data accurately and respond quickly because excessive treatment of fluid, electrolyte, or acid–base imbalance can result in the occurrence of the opposite condition (eg, overcorrection of hyponatremia may cause hypernatremia). Careful determination that treatment has been effective can facilitate moderation of treatment to prevent imbalances from toxicity. Examples of outcomes that may be useful in evaluating the patient's status include:

- Skin and mucous membranes (moist, good skin turgor with absence of edema)
- Circulatory status (blood pressure, pulse within normal range)
- Urinary output (minimum, 30 cc/h)

If goals and expected outcomes are not being met, the nurse must determine whether it is because the interventions are not effective, the goals or expected outcomes are inappropriate, or the patient is noncompliant. The nurse should then alter the plan of care as indicated with teaching or additional interventions.

Conclusion

Several key points should be noted from this chapter:

- Fluid balance is regulated by several mechanisms, including osmosis, the sensing of osmolality, the actual level of fluids in the body, the renin–angiotensin–aldosterone mechanism, the ANP mechanism, and the type of fluids introduced into the body.
- Electrolytes move between the various compartments and structures in the body by diffusion, facilitative diffusion, filtration, endocytosis, and exocytosis.
- A person may experience electrolyte and acid–base imbalances simultaneously.
- An acid is defined as any chemical that releases hydrogen ions, and a base is a substance that accepts hydrogen ions. A base is also called an alkali.
- The pH is the value that tells how much acid or base is in a solution. A pH of 7 is considered neutral. Values below 7 result in a state of acidosis, and values above 7 lead to a state of alkalosis.
- The lungs can facilitate short-term correction of acid–base imbalances. Prolonged acidosis may lead to respiratory failure because of respiratory exhaustion. The kidneys, on the other hand, provide a more complete and long-term resolution of acid–base imbalances.
- Food and fluid intake, drugs (prescribed, over the counter, recreational), various health alterations, and age all influence fluid, electrolyte, and acid–base balance.

- The primary North American Nursing Diagnosis Association (NANDA) nursing diagnoses for patient experiencing fluid imbalances are actual or risk for deficient fluid volume, excess fluid volume, and risk for imbalanced fluid volume.
- Monitoring the patient's weight, intake and output, laboratory results, and skin condition (eg, turgor, moistness) as well as monitoring for complications associated with prescribed treatment should all be included in the patient's plan of care.

REVIEW QUESTIONS

1. **A nurse suspects that a patient is dehydrated. To confirm this suspicion, the nurse might expect the patient's assessment to show what findings?**
   A. A decreased hematocrit level
   B. An increased urine specific gravity
   C. Moist mucous membranes
   D. Decreased skin turgor rebound

2. **The body responds to low body fluid levels and increased osmolality with what actions?**
   A. Diarrhea
   B. Diuresis
   C. Tears
   D. Thirst

3. **A patient with a chronic respiratory condition resulting in poor ventilation might demonstrate what diagnostic findings?**
   A. pH of 7.45 or lower
   B. pCO_2 of 45 or higher
   C. HCO_3 of 28 or lower
   D. pO_2 of 80 or higher

4. **A nurse suspects that a patient has a low sodium level. What data collected in the history would place the patient at risk for hyponatremia?**
   A. A report of watery stools six to eight times per day for 4 days
   B. A recent history of taking Milk of Magnesia for constipation
   C. A past pregnancy resulting in aldosterone deficit
   D. A recent episode of acute renal failure

5. **A patient has had 300–400 cc of urine output each hour over the past 26 hours. The nurse would look for what signs of a likely potassium imbalance?**

   A. Slow cardiac rhythm with a wide QRS complex on electrocardiography

   B. Increased respiratory rate with deep, regular breathing

   C. Fluid build-up in the extremities and pulmonary edema

   D. Irregular pulse rhythm with intermittent fibrillation

6. **Which of the following findings would require that the nurse slow the intravenous infusion rate to a "keep vein open" rate and notify the doctor?**

   A. Dry mucous membranes

   B. Weak pulse

   C. Neck vein distension

   D. Chills and fever

7. **A patient has been diagnosed with hypermagnesemia. Which of the following interventions would be appropriate for this patient?**

   A. Teach the patient about the correct use of antacids.

   B. Check the reflexes regularly if the patient is hospitalized.

   C. Monitor for signs of infection.

   D. A and B

   E. All of the above

8. **Which of the following interventions would be appropriate for a patient who is experiencing respiratory alkalosis?**

   A. Have the patient hold his or her breath for 5 seconds and then breathe quickly.

   B. Approach the patient in a calm matter.

   C. Administer bicarbonate as ordered by the doctor.

   D. All of the above

9. **Which of the following actions will limit the occurrence of tubing misconnections?**

   A. Trace the tubing to the point of insertion before starting the infusion.

   B. Use a Luer lock end exclusively.

   C. Standardize the location of tubing (eg, put all IV tubes on the right side of the bed and all others on the left side of the bed).

   D. A and C

10. **Which symptoms indicate a complication that is likely to occur with prolonged acidosis?**

    A. Cardiac dysrhythmia caused by hypokalemia

    B. Fluid overload caused by chloride reabsorption and intoxication

    C. Respiratory failure caused by workload on lungs

    D. Renal calculi caused by hypercalcemia attributable to protein release of Ca^+

ANSWERS

Routine Checkup 1

1. Interstitial, intravascular, transcellular.
2. False.
3. Buffer.
4. True.

Routine Checkup 2

1. Food and fluid intake
   Drugs
   Health alterations
   Age
2. True.
3. Acid–base imbalances.

Review Questions

1. B
2. D
3. B
4. A
5. D
6. C
7. D
8. B
9. A
10. C

References

Craven RF, Hirnle CJ: *Fundamentals of Nursing: Human Health and Function*, 5th ed. Philadelphia, PA: Lippincott, 2006.

Daniels R: *Nursing Fundamentals: Caring & Clinical Decision Making*. New York, NY: Delmar Thomson Learning, 2004.

Needham A: Comparative and Environmental Physiology. Acidosis and Alkalosis. 2004.

Pagana KD, Pagana TJ: *Mosby's Manual of Diagnostic and Laboratory Test*, 3rd ed. St. Louis, MO: Mosby Elsevier, 2006.

Potter PA, Perry AG: *Fundamentals of Nursing*, 6th ed. St. Louis, MO: Mosby Elsevier, 2005.

Saladin K: *Anatomy and Physiology: The Unity of Form and Function*, 4th ed. New York, NY: McGraw-Hill, 2007.

Additional Resources

eMedicine: *Metabolic Acidosis*. Available at http://emedicine.medscape.com/article/768268-overview.

eMedicine: *Respiratory Acidosis*. Available at http://emedicine.medscape.com/article/301574-overview.

Gondar Design Science: *Acids and Alkalis-The pH Scale*. Available at http://www.purchon.com/chemistry/ph.htm.

How Stuff Works: *Chemistry Connections: The Body's Buffer System*. Available at http://videos.howstuffworks.com/hsw/17357-chemistry-connections-the-bodys-buffer-system-video.htm.

Needham A (2004): *Comparative and Environmental Physiology Acidosis and Alkalosis*. Cited in online reference: Experts—Acidosis: Encyclopedia beta: http://en.allexperts.com/e/a/ac/acidosis.htm.

Resource Nurse: *Transfusion Basics*. Available at http://www.resourcenurse.com/feature_transfusion.html.

The Joint Commission: *Tubing Misconnections-A Persistent and Potentially Deadly Occurrence*. Available at http://www.jointcommission.org/SentinelEvents/SentinelEvent Alert/sea_36.htm.

Tuberose.com: Acid/Base Balance. Available at http://www.tuberose.com/Acid_Base_Balance.html.

Vision Learning: Acids and Bases. Available at http://www.visionlearning.com/library/module_viewer.php?mid=58.

Wikipedia: *Acidosis*. Available at http://en.wikipedia.org/wiki/Acidosis.

Wikipedia: *Metabolic Acidosis*. Available at http://en.wikipedia.org/wiki/Metabolic_acidosis.

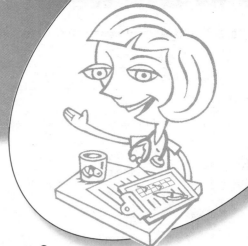

Chapter 15

Urinary Elimination

LEARNING OBJECTIVES

At the end of the chapter, the reader will be able to:

1. List the major structures of the urinary system.

2. Describe how the urinary system affects the proper functioning of other body processes.

3. Discuss factors that influence urinary elimination.

4. Discuss alterations in urinary elimination.

5. Define terms that may be used when describing manifestations of altered urinary elimination.

6. Describe six types of urinary incontinence.

7. Describe the three types of urinary tract infections.

8. Discuss information that should be collected during assessment of a patient experiencing alterations in urinary elimination.

9. Discuss nursing interventions that may be included when providing care for a patient who has altered urinary elimination.

KEY WORDS

Anuria	Nocturia
Cystitis	Oliguria
Diabetes insipidus	Polyuria
Diuretics	Pyelonephritis
Dysuria	Pyuria
Enuresis	Stenosis
Frequency	Urethritis
Hematuria	Urgency

Overview

The urinary system, which provides the means for removal of liquid waste from the body, consists of the kidneys, ureters, bladder, and urethra. It plays a key role in fluid, electrolyte, and acid–base balance. Urine is formed as waste products are filtered from the blood by the kidneys. Urine is then transported by way of the ureters to the bladder, where it is stored until it is excreted from the body via the urethra. Under normal circumstances, emptying of the urinary bladder is a voluntary action that relies partly on a properly functioning neurologic system.

Factors Influencing Urinary Elimination

Numerous variables influence the production and excretion of urine. The spectrum of influencing variables ranges from those that are a part of person's everyday activities to deviations that are related to health issues. For example, the kidneys regulate the amount of urine produced based on an individual's activity level and fluid intake. Thus, if a person engages in very strenuous activities that result in significant fluid loss (eg, sweating and rapid breathing) yet does not take in enough fluids to compensate for this loss, then the kidneys will reabsorb fluids to maintain balance, and urinary output will be decreased. Certain health deviations, such as hypotension, **diabetes insipidus** (inability to concentrate urine), and enlargement of the prostate gland, also alter urine production, urine excretion, or both. A discussion of additional factors that influence urinary elimination follows in the remainder of this section.

Age and Developmental Stage

Infants have immature kidneys with minimal ability to concentrate urine and lack of voluntary control of urinary elimination. Voluntary control is achieved during the toddler and preschool years. School-age children, teenagers, and adults have maximum urinary function. Older adults experience diminished urinary function that results in more instances of incontinence and an increased risk for urinary tract infections (UTIs). Anatomical and hormonal changes of pregnancy also alter urinary function.

NURSING ALERT

Developmental Tip
Although incontinence is a common finding among elderly individuals, it is *not* caused by aging. Incontinence is related to medical conditions.

Diet and Fluid Intake

Foods high in water content increase fluid in the body and those that contain caffeine may increase urinary elimination. Caffeine increases blood flow to the kidneys leading to the increased fluid in the bladder and the desire to urinate (diuretic effect). In contrast, foods that have a high level of sodium cause a decrease in urinary output. Also, the amount of fluids an individual takes in influences the amount and frequency of urinary elimination. Whereas decreased fluid intake results in decreased urinary elimination and frequency, increased fluid intake results in increased output and frequency.

Psychosocial Factors

A person's emotional state as well as sociocultural expectations may alter urinary elimination. Stress and anxiety may trigger an intense urge to void or may have the opposite effect by preventing relaxation of the muscles and sphincters responsible for emptying of the bladder. When and where it is appropriate to void is dictated by sociocultural rules; thus, an individual may refrain from voiding if the place and time are not considered to be appropriate. Position may also influence an individual's ability to void. Men are usually accustomed to standing to void and women usually sit to void; thus, using a bedpan may present a real challenge for a person who is unable to sit or stand to void. Additionally, adults as well as children sometimes ignore the urge to void because of being deeply engaged in their work activities or play, respectively.

> ### NURSING ALERT
>
> **Minimize Patient Stress**
> When introducing the bedpan to the patient, tell the patient that some of your patients found using the bedpan challenging to use. Identify the challenges and explain how "the other patients" overcame those challenges. In this way you are being proactive addressing a potential problem before the problem arises and you are in directly teaching the patient by telling the story on how to resolve common problems using the bedpan. You are also lowering the patient's stress level.

Health Alterations

Alterations in an individual's health status may impact urinary elimination. Some of the more common influencing factors include:

- **Fluid loss:** As stated previously, when the body losses excessive amounts of fluid, the kidneys respond by reabsorbing fluids and decreasing urinary output. Significant amounts of fluid may be lost when a person experiences vomiting, diarrhea, hemorrhaging, fever, or extensive burns.

- **Structural obstructions:** Tumors, prostatic hypertrophy, stenosis (or narrowing) of the ureters or urethra may all interfere with the outflow of urine. In addition to affecting voiding patterns, obstructions may lead to a backflow of urine into the kidney, resulting in kidney damage.

- **Decreased muscle tone:** Weak abdominal and perineal muscles impair bladder and sphincter control, which in turn results in urinary retention. Factors that contribute to decreased bladder tone include obesity, multiple pregnancies, pushing during childbirth, straining to have a bowel movement, long periods of immobility, prolonged catheterization, menopausal atrophy, and trauma.

- **Hypotension:** Urine production requires an adequate flow of blood to the kidneys. Individuals who have hypotension, or low blood pressure, experience a decrease in the flow of blood to the kidneys. This in turn results in decreased urine production. However, this is not the only consequence. Remember that urine is the means by which we rid the body of waste. Therefore, if the waste cannot be eliminated from the body, other problems may occur, including acid–base and electrolyte imbalances and toxicity (toxins are unable to leave the body).

- **Diabetes mellitus:** Persons with diabetes mellitus often experience **polyuria** (increase blood glucose levels signs an need to increase fluid intake to flush excess glucose), or excessive urine production. Additionally, persons with diabetes are at a greater risk for developing end-stage renal disease (damage to small blood vessels in the kidneys caused by diabetes prevents the kidneys from functioning properly).
- **Neurological injury:** Any condition that causes damage to the neurologic centers that control bladder function may result in urinary retention or urinary incontinence. Conditions such as strokes and spinal cord injuries are most often associated with such damage. Receptors detect the level of urine in the bladder. When the bladder fills with fluid, receptors signals the brain that it is time to urinate. Nerve damage disrupts the signal. The patient does not have the sense to urinate.

> **NURSING ALERT**
>
> **Monitor Bladder Content**
> Always monitor bladder content of patients who infrequently urinates since the sense to urinate may have been disrupted. Look for bladder distention, fluid input/output measurements, and use a bladder scan (if available) to estimate the volume of fluid in the bladder.

Medical and Surgical Interventions

Various medications may alter urinary elimination. Some such as antidepressants, antihistamines, and narcotics cause urinary retention. Others, such as **diuretics**, increase urinary output. There are also some medications that change the color of urine. For example, rifampin, a medication used to treat mycobacterium infections, causes a red-orange discoloration of urine.

> **NURSING ALERT**
>
> **Urine Discoloration**
> To prevent unnecessary worry, always inform the patient of urine color changes that may be associated with a medication that has been prescribed by the doctor.

Reproductive, intestinal, and urinary surgical procedures may increase the risk for urinary retention during the postoperative period. This is mainly the result of tissue edema. Additionally, medications that are used to control pain (narcotics and anesthetics) may alter urinary muscle contractility and glomerular filtration, thereby decreasing urinary output.

ROUTINE CHECKUP

1. Foods high in water content and those high in _____ may increase urinary elimination.

Answer:

2. The nurse should inform the client that certain medications such as rifampin might change the color of his or her urine. True/false?

Answer:

Alterations in Urinary Elimination

One of the main gauges of normal urinary function is the characteristic of the urine produced. The amount of urine contained in a single voiding ranges between 250 and 400 mL. Daily amounts vary depending on the age of the individual. Newborns usually average 500 mL/day, whereas adults average 1500 mL/day. Urine amounts of less than 30 mL/hr signify a problem with urinary function. Urine is usually a straw color and clear and has a faint odor. Alterations in urinary function are usually related to retention, incontinence, or infections. Manifestations of alterations in urinary function involve changes in the amount of urine produced, changes in urinary elimination patterns, and changes in the characteristics of urine (Table 15–1).

TABLE 15–1 Terms Related to Altered Urinary Function

Term	Definition
Polyuria	Excessive amounts of urine (>2500 mL in 24 hours)
Oliguria	Decreased amount of urine (<500 mL in 24 hours)
Anuria	Urine output <100 mL in 24 hours
Frequency	Voiding in very short intervals
Urgency	A strong sensation to empty the bladder regardless of the amount of urine or fullness of the bladder
Nocturia	Having to void during usual sleep hours
Enuresis	Involuntary voiding without cause after the age at which voluntary control should have been achieved
Dysuria	Painful urination
Hematuria	Blood in the urine
Pyuria	Pus in the urine

> **NURSING ALERT**
>
> **Urinary Output**
> The volume of urine excretion is influenced by the amount of fluid ingested by the patient and the activity of the patient (a runner will have lower urine output until the runner is rehydrated).

Urinary Retention

Urinary retention, or inability to empty the bladder, occurs for one of two reasons. Either the person is unable to sense that the bladder is full or there is an inability to sufficiently relax the urethral sphincter to allow complete emptying of the bladder. A patient who has urinary retentions manifests the following signs and symptoms:

- Inability to void or voiding small frequent amounts (25–50 mL every 2–3 hours)
- Discomfort over the pubic area
- Palpable bladder distension over the suprapubic area
- Significant mismatch between fluid intake and urine output

If urinary retention is not corrected, it may lead to loss of bladder tone, UTIs, and damage to the kidneys because of a backflow of urine.

Urinary Incontinence

Urinary incontinence is the inability to control bladder emptying. It may be temporary or chronic and occurs for various reasons. Table 15–2 summarizes the different types of urinary incontinence. A patient who has urinary incontinence may not disclose this to the doctor because he or she may be embarrassed. Additionally, the individual may refrain from activities that involve interaction with others for fear of having urine leakage or an odor that others may notice. Patients experiencing chronic incontinence may also experience skin breakdown.

> **NURSING ALERT**
>
> **The Patient Feel Comfortable**
> Anticipate urine incontinence with patients who have a medical condition that normally leads to incontinence. Tell the patient the story about your "other patient" who started to lose control of his bladder and how he managed the challenges of urinary inconstancy. Doing this acknowledges that the patient isn't the only one who experienced urinary incontinence. Furthermore, you are sharing how your "other patient" dealt with all the social situations.

TABLE 15–2 Types of Urinary Incontinence

Type	Description	Related Factors
Functional	Involuntary voiding in a person who has normal bladder and sphincter control	• Cognitive and sensory impairment • Motor impairment • Environmental constraints
Overflow	Leaking urine from an overfilled bladder	• Enlarged prostate gland • Uterine prolapse • Diabetes • Spinal cord injury • Certain medications
Reflex	Involuntary voiding at a predictable time caused by a person's inability to sense that the bladder is full	• Neurologic dysfunction (stroke, spinal cord injury, brain tumors)
Stress	Involuntary loss of <50 mL of urine secondary to a sudden increase in intraabdominal pressure (eg, coughing, laughing, sneezing)	• Weak pelvic floor muscles • Obesity • ↓ Estrogen levels • Pregnancy and childbirth trauma • Certain medication
Urge	A strong sensation to void, but the person cannot delay voiding until he or she reaches the bathroom; the amount of urine voided varies	• Diuretics • Caffeine and alcoholic beverages • UTI • ↑ Fluid intake • Catheterization or bladder irritation
Mixed	A combination of any of the above described types of incontinence	• Depends on the type of incontinence the patient is experiencing

Urinary Tract Infections

UTIs are the second most common type of infection in the body. They most often affect the lower urinary tract because microorganisms have easier access to the structures of the lower tract via the urethral meatus (Box 15–1). The most common organism causing UTIs is *Escherichia coli*, which is normally found in the rectum. Women tend to have UTIs more often than men possibly because of the close proximity of the vagina and the rectum to the urethral meatus. Signs and symptoms of a UTI include dysuria, hematuria, frequency, and urgency. If

> **Box 15–1**
> **Urinary Tract Infections**
>
> - **Urethritis:** Infection of the urethra
> - **Cystitis:** Infection of the bladder
> - **Pyelonephritis:** Infection of the kidneys

the infection becomes more severe, especially those that affect the kidneys, the patient may also experience fever, chills, nausea, and vomiting.

> **NURSING ALERT**
>
> **UTI in Elderly**
> Older adults may not display the classic symptoms of a UTI. A UIT may present as behavioral symptoms (ie, confusion).

Urinary Diversions

Urinary diversion involves the rerouting of the ureters to the abdominal wall for excretion of urine from the body. Diversion may be temporary or permanent depending on the underlying reason for the procedure. Patients who require a urinary diversion lose their ability to control urine elimination and may experience problems with skin breakdown as well as altered body image.

The Nursing Process and Urinary Elimination

Information presented to this point in this chapter forms the basis for application of the nursing process for patients experiencing alterations in urinary elimination. Having knowledge of what factors influence urinary elimination as well as possible alterations that can occur provide the foundation for:

- Assessment of the patient's needs through the collection of data, including the history, physical examination, laboratory tests (Table 15–3), and diagnostic tests
- Identification and prioritizing nursing diagnoses
- Identification of goals and expected outcomes
- Planned interventions
- Implementation of the plan of care
- Evaluation of whether the plan is effective and if modifications are required

TABLE 15–3 Urine Specimen Collection		
Test	Description	How to Collect
Random urine	Clean but not sterile specimen collected for routine urinalysis	• Can be collected from normal voiding, catheter, urinal, or bedpan directly into a clean specimen cup • Should not be contaminated with feces
Clean catch or midstream	Sterile specimen collected for culture and sensitivity test	• Collected in sterile specimen cup • Urinary meatus should be cleansed with sterile wipe when collecting voided specimen • Can be collected from a port on the catheter tubing using aseptic technique, sterile needle, and sterile syringe • Sterile technique should be maintained when transferring the specimen from the syringe to the sterile specimen cup
24-hour	Specimen collected to measure quantity of a particular substance in urine within a prescribed time frame	• Patient is instructed to void, discard the urine, record the time, and collect all urine in provided container over the next 24 hours • It is important to start as described and stop exactly when the time period is up • If urine is accidentally discarded during the time period, the test must be restarted with a new container • The specimen may or may be not be required to be kept on ice depending on the type of test; instruct the patient to follow the directions carefully

Table 15–4 summarizes each component of the nursing process for a client experiencing alterations in urinary elimination. The remainder of this section is devoted to taking a closer look at selected nursing interventions for clients experiencing alterations in urinary elimination.

Nursing Interventions

A variety of interventions may be used to assist patients to maintain normal urinary elimination patterns or to address alterations in urinary elimination. Patients need to be educated on ways they can promote normal urinary elimination (eg, adequate fluid intake, allowing adequate time for voiding,

TABLE 15–4 Urinary Elimination and the Nursing Process

Assessment	Nursing Diagnosis	Planning	Implementation
History (Ask About) • Usual voiding pattern (amount, how often, time of day) • Changes in voiding (eg, urgency, burning, frequency) • Other health deviations (eg, diabetes, pregnancy, prostatic hypertrophy) • Medications • Diet and fluid intake **Physical (Observe)** • Hydration status • Urine characteristics • Bladder distention • Cognitive, sensory, or motor changes **Laboratory and Diagnostic Tests** • Urinalysis • IVP • Cystoscopy	• Impaired urinary elimination • Urinary retention • Urinary incontinence (functional, reflex, stress, total, urge) **Related Diagnoses** • Risk for imbalanced fluid volume • Risk for infection • Deficient knowledge • Risk for impaired skin integrity • Impaired social interaction • Risk for situational low self-esteem	Goals and outcomes will vary depending on the specific nursing diagnoses and priorities identified. Examples of goals include • Patient will be able to voluntarily control voiding • Skin will remain intact • Patient will be free of infection • Patient will demonstrate knowledge (specify information to be gained). Note: Goals and outcomes should specify who, what, when, and how as appropriate. Interventions are also planned during this phase of the nursing process.	The planned interventions are put into action during this phase. Examples of interventions include: **HEALTH PROMOTION** **Patient Teaching** • Effects of caffeine and alcohol • Fluid requirements and importance of adequate intake • Ways to prevent UTIs • Exercises to improve abdominal and perineal muscle tone (Kegel exercises) **Promoting Normal Voiding** • Privacy, positioning, and so on **ALTERED ELIMINATION** • Bladder training • Catheterization • Dialysis • Home care

The effectiveness of the plan of care evaluated after implementation, however, should be integrated throughout all phases of the nursing process. Evaluate data collected during assessment, evaluate accuracy of nursing diagnoses and order of priority, evaluate accuracy of goals and appropriateness of outcomes, and evaluate proposed interventions. Make adjustments as necessary and reevaluate.

maintaining good muscle tone). Additionally, patients may sometimes be required to perform certain treatments themselves. In this case, the patient should be taught how to perform the procedures, including adaptations that may be required. Special emphasis should be placed on preventing infections.

NURSING ALERT

CAUTI

Catheter-Associated Urinary Tract Infection (CAUTI) is the most common infection in a hospital and is easily prevented by frequently cleaning the area around the catheter. Patients who experience a CAUTI is at a serious risk for kidney infections because the UTI may be undiagnosed (no burning sensation when urinating).

Catheterization (Box 15–2)

The different types of catheters are:

- **Condom catheter:** An external device that consists of a condom, tubing, and a drainage bag. The condom is secured to the shaft of the penis using a special adhesive. To prevent constriction of the penis, the adhesive should be applied to the shaft of the penis in a spiral fashion. The condom is then rolled over the shaft of the penis. The tubing is attached to the end of the condom on one end and to the drainage bag on the opposite end. The condom catheter should be changed frequently, and the penis should be observed for skin breakdown.

- **Straight catheter:** A device used to obtain sterile urine specimens, assess for residual urine volume, and relieve bladder distention. Intermittent catheterization with a straight catheter may also be used to manage patients experiencing neurologic damage that affects bladder function. The primary risk of catheterization is infection and tissue trauma. Regardless of the underlying reason for catheterization, a physician's order is required.

- **Indwelling catheter:** An indwelling catheter is different than a straight catheter in that it has an inflatable bulb that is filled with water to hold it in place for as long as the catheter is to remain in the bladder. The catheter is attached to a closed-system drainage bag and emptied as necessary. Just as with straight catheterization, indwelling catheterization requires a physician order and is associated with a risk of infection. Indwelling catheterization may be required postsurgically and for patients with long-term disorders such as spinal cord injuries, stroke, or paralysis.

Bladder Training

Bladder training is an intervention used to assist incontinent patients to regain control over bladder emptying. It requires the patient to:

- Have an adequate intake of fluids.
- Establish a voiding pattern with the goal of gradually increasing the interval between voiding and the volume of urine that the bladder can hold.

BOX 15–2
Procedure Tip: Female Urinary Catheterization

Insertion of the catheter during female urinary catheterization can be very challenging. To assist with successful insertion, the following tips are provided:

Tip	Rationale
• Have confidence in your ability to successfully perform the procedure.	• If you begin the procedure doubting yourself, you are more likely to fail.
• Review a diagram of the female perineum, paying particular attention to the location of the urethral meatus and the vagina. 	• Provides you with mental picture for comparison to what actual patient's perineum should look like.
• During the step when perineal care is performed, carefully inspect the patient's perineum and locate the vagina and urethral meatus.	• The actual patient's perineum may not look exactly like textbook picture (eg, aging variation or changes during labor and delivery). Locating the landmarks before actual catheterization increases the likelihood of successful catheterization.
• If at any time during the procedure any component of the sterile field is contaminated, stop the procedure and reestablish the sterile field.	• Catheterization procedure places patient at a greater risk for UTIs. If the catheter is contaminated, the likelihood of the patient's developing a UTI is increased even more.

- Schedule bathroom visits.
- Delay urination until there is a feeling to urinate.
- Suppress the urge to void at times that are not in line with the schedule.
- Be patient because the process takes time to work.

Keeping a bladder diary, performing pelvic strengthening exercises, and using distractions are all strategies that may assist clients to be successful with the bladder-training program.

> **NURSING ALERT**
>
> **Kegel Exercise**
> The Kegel exercise strengths the muscles used to start and stop urination. First, squeeze and hold the contraction of muscles used to stop urinating for 5 seconds and then relax for 5 seconds. Gradually increase this to 10 seconds. Perform the Kegel exercise daily.

Conclusion

Urinary elimination is the primary means for ridding the body of fluid waste. Key concepts presented in this chapter on urinary elimination include:

- The urinary system plays an important role in maintaining fluid, electrolyte, and acid–base balance.
- Many variables influence urinary elimination, including diet, fluid intake, activity level, age and developmental stage, psychosocial factors, health deviations, and medical and surgical interventions.
- Urinary retention, urinary incontinence, and UTIs are the three most common urinary elimination alterations.
- Urinary incontinence may be temporary or chronic and may come in various forms, including stress incontinence, urge incontinence, reflex incontinence, overflow incontinence, functional incontinence, and total incontinence.
- Patients may experience physical and psychosocial consequences as a result of alterations in urinary elimination.

REVIEW QUESTIONS

1. **A patient who experiences an alteration in urinary elimination may experience:**
   A. Fluid imbalances
   B. Electrolyte imbalances
   C. Acid–base imbalances

    D. A and B

    E. All of the above

2. Which of the following factors may cause incontinence?

    A. Aging

    B. Catheterization

    C. Weak perineal muscles

    D. B and C

    E. All of the above

3. _____ incontinence is defined as involuntary voiding in a person who has normal bladder and sphincter control.

    A. Functional

    B. Overflow

    C. Reflex

    D. Stress

    E. Urge

4. Which of the following terms is used to describe an infection of the kidney?

    A. Cystitis

    B. Pyelonephritis

    C. Ureteritis

    D. Urethritis

5. A patient with a UTI may present with all of the following signs and symptoms EXCEPT:

    A. Anuria

    B. Dysuria

    C. Hematuria

    D. Pyuria

6. A 24-hour urine specimen has been ordered. Which of the following instructions would best ensure that the patient collects the specimen correctly?

    A. Void, pour urine into the provided container, note the time, and collect urine for the next 24 hours.

    B. Void, discard the urine, note the time, and collect all urine from this point on in the provided container for the next 24 hours.

    C. Notify the physician if any urine is accidentally discarded during the 24-hour period because the test will have to be restarted.

    D. A and C

    E. B and C

ANSWERS

Routine Checkup

1. Caffeine.
2. True.

Review Questions

1. E
2. D
3. A
4. B
5. A
6. E

References

Craven RF, Hirnle CJ: *Fundamentals of Nursing: Human Health and Function*, 5th ed. Philadelphia, PA: Lippincott, 2006.

Daniels R: *Nursing Fundamentals: Caring & Clinical Decision Making.* New York, NY: Delmar Thomson Learning, 2004.

Potter PA, Perry AG: *Fundamentals of Nursing*, 6th ed. St. Louis, MO: Mosby Elsevier, 2005.

Additional Resources

Medline Plus: *Urinary Incontinence.* Available at http://www.nlm.nih.gov/medlineplus/urinaryincontinence.html.

National Kidney and Urologic Diseases Information Clearinghouse: *Urinary Tract Infections in Adults.* Available at http://kidney.niddk.nih.gov/Kudiseases/pubs/utiadult/.

National Kidney and Urologic Diseases Information Clearinghouse: *Urologic Diseases Dictionary Index.* Available at http://kidney.niddk.nih.gov/kudiseases/pubs/udictionary/index.htm.

National Kidney and Urologic Diseases Information Clearinghouse: *Your Urinary System and How It Works.* Available at http://kidney.niddk.nih.gov/kudiseases/pubs/yoururinary/.

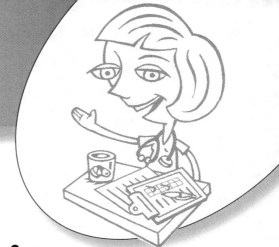

Chapter 16

Bowel Elimination

LEARNING OBJECTIVES

At the end of the chapter, the reader will be able to:

1. Briefly describe the digestive process.

2. Discuss factors that influence bowel elimination.

3. Discuss five major alterations in bowel elimination.

4. Differentiate between and an ileostomy and a colostomy.

5. Discuss the impact of the location of an ostomy on the consistency of the stool.

6. Discuss information that should be collected when assessing a patient who is experiencing an alteration in elimination.

7. Describe complications that may occur as a result of tests that require the use of barium.

8. Discuss patient teaching that should be provided for patients having a Hemoccult test.

9. Discuss psychosocial consequences that may occur as a result of alterations in bowel elimination.

10. Discuss nursing interventions that may be included when providing care for a patient who is experiencing alterations in bowel elimination.

KEY WORDS

Belching	Flatulence
Bowel diversion	Flatus
Colon	Hemorrhoids
Colostomy	Ileoanal pouch
Constipation	Ileostomy
Defecation	Kock continent ileostomy
Diarrhea	Ostomy
Endoscopic	Peristalsis
Fecal diversion	Resection
Fecal impaction	Stoma
Fecal incontinence	

Overview

Solid waste is removed from the body by way of the gastrointestinal (GI) tract. Major structures of the GI system include the mouth, esophagus, stomach, small intestines, and large intestines. Food is usually ingested via the mouth, where the digestive process begins. It then travels to the stomach by way of the esophagus. The digestive process continues in the stomach, where food is changed into a liquid consistency. From the stomach, food enters the intestine, where absorption of most nutrients takes place. What remains after absorption in the small intestine travels to the **colon** or large intestines, where water absorption occurs; leaving a formed soft stool that is eventually evacuated from the body through the anus.

Factors Influencing Bowel Elimination

Bowel elimination patterns are very individualized. Some people may have a bowel movement every day, but others may skip a day or two. The constant factors that are characteristics of bowel elimination are (1) "normal stools" are usually brown and formed and (2) beyond infancy and the toddler years, an individual can control when he or she has a bowel movement. Multiple variables influence a person's bowel elimination pattern. Everyday practices such as what foods a person eats, whether the person leads an active or sedentary lifestyle, and his or her beliefs about the need for privacy for bowel elimination have some influence over the individual's bowel elimination pattern. The growing fetus as well as hormonal changes of pregnancy may make it difficult for pregnant women to have bowel movements. Certain diagnostic procedures, treatments, and medications may alter bowel elimination as well. These and other influencing factors are briefly discussed in the remainder of this section.

NURSING ALERT

Stool colors can be used as a sign of a GI problem. Further testing is necessary to diagnose a GI problem.

Shades of Brown: Normal

Green: Increase ingestion of food with green food coloring, green leafy vegetables, iron supplements. Food may be moving too quickly through the intestine for bile to completely breakdown the food.

White, light or clay color: Missing bile in the stool resulting from a bile duct obstruction or from medication such as bismuth subsalicylate (Pepto-Bismol, Kaopectate).

Yellow: Greasy foul smelling stool indicates excess fat in the stool resulting from malabsorption disorder (celiac disease).

Black: Upper gastrointestinal tract bleeding might be the cause but it can also be from iron supplements, bismuth subsalicylate (Pepto-Bismol, Kaopectate). And even black food (licorice).

Bright red: Lower gastrointestinal tract bleeding might be the cause (rectum, hemorrhoids) but it can also be from beets, cranberries, and red colored food.

Age and Developmental Stage

The most notable variations in bowel elimination occur at the two extremes of age (infancy and old age). At birth, digestive processes are immature. Food passes through the GI system rather rapidly, and complex foods are not tolerated well. The muscles and sphincters that allow voluntary bowel elimination are also immature. Thus, stools are soft, without form, and occur randomly (usually somewhere around mealtimes). Changes that occur in the GI tract as well as changes in the function of other body systems of elderly individuals may lead to changes in bowel elimination patterns. It is important for nurses to educate elderly patients about these changes and about ways to minimize adverse effects of the changes. For example, a normal change that occurs with aging is decreased intestinal motility. Patients need to know that a decrease in the number of stools that they are having do not necessarily mean that they are experiencing constipation. Instead, patients should be taught the importance

TABLE 16–1 Food Intolerances		
Intolerance	Food Triggers	Manifestations
Lactose intolerance	Milk and milk products	Diarrhea Distension Cramping
Gas-producing foods	Beans, onions, cabbage, and so on (varies from individual to individual)	Belching Flatus Distension
Spicy foods	Peppers and other hot spices	Indigestion Cramping Diarrhea
Gluten intolerance	Wheat, barley, and rye	Distension Bulky, greasy stools

of drinking sufficient amounts of fluid, eating fiber-rich foods, and being active to prevent the occurrence of **constipation** (hard, dry, infrequent stools that are difficult to evacuate from the intestinal tract) that may occur secondary to decreased intestinal motility.

Diet and Fluid Intake

Food choices, the frequency of food intake, and food intolerances (Table 16–1) influence the frequency as well as the consistency of bowel movements. Individuals who eat regularly, include foods rich in fiber (eg, vegetables, fruits, and grains), and have an adequate fluid intake usually have a regular bowel elimination pattern, and their stools are usually soft and formed. The opposite is true for those who do not consume fiber-rich foods and adequate fluids on a regular basis. These individuals are more likely to pass hard, dry stool on a less frequent basis. They are more likely to complain of discomfort and may even develop **hemorrhoids** (distended veins in the rectum and anus).

NURSING ALERT

NonMedication Treatment for Constipation
Increase intake of fiber and fluids and mobility are nonmedication treatment for constipation. Undigested fiber (indigestible part of plants) creates the bulk of stool that assists the intestine to expel waste from the body.

Activity and Exercise

Physical activity and exercise increase muscle tone and **peristalsis** (wave-like contractions of a structure, such as the intestines, that propel content forward), which in turn promotes regular bowel elimination and prevents constipation. Person who leads a sedentary lifestyle and those who are incapable of being active or mobile because of physical limitations are more likely to experience problems with bowel elimination.

Psychosocial Factors

A person's bowel elimination habits may be influenced by changes in his or her daily routine. For example, a person who goes on vacation may have to alter his or her eating pattern, which may in turn alter his or her elimination pattern. Likewise, a person who is hospitalized and confined to bed may find it difficult to have a bowel movement because of lack of privacy and the inability to assume the squatting position (the normal position for bowel elimination). A person may choose to delay bowel elimination when in public places such as at school or in shopping malls because of perceptions about cleanliness or the fear of embarrassment because of the odor associated with bowel elimination. A person's emotional state may also cause changes in bowel elimination patterns. Feelings of anxiety and fear may cause the person to have diarrhea; constipation has been associated with chronic depression. Having an awareness of all of the above-mentioned factors is very important. The nurse should ask questions to ascertain what influencing variables may be altering an individual's usual elimination pattern, and the plan of care should include provisions for these findings.

Medical and Surgical Interventions

Diagnostic test, medications, and surgical interventions may all alter bowel elimination:

- **Diagnostic tests:** GI tests that require the ingestion of barium or a barium enema may cause alterations in bowel elimination. Barium is a white, chalky substance that helps with visualization of the GI tract during radiologic (x-ray) procedures. A person who has had a procedure requiring the use of barium will have white to tan colored stools until all of the barium is evacuated from the GI tract. Also, if the barium does not pass through the GI tract in a timely manner, it will harden just like plaster hardens in a mold and will cause **fecal impaction** (a collection of hardened stool in the large intestines). Persons who have **endoscopic** procedures (insertion of a small, flexible tube into the body cavity to visualize the internal structure), especially those involving the lower GI tract, may have gas and loose stools for a short period of time after the procedures. Gas and loose stool occur as a result of (1) bowel cleansing to remove stool and improve visualization of the inside of the colon, (2) the injection of gas to distend the colon and improve visualization inside the folds of the colon, and (3) manipulation of the scope while inside the colon.

> ### NURSING ALERT
>
> **Barium Enema After Care**
> When a barium enema is performed, impaction can occur if the barium is not passed. A cleansing enema may be ordered to prevent this occurrence.

- **Surgical procedures:** Abdominal surgery affects the muscles that are used to assist with **defecation**, or evacuation of stool from the rectum. General anesthetic agents slow intestinal motility, which in turn may delay fecal elimination. Stool softeners and laxatives may be used to reestablish normal bowel elimination. Postsurgical pain as well as narcotic medications used for pain control may also inhibit bowel elimination.

- **Medications:** Some medications are intentionally given to a patient to promote normal bowel elimination. Laxatives, cathartics, and stool softeners, which are given to promote bowel evacuation, should be given with caution to prevent unwanted and unintended effects (eg, dependency, diarrhea, dehydration). An individual may be taking other medications that cause alterations in bowel elimination as a side effect. Some medications may cause diarrhea, and others may cause constipation (Box 16–1). For example, a patient who is taking an antibiotic for an infection may experience diarrhea as a side effect.

> ### NURSING ALERT
>
> **Opioid Substance Abuse**
> Patients who abuse opioid usually experience chronic constipation called opioid-induced constipation (OIC). Opioids decrease time for food to pass through the intestine causing a reduction in digestive secretions and a decrease in the urge to defecate. Large doses of opioids may result in partially paralyzing the GI tract (gastroparesis). The practitioner should anticipate OIC and prescribed a treatment to minimize or prevent occurrence of OIC.

BOX 16–1

Medications Associated with Constipation

- Pain medications (especially narcotics)
- Antacids (aluminum and calcium based)
- Blood pressure medications (calcium channel blockers)
- Iron supplements
- Diuretics
- Antispasmodics

- Antidepressants
- Anticonvulsants
- Antiparkinson drugs

 ROUTINE CHECKUP 1

1. A person who goes for 2 to 3 days without having a bowel movement is most likely experiencing constipation. True/false?

Answer:

2. Briefly describe two psychosocial factors that may cause a person to experience an alteration in bowel elimination.

Answer:

_____

_____

_____

Alterations in Bowel Elimination

The most common manifestations of alterations in bowel function are constipation, diarrhea, and **flatulence** (or gas accumulation). In some instances, an individual may develop an impaction from unrelieved constipation. Some diseases such as cancer, Crohn's disease, and ulcerative colitis may require a patient to have a temporary or permanent bowel diversion.

Constipation

Constipation occurs when stool remains in the colon for extended periods of time, allowing excess water to be absorbed from the contents. The stool becomes hard, dry, and difficult to pass. It is important not to automatically assume that a person is constipated because of infrequent bowel movements. Normal elimination patterns vary from person to person. One individual may have a bowel movement every day, but another may have bowel movements every 2 to 3 days. If both individuals have soft, firm stools, neither is experiencing constipation. However, if the stool of the person who is having bowel movements every 2 to 3 days is hard, dry, and difficult to pass, then that person is experiencing constipation.

> **NURSING ALERT**
>
> **Constipation Precaution**
> Straining associated with constipation can be dangerous for patients who have cardiovascular disease:
>
> Straining → Vagal stimulation → Dysrhythmias

Impaction

If constipation is not resolved, then an impaction will occur and may possibly require manual removal because the patient will not be able to pass the stool under his or her own power. The nurse should suspect an impaction if:

- The patient has not had a bowel movement for several days.
- Rectal fullness accompanied by unsuccessful attempts to have a bowel movement.
- There is involuntary seepage of loose stool from the rectum.

Diarrhea

Diarrhea is the passage of loose or watery stools, usually on a frequent basis. It occurs because the food content passes through the GI tract too fast for nutrients and water to be absorbed adequately. This may happen for a number of reason, including food intolerances, stress and anxiety, laxative misuse, and inflammatory disorders of the GI tract. Diarrhea stools are usually acidic and may cause irritation, pain, and bleeding in the perianal area. They are accompanied by a strong urge to pass stool. Diarrhea may also be accompanied by abdominal cramping.

> **NURSING ALERT**
>
> **Diarrhea Precautions**
> The nurse should monitor patients who have persistent diarrhea for signs of dehydration.

Fecal Incontinence

Fecal incontinence is different than diarrhea. It is an involuntary elimination of stool and is often associated with the presence of neurologic or mental impairment (eg, stroke, paralysis, confusion, disorientation). A person who has diarrhea may experience fecal incontinence if he or she cannot control the strong urge to evacuate the rectum that often accompanies diarrhea.

Flatulence

Flatulence is the accumulation of gas in the GI tract. Gas that accumulates in the GI tract is either eliminated from the mouth (**belching**) or from the anus (**flatus**). If the flatulence is not eliminated from the GI tract, it may cause abdominal distension, pain, and cramping. Gas in the digestive tract comes from two sources: (1) swallowed air and (2) undigested food breakdown by harmless bacteria that normally live in the colon. Excessive air swallowing usually occurs as a result of:

- Rapid food and fluid intake
- Chewing gum
- Smoking
- Wearing loose dentures
- Drinking carbonated drinks

Carbohydrates may not be digested before entering the large intestine. If this is the case, then bacteria normally found in the large intestine break down the carbohydrates and produce gas in the process. Foods containing carbohydrates that produce gas in one individual may not necessarily produce gas in another person. One possible explanation for this phenomenon is the belief that other bacteria reside in the colon that are capable of destroying residual gas from carbohydrate breakdown. Gas accumulates in the colon when the bacteria responsible for carbohydrate breakdown outnumber those that destroy the gas produced from carbohydrate breakdown.

Dietary selections may cause flatulence such as beans, cabbage, broccoli, and fruit juices (high in fructose or sorbitol) because they can take a long time to digest and may not be fully absorbed. Food that is incompletely digested moves from the intestine to the colon where bacteria in the colon break down the food releasing gases (flatulence). Flatulence may also be an indicator of a digestive problem such as irritable bowel syndrome (IBS), lactose intolerance, gastroenteritis, dumping syndrome, ulcerative colitis, and celiac disease.

Bowel Diversions

Some disorders of the GI tract require the removal of portions of the small or large intestines (or both). In such a case, a temporary or permanent bowel diversion will be created. **A bowel diversion**, also referred to as a **fecal diversion**, requires that a segment of the small or large intestines be brought through the abdominal wall, creating an alternate route for evacuation of fecal material from the intestinal tract. The actual opening is called a **stoma** or **ostomy**. When the ostomy is created from the small intestines, it is called an **ileostomy**, and when it is created from the colon or large intestines, it is referred to as a **colostomy** (Figure 16–1).

Temporary ostomies are performed when reconnection or **resection** can be performed and normal bowel elimination can be reestablished. Permanent ostomies are required when a segment of the intestines has to be removed and resection is not possible. The consistency and content of the stool evacuated through the ostomy depend on the location of the stoma. The more distal the stoma is, the more formed the stool will be. Therefore, whereas ileostomy stool content is liquid, stool content of descending and sigmoid colostomies is more formed. Still, in both instances, an external collection bag is usually required. Skin care, diet modifications, application of a pouch device, colostomy irrigation, and recognizing complications are topics that need to be covered with patients who have ostomies. The nurse should also be aware of the psychological impact of having an ostomy. Patients may have problems with poor self-esteem or altered body image and may avoid social interaction.

> ### NURSING ALERT
>
> **Psychosocial Considerations for Ostomy Patients**
> Patients who have ostomies should be monitored closely for signs of depression and isolation that may occur secondary to a perceived change in body image. Training and encouraging the patient to care for the ostomy himself gives the patient autonomy and may reduce depression as living with an ostomy becomes part of the patient's daily routine.

Alternative procedures are now available for some patients who would otherwise require a permanent ileostomy. Both procedures afford the patient more control over bowel elimination. The **ileoanal pouch** involves the creation of a stool collection reservoir using the distal end of the ileum.

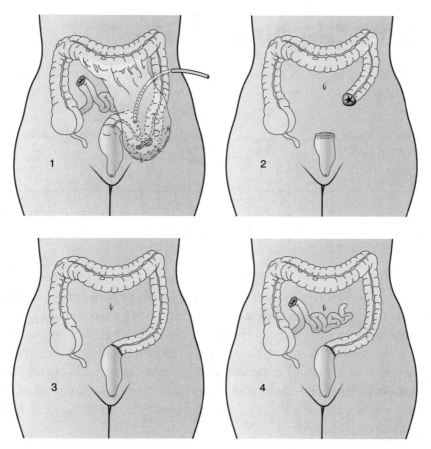

FIGURE 16-1 • A colostomy is a bowel diversion from the ascending colon, transverse colon, or descending colon depending on the underlying cause for the colostomy. (Reproduced with permission from Kasper DL et al (eds). *Harrison's Principles of Internal Medicine*, 19th ed. New York: McGraw-Hill; 2015, Fig 353-3.)

The reservoir or pouch serves the same purpose as the rectum. The ileoanal pouch is attached to the patient's anus, and stool is evacuated at will through the anus. The patient may still require a temporary ileostomy to allow the connection sites in the pouch to heal. The **Kock continent ileostomy** is also created by forming a pouch from the distal end of the ileum. However, in this procedure, the patient will have a stoma. The stoma contains a valve that can be drained with an external catheter, thus affording the patient control over bowel evacuation and eliminating the need for a drainage bag.

ROUTINE CHECKUP 2

1. Foods that cause gas in one person may not necessarily cause gas in another person. True/false?

Answer:

2. A stoma that is _____ in color should be reported immediately because it indicates circulation impairment.

Answer:

The Nursing Process and Bowel Elimination

Assessment

Assessment of bowel elimination patterns can be tricky. Most patients consider this to be a rather private topic and are sometimes embarrassed to disclose information about their normal bowel elimination patterns. The nurse must establish good rapport with the patient and rely on keen observational skills to ensure that information obtained truly reflects the patient's current bowel elimination pattern. The assessment database should include information derived from the nursing history, laboratory and diagnostic test results, and the physical examination.

> **NURSING ALERT**
>
> **Bowel Elimination is an Uncomfortable Discussion Topic**
> Few patients want to have a discussion about their bowel elimination so expect the patient to be hesitant speaking about this topic with a nurse (a stranger). Begin your assessment with questions about the patient's dietary intake then ask questions as you talk through the digestive process (ie, mouth, esophagus, stomach, and intestine). The patient has time to anticipate questions about bowel elimination and will be in a better frame of mind to respond.

Nursing History

When collecting the nursing history, ask the patient about:

- Usual bowel elimination pattern (how often, color, consistency, odor)
- Recent changes in frequency and consistency
- Lifestyle information (diet, fluid intake, exercise, stressors)

- Use of assistive aids (laxatives, enemas)
- Current medications
- Medical history (inflammatory bowel disease, cancer, neuromuscular disorders)

Diagnostic Test and Procedures

Examples of laboratory and diagnostic test include:

- Hemoccult test (Box 16–2)
- Stool cultures
- Upper GI series (radiography of the upper GI tract using barium)
- Barium enema (radiography of the lower GI tract using barium)
- Endoscopy and colonoscopy

Physical Examination

During the physical examination:

- Observe the condition of the patient's mouth (note any tooth decay or mouth lesions).
- Assess the abdomen.

  - Observe for distension and possibly measure abdominal girth.
  - Auscultate bowel sounds (always auscultate before palpating) (Figure 16–2).
  - Palpate the abdomen for masses and observe for signs of discomfort.
  - If the patient has a bowel diversion, observe the condition of the stoma.

BOX 16–2
Hemoccult Testing

To prevent a false-positive result, the patient should be instructed to avoid the following for 3 days before Hemoccult is performed:

- Red meats
- Vitamin C (>250-mg doses)
- Aspirin
- Nonsteroidal antiinflammatory medications

Recommended that test be repeated three times before confirming GI bleeding.

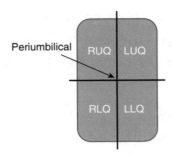

FIGURE 16–2 · Auscultate bowel sounds from the right lower quadrant clockwise to the left lower quadrant.

Nursing Diagnosis

Nursing diagnoses directly related to bowel elimination as well as those that relate to other physical and psychosocial issues experienced by the patient should be included. Examples of nursing diagnoses include:

- Bowel incontinence
- Constipation, risk for constipation, perceived constipation
- Diarrhea
- Risk for impaired skin integrity
- Risk for deficient fluid volume
- Deficient knowledge
- Disturbed body image
- Impaired social interaction

Planning

Identifying goals and expected outcomes, setting priorities, and planning interventions are all included in the planning phase of the nursing process. The goal of care is to return the client to a normal bowel elimination pattern. However, it is important to develop goals and outcomes that are realistic for the client and his or her unique situation. There may be some situations where returning the patient to his or her normal pattern of bowel elimination is not desired (it may have been an unhealthy pattern) or not realistic. For example, a patient who has been diagnosed with colon cancer and who has to have a permanent colostomy will not be able to reestablish his or her usual bowel elimination pattern. Instead, it is appropriate to work together with the patient to identify ways to ensure that the required changes minimally impact how he or she is accustomed to living (eg, shopping, traveling, socializing).

Implementation

Interventions may be directed toward preventing bowel elimination problems or toward resolving alterations in bowel elimination.

Health Promotion Interventions

Depending on the information provided by the patient during the assessment, it may be necessary to teach the patient about practices that will promote a healthy bowel elimination pattern. The patient should be encouraged to include fiber in the diet, drink plenty of fluids, allow time for bowel elimination, and identify ways to effectively cope with stress. The patient should also be informed of the effects of alcohol and tobacco on bowel elimination (chronic use can cause diarrhea). When it is necessary for a patient to be hospitalized or for a patient who resides in an extended care facility, the nurse should ensure that privacy needs are met and should remember that positioning plays an important role in the patient's ability to defecate.

Altered Elimination Interventions

The following are interventions that may be used for a patient who is experiencing alterations in bowel elimination:

- **Medications:** Laxatives and cathartics may be given for constipation, and antidiarrheal agents may be given for diarrhea. The nurse should monitor for dependence.
- **Enema:** Used for temporary relief of constipation. May also be used as preparation for GI tests.
- **Digital removal of stools:** Used when a patient has an impaction. Caution must be taken to avoid perforation of the rectum. *A physician order is required.*
- **Rectal tube:** Used to relieve gas.
- **Nasogastric intubation:** Used to relieve pressure caused by the accumulation of fluids and air. Intubation may also be used for feeding patients and to irrigate the stomach. The nurse should always check for tube placement after insertion and whenever the tube is repositioned. The most accurate way to check placement of the tube is by radiography.

> **NURSING ALERT**
>
> **Nasoenteric Tube Placement**
> If a nasoenteric tube is ordered for feeding purposes, correct placement should be confirmed by radiography before any feeding is initiated.

- **Ostomy care:** Ostomy care involves three components (Box 16–3):

  1. **Assessment of the stoma:** The stoma color ranges from pink to red. Bluish discoloration (cyanosis) is a sign of poor circulation and should be reported.

  2. **Pouch application and skin care:** The skin should be cleansed and prepped to provide a good seal when the pouch is applied. There are various types of pouches; the enterostomal nurse usually assists the patient in selecting the pouch that best meets his or her needs.

  3. **Management of stool characteristics:** Teach the patient to observe the effects of foods on the consistency and odor of stool and to make adjustment accordingly. This will also help with establishing a regular bowel elimination pattern for certain types of ostomies.

BOX 16–3
Procedure Tip: Stoma Care

Key goals of stoma care include:
1. Prevent leakage
2. Prevent skin breakdown
3. Recognize complications early on

Tip	Rationale
• Observe the color of the stoma. It should be red to pink. *It should not be bluish.*	• A bluish discoloration suggests compromised circulation and needs to be reported immediately.
• Clean the skin thoroughly and allow to dry before applying the drainage bag.	• Promotes a secure seal with the skin and prevents leakage of stool, which can be highly irritating to the skin.
• Select a drainage bag with an opening that properly matches the size of the stoma. Some bags come with a precut opening, but others require the opening to be cut.	• An opening that is too large will allow stool to come in contact with the skin surrounding the stoma and may cause skin irritation and breakdown.
• Teach the patient how to properly care for the stoma at home (application of drainage bag, skin care, and signs of complications).	• Promotes achievement of key goals of stoma care.

- **Bowel training:** Bowel training is most beneficial for patients who are recovering from neurologic disorders and still maintain some muscular control over bowel evacuation. The patient attempts to establish set times for elimination. This may require diet adjustments and medications. The program takes time to work and requires patience and diligence.

Conclusion

Key concepts presented in this chapter include:

- Bowel elimination patterns vary widely from individual to individual.
- Age, diet, fluid intake, level of activity, health status, and emotional state all influence an individual's bowel elimination pattern.
- Alterations in bowel elimination include constipation, diarrhea, flatulence, fecal incontinence, and bowel diversions.
- Common diagnostic tests that may assist in identifying underlying causes of alterations in bowel elimination include Hemoccult test, stool cultures, upper and lower GI series, and endoscopic procedures.
- Alterations in bowel elimination may cause patients to experience altered body image and impaired social interaction.
- Nursing interventions related to bowel elimination are directed toward promoting health; correcting alterations in bowel elimination when possible; and restoring the patient to his or her optimal level of functioning, which may or may not be the same as that experienced before the alteration in bowel elimination.

REVIEW QUESTIONS

1. **All of the following may occur as a result of diarrhea EXCEPT:**
   A. Bleeding
   B. Hemorrhoids
   C. Irritation
   D. Pain

2. **Which of the following contribute(s) to the occurrence of gas?**
   A. Eating too fast
   B. Loose dentures
   C. Smoking

    D. A and C

    E. All of the above

3. **Which of the following findings suggest that a patient is experiencing an alteration in bowel elimination?**

    A. Stool frequency of every 2–3 days

    B. Brown-colored stool

    C. Hard and dry stool

    D. A or C

    E. All of the above

4. **Which of the following instructions should be given to the patient who is to have a Hemoccult stool test?**

    A. Do not take aspirin for 3 days before the test.

    B. Do not eat red meat for 3 days before the test.

    C. Do not take more than a 250-mg dose of vitamin C for 3 days before the test.

    D. A and C

    E. All of the above

5. **Patients who are lactose intolerant should avoid which of the following foods?**

    A. Beans

    B. Wheat bread

    C. Eggs

    D. Ice cream

    E. C and D

6. **When performing the physical exam for a patient who is experiencing an alteration in elimination, the nurse should:**

    A. Check the condition of the patient's teeth.

    B. Observe for abdominal distension.

    C. Listen for bowel sounds.

    D. Palpate the abdomen.

    E. All of the above

ANSWERS

Routine Checkup 1

1. False.

2. Any two of the following four:

   Changes in a person's eating patterns with subsequent changes in elimination while on vacation.

   Hospitalized patients may find it difficult to have a bowel movement because of lack of privacy and the inability to assume the squatting position (the normal position for bowel elimination).

A person may choose to delay bowel elimination when in public places because of perceptions about cleanliness or the fear of embarrassment.

A person's emotional state may also cause changes in bowel elimination patterns. Feelings of anxiety and fear may cause the person to have diarrhea; constipation has been associated with chronic depression

Routine Checkup 2

1. True.
2. Bluish.

Review Questions

1. B
2. E
3. C
4. E
5. D
6. E

References

Craven RF, Hirnle CJ: *Fundamentals of Nursing: Human Health and Function*, 5th ed. Philadelphia, PA: Lippincott, 2006.

Daniels R: *Nursing Fundamentals: Caring & Clinical Decision Making*. New York, NY: Delmar Thomson Learning, 2004.

Potter PA, Perry AG: *Fundamentals of Nursing*, 6th ed. St. Louis, MO: Mosby Elsevier, 2005.

Additional Resources

American Cancer Society: *Colostomy Guide*. Available at http://www.cancer.org/docroot/CRI/content/CRI_2_6x_Colostomy.asp?sitearea=&level=.

American Cancer Society: *Ileostomy Guide*. Available at http://www.cancer.org/docroot/CRI/content/CRI_2_6x_Ileostomy.asp.

Family Doctor: *Elimination Problems*. Available at http://familydoctor.org/online/famdocen/home/tools/symptom/532.html.

The J-Pouch Group: *Living with Your J-Pouch*. Available at http://www.j-pouch.org/illustratedpouch/index.html.

Medline Plus: *Colostomy*. Available at http://www.nlm.nih.gov/medlineplus/tutorials/colostomy/htm/index.htm.

Medline Plus: *Ostomy*. Available at http://www.nlm.nih.gov/medlineplus/ostomy.html.

National Digestive Diseases Information Clearinghouse: *What Causes Constipation?* Available at http://www.digestive.niddk.nih.gov/ddiseases/pubs/constipation/index .htm#what.

National Digestive Diseases Information Clearinghouse: *What Causes Gas?* Available at http://digestive.niddk.nih.gov/ddiseases/pubs/gas/#cause.

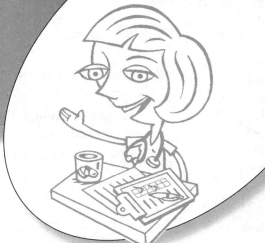

Chapter **17**

Psychosocial Needs

LEARNING OBJECTIVES

At the end of the chapter, the reader will be able to:

1. Differentiate between self-concept and self-esteem.
2. Discuss identity, body image, and roles as components of self-concept.
3. Discuss factors that influence self-concept.
4. Describe manifestations of altered self-concept.
5. Identify factors that influence role and relationship.
6. Discuss alterations in roles and relationships.
7. Differentiate between gender, gender role, and sexual orientation.
8. Discuss factors that may influence a person's sexuality.
9. Contrast spirituality with religion.
10. Discuss variables that may influence a person's spirituality.
11. Discuss stress, sources of stress, and stress response.
12. Describe stress, coping, and adaptation.
13. Discuss factors that may influence how a person handles loss and expresses grief.
14. Compare and contrast grief models.

15 Differentiate between effective therapeutic communication techniques and communication blocks.

16 Discuss interventions that may be called upon to meet the patient's psychosocial needs.

17 Understand the importance of stress and coping when caring for patients.

18 Discuss behavioral health and behavioral health disorders.

KEY WORDS

Abnormal behavior	Normal behavior
Adaptation	Personality disorders
Body image	Psychotic disorders
Coping	Religion
Distress	Role
Gender	Role performance
Gender role	Self-concept
Hermaphrodites	Self-esteem
Identity	Sexual orientation
Intersexed	Stress
Libido	

Overview

Many topics have been discussed throughout this textbook, and each has in some way touched on the psychosocial needs of patients. The discussions have ranged from the relationship between basic physiological functions and psychosocial factors (eg, excitement elevates the blood pressure) to the impact of physiological function on an individual's psychosocial well-being (eg, altered body image or sexuality related to the presence of an ostomy). This chapter differs from previous chapters because the spotlight here is on the psychosocial needs of the patient. The chapter includes a discussion of self-concept, family roles and relationships, sexuality, human spirituality, stress, loss, grief, and coping. A brief discussion of each of these concepts will be presented. The nursing process will serve as the platform for discussing how to best meet the psychosocial needs of patients.

Self-Concept

Self-concept is defined as the way an individual *thinks* of him- or herself (eg, smart, dumb, tall, short, mild-mannered, assertive). **Self-esteem** relates more to how a person *feels* about him- or herself (eg, good, bad, like, dislike). All of us experience periods of time when we have a low self-esteem. However, a person's core self-esteem (low or high) is stable over time and is a better indicator of how a person truly *feels* about him- or herself. Individuals are not born with a self-concept or self-esteem; both develop over the course of a lifetime and are influenced by many variables. An individual's self-concept is very important because it significantly influences interpersonal interactions and the person's ability to form healthy relationships.

Components of Self-Concept

Identity, body image, and role (role performance) all help to define a person's self-concept and core self-esteem. Each plays a unique role.

- **Identity** is the organizing principle of the self, the awareness that one is a distinct individual separate from others. Initially, individuals rely on others to define who they are. Parents strongly influence their children's identity in the early years. However, as children grow older and begin to interact with individuals other than their parents, they develop different reference points or expand the boundaries for defining who they are. Adolescent identity, in particular, is strongly influenced by peers (people who they perceive to be very similar to them). Eventually, an individual will participate in a self-evaluation process and further define who she or he is. The outcome of the self-evaluation and the resulting establishment of his or her unique identity will be more than the sum of parents, peers, and other influences.

- **Body image** is an individual's description of his or her physical body (eg, weight, height, body shape, skin color). Furthermore, a person develops perceptions about his or her physical make-up. A person may perceive him- or herself to be feminine, masculine, strong, weak, pretty, or ugly. Positive perceptions of body image contribute to the establishment of a positive self-concept as well as high core self-esteem. Conversely, negative perceptions of body image contribute to poor self-concept and low core self-esteem.

- A **role** is "an expected behavior in a given individual." Roles may be ascribed or forced, in which case the individual has no control over being in the role (eg, sister, child), or roles may be assumed. Assumed roles may or may not be by choice (eg, husband, mother, nurse, politician). **Role performance** is an individual's perception of his or her success in performing a certain role. A person's self-concept is influenced in a positive way when the individual perceives success in his or her role performance. The opposite effect occurs when an individual believes he or she has failed to successfully function in a particular role.

Influencing Factors

Multiple variables can influence a person's self-concept. Examples of influencing factors include:

- **Cultural expectations:** Physical characteristic such as large size may be viewed negatively in one culture and completely acceptable or even desired in another culture.

- **Developmental stage:** The self-concept evolves over the life span and is influenced by developmental tasks unique to the various developmental stages. For example, toddlers are tasked with establishing a sense of autonomy and do so by experimenting with their environment. If the toddler is allowed to explore the environment, he or she will feel confident and begin establishing a sense of confidence. On the other hand, if the toddler is constantly told "no" and not allowed to explore the environment, then he or she may develop feelings of shame and doubt.

- **Past experiences:** Whereas successful past experiences build a positive self-concept, repeated instances of failure lead to the formation of a negative self-concept and poor self-esteem.

- **Health deviations:** Illnesses, surgery, and trauma may change an individual's outward appearance or functional capacity. Changes in appearance may cause the individual to feel shame, withdraw, and develop poor self-esteem. Changes in functional capacity may require role changes, affect an individual's ability to be self-sufficient, and may change relationships, all of which may lead to a negative self-concept and poor self-esteem.

Alterations in Self-Concept

Altered self-concept may be manifested by a person's failure to perform self-care activities. The individual may demonstrate poor hygiene, inappropriately expose or conceal his or her body, deny health concerns, become noncompliant with recommended treatments, or even refuse to participate in planning her or his own care. A patient with an altered self-concept may also exhibit anxiety, depression, and self-destructive behaviors such as drug abuse and overeating. He or she may also withdraw from social interactions.

Families, Roles, and Relationships

The nurse working with individual clients must consider their roles and relations within social networks. There are varying types of social networks. The family is one such network. The family is a social group whose members share common values, occupy specific positions, interact over time, and have diverse strengths and needs. Not all families are alike; in fact, there are numerous types of family structures, including nuclear, single parent, blended, cohabitated, extended, and communal (Figure 17–1). Family function may differ in each type family, but almost all families include the basic functions of

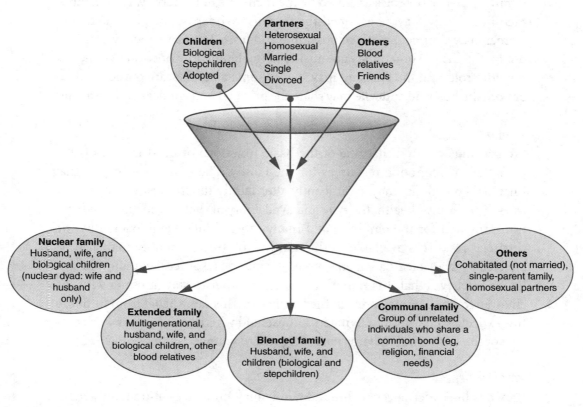

FIGURE 17–1 · Schematic diagram of family structures.

meeting physical and economic needs, sexual intimacy, reproduction, education, socialization, nurturing, and support. It is also important for healthcare workers to keep in mind that informal families (ie, those not established through marital ties and blood relationships) also exist and serve some of the same functions as a formal family structure.

Influencing Factors

Factors influencing family roles and relationships include values and beliefs system, finances, past experiences, and health alterations as well as other life stressors.

Values and Beliefs

The values and belief systems of a group of people may influence how individuals grow and function in society as well as what roles are acceptable or not both within and outside of the family. In some societies, gender and position in the family influence the roles assumed by the members of the family. For example, men in a family may be ascribed the role of provider or "breadwinner," and women may assume the role of providing childcare. In today's society, this may not be the case. Women may go outside of the family to work and assume the provider role, and the husband may stay at home and take care of the children or both the husband and wife may share the provider and childcare roles equally.

Finances

We previously stated that one of the basic functions of most families is the provision of economic resources for the family. Therefore, it is logical that financial constraints may significantly alter family function as well as family roles. The family's health, the type and availability of shelter, the type of education provided for the children, and many other things are impacted by the financial resources available to the family. Roles in the family may also be affected by available financial resources. Economic resources may allow a family who believes that it is important for the mother to stay at home with the children to do so or may prevent the family with this same belief from fulfilling this expectation. Children living in a household where both parents work outside of the home may serve as parent figures to younger siblings.

Past Experiences

Previous life experiences within the family may influence future family function and relationships. Individuals who as children were accustomed to sitting down at the table and eating together may continue the tradition in their families and may demonstrate better communication and problem-solving skills than those who infrequently see each other. On the other hand, a person growing up in an environment of abuse may become an abuser, may shy away from relationships, may accept abuse as a normal part of relationships, or may seek out resources to build healthy relationships.

Crisis Situations

Loss of a family member, loss of employment, involvement in accidents or disasters, and illnesses (both acute and chronic) are all potential family crisis situations. Temporary changes in family roles or the assumption of additional roles may be required by any one of the above-mentioned situations. How well the family adapts will depend on the available support system that is in place and the coping skills of individual family members. Chronic illnesses may have a long-lasting, profound effect on the family. Many adjustments may be required. In some instances, families cannot withstand the stress. In such cases, divorce is usually the resulting outcome.

Alterations in Roles and Relationships

Changes necessitated by any of the above-identified influencing factor may result in various alterations in roles and relationships (Box 17–1). Examples of alterations that may occur include:

- **Separation and divorce**, although not the most desirable choice, is sometimes a necessary choice. Regardless of the motive for separation or divorce, the outcome almost always requires role adjustments.
- **Abuse** may be physical, sexual, or emotional. It may be directed toward children, husbands, wives, parents, or other extended family members

---

BOX 17–1
Role Disorders

The nurse should carefully assess for the presence of role strain and role conflict when there have been changes in normal family function.
- **Role strain:** Perceived or actual inability to perform the expectations of a role
- **Role conflict:** Occurs when an individual is functioning in roles that are incompatible with each other
- **Role confusion:** Occurs when there is uncertainty about what role to assume

(eg, grandparents). All forms of abuse may have devastating, long-lasting effects. In some instances, abuse can be resolved, and the family can be salvaged. In other instances, this may not be possible, and in extreme cases, the outcome may even be the death of the abused or neglected individuals.

- **Depression, developmental deviations, and social isolation** are also potential manifestations of altered roles and relationships. Individuals who are forced into role changes because of the loss of a job or retirement may exhibit depression. A lack of parental bonding may cause failure to thrive and developmental delays in children. Abuse and other forms of family dysfunction may impede mastery of developmental tasks by individual family members. For example, constant negative feedback about behavior in a preschooler may lead to feelings of guilt instead of initiative. Families or individual family members may not interact with others out of embarrassment about their financial status, as a means of hiding the presence of alcoholism or domestic violence, or out of fear of rejection or ridicule by outsiders. In other instances, isolation may not be by choice. For instance, isolation may be the result of discrimination, incapacitating illnesses, or forced job relocation.

✔ ROUTINE CHECKUP 1

1. Self-esteem is how a person thinks of him- or herself, and self-concept is how a person feels about him- or herself. True/false?

Answer:

2. List four types of family crises that may alter the roles of family members.

Answer:

_____

_____

_____

_____

Human Sexuality

Sexuality is a physiological, psychological, and social experience. It is a basic, "completely normal" part of being human. A wide range of topics may be

BOX 17–2
Components of Sexuality

Gender
- Male
- Female
- Intersexed

Gender role
- Masculine
- Feminine
- Transgendered

Sexual orientation
- Heterosexual (straight)
- Homosexual (gay or lesbian)
- Pansexual (bisexual)

included in a discussion of human sexuality. The discussion may be as basic as discussing the physiology of human reproduction or as complex as discussing sexual role expectations (Box 17–2). The promotion of sexual health, likewise, requires the nurse to address any physiological, psychological, and social concerns expressed by the patient. To effectively identify and respond to the patient's needs, the nurse must first establish a rapport and a trusting relationship with the patient. The remainder of this section includes a discussion of basic concepts related to human sexuality, influencing factors, and common alterations.

NURSING ALERT
Nonjudgmental Discussion of Sexuality
The nurse should take an open approach when discussing sexuality with the patient. No assumptions or judgments should be made about the patient's gender role or sexual orientation.

Basic Concepts

Gender is defined by the biologic sex of an individual—male, female, or intersex. **Intersexed** individuals (referred to by some people as **hermaphrodites**), are born with a combination of male and female sex organs. **Gender role** is the masculine or feminine role adopted by a person and is partially defined within the individual's cultural and social context. **Sexual orientation** refers to the affection and sexual attraction of one person to another. Persons with a heterosexual orientation are attracted to the opposite gender (eg, male to female or female to male). On the other hand, individuals who are homosexual are attracted to persons of the same gender (eg, male to male or female to female). Some people have a bisexual orientation and are equally attracted to one gender as they are to the other. During the course of performing assessments and providing patient care, nurses may encounter individuals with any one of the above-described sexual orientations. In any case, the nurse should not make any assumptions. Instead, the nurse should make general references to the patient's significant other; allowing the patient to specifically define the gender and nature of the relationship with the individual.

Influencing Factors

A number of variables influence an individual's sexuality as well as his or her sexual health. A person's physical and psychological status, his or her use of drugs (prescribed and recreational) and alcohol, and medical interventions (eg, surgery, radiation therapy) as well as cultural and societal expectations all have the potential to impact an individual's sexuality.

Health Factors

A wide gamut of health alterations may affect sexuality or sexual health. Changes in the secretion of hormones that control sexual function (eg, testosterone, estrogen, progesterone) may lead to problems with gender determination, sexual intercourse, and reproduction. Each of these issues can also cause psychosocial issues (eg, self-esteem, self-concept, and gender role issues). Hormonal changes also occur as a part of the normal aging process, particularly in women. The nurse must understand that the patient's expectations regarding sexuality and intimacy may not necessarily change; thus, the nurse has the challenge of assisting the patient to identify ways to meet his or her sexual needs within the context of the hormonal changes.

Systemic disorders such as diabetes, hypertension, and heart disease may interfere with sexual function and influence sexuality because of both the physiological impact as well as the psychological impact. For instance, a person with heart disease may have erectile dysfunction secondary to circulatory problems but may also be afraid to have sexual intercourse because of the fear of having a heart attack because of physical exertion. Other disorders such as arthritis, paralysis, or physical disabilities may cause physical limitations that interfere with an individual's ability to engage in sexual intercourse. Pain is another phenomenon that may limit a person's capacity to engage in sexual intercourse. Each of these situations not only has the potential to limit a person's physical capacity for sexual intercourse but also may impact other components of sexuality, including gender role identity (masculinity or femininity), the ability to maintain or develop affectionate relationships, and the ability to meet role expectations set by their culture and society.

Sexually transmitted diseases (STDs) may have an impact on a person's sexuality in multiple ways. An STD may incapacitate the person to the point that he or she is unable to have sexual intercourse. It may also inhibit a person or his or her partner from engaging in sexual intercourse because of the fear of transmitting or contracting the disease. Additionally, a person with an STD may be ostracized, which may interfere with her or his ability to form affectionate or intimate relationships with others. Patient education is a key component of minimizing the negative impact of an STD on sexuality. The approach should be twofold: (1) the nurse should seek out opportunities to educate patients and other members of the community on how to protect themselves from STDs and (2) the nurse should teach patients with STDs how to prevent transmission as well as discuss with them other components of achieving and maintaining healthy intimate relationships.

Drugs and Medications

Prescribed medications as well as recreational drugs, including alcohol, may influence a person's sexuality. The influence may be direct or indirect. For example, an antihypertensive medication may contribute to erectile dysfunction, which directly affects a person's ability to have sexual intercourse. On the other hand, a woman may develop a yeast infection and subsequent body odor after taking an antibiotic; this may impact her ability to be sexually appealing (indirect influence). Other examples of how drugs and medications influence sexuality and sexual health are as follows:

- Interfere with an individual's ability to make a sound decision to engage in or not to engage in sexual intercourse because of altered mental status (alcohol intoxication, date rate drugs); may cause a decreased **libido** or desire to have sex
- Interfere with a person's ability to achieve an erection, orgasm, or ejaculate and associated feeling of inadequacy
- Cause dryness and pain

Therapeutic Interventions

Any major surgical procedure has the potential to temporarily alter a person's ability and desire to engage in sexual intercourse. In such cases, there are usually no long-lasting consequences. To the contrary, surgical interventions such as hysterectomies, mastectomies, and colostomies have the potential to have long-standing adverse consequences, especially without proper intervention. Some people have misconceptions about the effect of a hysterectomy or mastectomy on a woman's femininity. Likewise, the same is true about unfounded beliefs regarding a person's sexuality when he or she has a colostomy. There is no physiological reason that any one of the above-mentioned situations should cause a change in an individual's sexuality, but the presence of outward changes in the body, as is the case with a mastectomy or colostomy coupled with low self-esteem and strong cultural or societal influences make it difficult to convince the patient otherwise. Nurses and other healthcare team members should clarify misconceptions, help the patient identify ways to enhance his or her sexuality, actively listen to patient's concerns as well as assist him or her to work through feelings related to sexuality, and make referrals as needed when specialized assistance is required.

Psychosocial Factors

Family beliefs, religion, cultural and societal expectation, a person's self-concept, and past experiences all influence how an individual defines and expresses his or her sexuality. For example, two individuals may label a particular style of dress totally different depending on what is considered acceptable within his or her family, culture, religion, or society. One individual may perceive the dress style to be promiscuous, but the other individual may perceive it as totally acceptable and appropriate. Another example may be the meaning assigned to two men kissing. In some cultures, this is acceptable, but in other cultures, it is labeled "inappropriate."

A person's past experiences may also influence his or her sexuality. Persons who have been sexually abused may withdraw from intimate relationships, may become sexually promiscuous, or may become abusers themselves. The physical environment as well as the context of an individual's environment may have an impact on sexuality. For example, hospitalized patients and patients residing in long-term residential settings may not be afforded an environment conducive to free sexual expression or may feel uncomfortable expressing affection to significant others in this setting. Concerns regarding contracting an STD or becoming pregnant may lead to alterations in sexual intimacy as well. Also, whether or not open discussion of sexuality is permitted can be considered an environmental influencer on sexuality.

Alterations in Sexuality

Alterations in sexuality may be physiological or psychosocial in nature. Alterations may occur as a result of any of the above-mentioned influencing factors (individually or in combination). Examples of alterations in sexuality include:

- **Dyspareunia**, or painful intercourse, may be associated with vaginal dryness secondary to inadequate sexual arousal, estrogen deficiency, and certain types of medications such as antihistamines. Infections and barrier contraceptive devices may also cause irritation and pain.

- **Erectile dysfunction**, also referred to as **impotence**, is the inability to achieve or maintain erection of the penis. Cialis, Levitra, and Viagra are medication currently available to treat erectile dysfunction. Surgical intervention and counseling are also treatment options for erectile dysfunction.

> **NURSING ALERT**
>
> **Avoid Medication**
> Cialis, Levitra, and Viagra are contraindicated in men who take nitrates, use nitrate patches, take blood thinners, or take certain alpha blockers.

- **Ejaculatory dysfunction** is the inability to ejaculate (a rare occurrence) or premature ejaculation (more common). Premature ejaculation is determined subjectively and depends on the perception of whether or not sexual satisfaction is achieved. Anxiety is thought to contribute to ejaculatory dysfunction.

- **Orgasmic dysfunction**, or difficulty achieving a satisfying orgasm, may occur in either gender but is more commonly reported as a problem by women. The physical build of women as well as the inhibition to explore means for achieving an orgasm may contribute to orgasmic dysfunction.

- **Vaginismus** is a reflexive tightening of the muscle surrounding the vaginal opening that makes penetration difficult and very painful. This usually takes place in the absence of any underlying physical or structural deviations.

Spirituality

Spirituality is an abstract concept that is best defined individually for each person. Although there is a lot of variation in how spirituality is defined, most would agree that it is a central theme interwoven into how individuals characterize the quality of their lives as well as their life purpose. It is also a resource called upon to:

- Guide daily living.
- Guide interactions with others.
- Promote a feeling of security, safeness, strength, and hope, especially during crises.

For nurses and other members of the healthcare team to provide holistic care to patients, each member must acknowledge that spirituality is a "real" and legitimate aspect of a person's health and likewise the plan of care. Team members must also understand that spirituality and religion are *not* synonymous. **Religion** is more accurately described as a formalized system of beliefs and rituals shared by a group of people. Thus, religion may or may not be a part of an individual's spiritual dimension, and asking a person about his or her religious preferences (which is too often labeled as a spiritual assessment) will not adequately address the person's spiritual needs.

Influencing Factors

Spirituality evolves over time from the early childhood years all the way through adulthood. It may be redefined numerous times over the course of a person's lifetime depending on family values, cultural values, and life experiences. What is acceptable or unacceptable within the context of a person's family or culture usually exerts a strong influence on how a person defines his or her spiritual dimension (eg, whether the person calls upon a higher being for help or strictly relies on concrete resources such as medicine, money, and so on). Past experiences may also influence a person's spirituality. For example, a person who experienced a tragedy in the past and who prayed about it and had a positive outcome may call upon prayer in future situations when stress or tragedy is encountered. On the other hand, an individual who did not have a positive outcome may feel hopeless early on and may not even seek sources for achieving a positive outcome.

✔ ROUTINE CHECKUP 2

1. Sexuality is a(n) _____, _____, and _____ experience.

Answer:

2. Levitra, Cialis, and Viagra are contraindicated in men who are also taking a nitrate, a blood thinner, or certain α blockers. True/false?

Answer:

3. *Spirituality* and *religion* are synonymous with one another. True/false?

Answer:

Stress, Loss, Grief, and Coping

Stress, loss, and grief are universal experiences that will inevitably occur during a person's life. The mere nature of healthcare almost guarantees that you as a nurse will encounter patients experiencing some type of stress, loss, and grief.

Stress and Coping

Stress is a condition that occurs when a person encounters physical or social stimuli (stressors) that are perceived as challenging. Some of these stressors, although temporarily uncomfortable, actually result in positive outcomes and growth. For example, a student who is working on a math problem may become very frustrated, but if the student is able to successfully solve the math problem, then he or she will be able to use this new skill to solve future problems that may even be at a higher level of difficulty. When an individual is able to successfully manage a stressor, he or she is said to be **coping** with the stressor. The outcome of successfully coping with challenging stimuli is called **adaptation** or adjustment. When an individual has inadequate resources or limited or ineffective coping strategies, he or she may not adapt and instead may experience **distress** or bad stress. Individuals who do not have effective coping strategies may also use defense mechanisms to deal with stressors (Table 17–1).

What is perceived as stress and how an individual manages stress are influenced by values engrained in an individual through his or her family, culture, and even society as a whole. Also, previous encounters with stress as well as success and failure with dealing with stress shape how a person adapts to stressful life events.

TABLE 17−1 Defense Mechanisms

Defense Mechanism	Description
Denial	Refusing to believe or accept something as being true Example: An expectant mother's refusal to believe that she is no longer pregnant after a spontaneous abortion
Displacement	Transferring emotions away from the person or situation that provokes the emotion to someone or something that is less threatening Example: Lashing out at a coworker when you are actually angry at your boss for something he or she did
Introjections	Boundary distortion characterized by an individual's taking on the traits of someone or something external to him or her Example: A person becomes aggressive to deal with feelings of powerlessness evoked by an external aggressor
Projection	Boundary distortion characterized by an individual attributing his or her own thoughts, emotions, characteristics, or motives to another Example: An abusive husband who manipulates his wife into believing that she is the person responsible for their marital problems
Rationalization	Convincing oneself that no wrong was done through the use of faulty reasoning Example: A person overeats and justifies the behavior by saying that it was acceptable because it was a special occasion
Regression	Return to behavior more appropriate to an earlier stage of development Example: An adult who throws a temper tantrum to get his or her way
Repression	Involuntarily immersing something in the subconscious or unconscious level of thought Example: Pushing memories of a divorce out of your mind yet at the same time that experience may be affecting the current relationship you are in
Suppression	Very similar to repression, but with suppression, there is a *conscious* (voluntary) decision to push a thought into the subconscious Example: Conscious decision to deny positive HIV status as evidenced by answering "no" to questions regarding HIV status and refusing to fill medication prescriptions
Sublimation	Channeling of socially unacceptable impulses into socially acceptable activities Example: Punching a boxing bag instead of a person
Reaction formation	Expression of a feeling that is the opposite of one's authentic feeling or of feeling that would be appropriate in the situation Example: Being nice to someone when you actually despise the person

Loss and Grief

A loss occurs when something is taken away. The loss may be tangible or physical (eg, loss of a house, money, a spouse, a child, a pet) or it may be intangible (eg, loss of companionship, status, freedom). The loss may evoke some level of stress depending on its value to the person experiencing the loss. Grieving is a normal process or coping strategy for dealing with a loss. Several models are available to describe the grieving process; however, there is no right or wrong way to grieve, and there is not a set time frame allotted for grieving (Table 17–2).

The same influencing factors mentioned in the discussion of stress (ie, family, culture, and past experiences) are also applicable to loss and grieving. For example, the loss of a pet may be devastating to one person and no big deal to another depending on the value assigned to having a pet by the family. One family may consider a pet to be a member of the family, and the

TABLE 17–2 Grieving Models		
Model	Stages	Timeline
Engel's model	Shock and disbelief Developing awareness Restitution Resolving the loss Idealization Outcome	≥1 year for grief resolution
Parkes' model	Numbness Yearning Disorganization Reorganization	≥2 years for grief resolution
Grief cycle model	Shock Protest Disorganization Reorganization	Time varies
Kubler-Ross' stages of dying	Denial Anger Bargaining Depression Acceptance	

other family may consider the pet to be a replaceable possession. Also, one family or culture may encourage free expression of sadness such as crying by all members regardless of gender, but another family or culture may strictly prohibit any emotional displays by certain genders. A person's spirituality may also influence how he or she copes with a loss. A person who believes that there is a higher being and that a lost loved one goes on to experience eternal life with this higher being may be able to accept the loss more readily than someone who believes that death is final and the loss is permanent.

The Nursing Process and Meeting Psychosocial Needs

The nursing process is the instrument that nurses use to effectively identify and address patients' psychosocial needs. This section looks at each component of the nursing process as it relates to psychosocial needs.

Assessment

The establishment of a trusting relationship with patients is especially important when assessing their psychosocial needs. Just as important is the nurse's awareness of his or her own value system as it relates to each psychosocial component. Patients are less inclined to freely share information about their self-perception, sexuality, and spiritually. This is even more true when the patient has a poor self-concept or fears that the nurse will judge her or him negatively regarding his or her sexuality or spirituality. The use of open-ended questions will increase the likelihood of the nurse obtaining more complete and accurate information. Closed-ended questions will allow the patient to simply answer in "yes" or "no.".

A comprehensive assessment of the patient's psychosocial status hinges on a combination of asking the right questions as well as correctly reading nonverbal cues provided by the patient. The use of open-ended questions will yield more information than questions that can be answered with yes or no responses. It is also advisable to start with less personal questions and progress to more intimate questions. In addition to asking questions to determine the patient's psychosocial status, the nurse should also collect information about the patient's support system and resources available to the patient. Influencing factors as well as usual manifestations of alterations in psychosocial function discussed throughout this chapter should be used as a guide for determining what specific information needs to be gathered during the psychosocial assessment.

Nursing Diagnoses

There is a high likelihood that the nurse will frequently interact with patients who have psychosocial needs either as primary needs or secondary to their physiological needs. Of course, there is a large list of nursing diagnoses that may be applicable. Examples of some of the more common nursing diagnoses are:

- Self-esteem, low
- Body image disturbances
- Identity, disturbed personal
- Caregiver role strain
- Family processes, interrupted
- Role performance, ineffective
- Sexuality pattern, ineffective
- Spiritual distress
- Coping, ineffective
- Grieving, dysfunctional

Planning

After diagnoses have been identified and prioritized, the nurse, in collaboration with the patient, establishes *realistic* goals to resolve or adequately control the identified psychosocial issues. A key part of the success of the plan is integration of resources identified during assessment process. This is especially important because in many instances, part of the problem is related to the patient's failure to reach out and use available resources and support systems.

Implementation

Interventions directed toward addressing psychosocial needs of patients can be grouped into the categories of therapeutic communication, education, and resource and support system identification.

Therapeutic Communication

Therapeutic communication can be accomplished by actively listening to patients and encouraging them to freely express their feelings. Refer to

Chapter 3 (Table 3–1) for additional techniques that promote therapeutic communication. Sometimes allowing the patient to freely express his or her feelings is all that is needed. In other instances, it is the first step toward resolution of issues. After the issue has been laid out on the table, then a problem-solving strategy can be identified. It is important for the nurse to avoid actions that block open communication. Examples of communication blocks include:

- False reassurance
- Minimizing the importance of information shared by the patient
- Shifting the focus to yourself or changing the subject
- Stereotyping or judging
- Giving advice or communicating opinions

Education

Education may range from teaching patients about very concrete concepts (eg, reproduction, how to perform self-examinations, parenting skills) to clearing up misconceptions that may be the source of feelings of inadequacy and stress. The nurse may also assist the patient with recognizing triggers or teaching the patient coping strategies. In many instances, teaching is most effective when the patient's significant other, family members, and other individuals of interest are involved because the source of concern may be grounded in perceptions held by these individuals.

Resource and Support System Identification

The nurse plays a key role in helping the patient to define his or her support system. Initially, the patient may indicate that he or she does not have anyone that he or she can call upon for support. But after further exploration, the patient is actually able to identify persons that can serve as a support system. In many cases, the problem may be have been that the patient was concerned about imposing on others or had a misperception that the support system could only be family members or blood relatives. The nurse can also be instrumental in identifying community resources (eg, support groups, shelters, churches, financial resources).

Stress and Coping

Stress occurs when a situation may cause an adverse consequence for a person such as tasking the NCLEX. Coping is how a person responds to stress. There are levels of stress based on the perceived adverse consequence. For example, there is a level of stress when you prepare for your pharmacy exam. There is a higher level of stress when you administer a medication to a patient during a clinical rotation under direct supervision of your clinical instructor. And an even higher level of stress is experienced when you administer medications to patients by yourself during your first day as a new nurse because there is no one who prevents you from making a medication error and injuring the patient.

Stress is exhibited as anxiety. Mild anxiety appears as having slight fear but the person remains in self-control and remains in touch with reality. Moderate anxiety appears as mistrustful that leads to distorted reality, increased fear that has the person challenges authority. Severe anxiety appears as irrational behavior with no sense of reality. The person is out of control, hostile and acts out.

How well a person copes with a stressful situation determines the level of anxiety that the person displays. Typically a person has a high level of anxiety if the person has not confronted the stressful situation previously. Anxiety decreases as the person's coping skills improve when dealing with the stressful situation more often. That is, the more you administer medications by yourself the more you learn to cope with the stress and your anxiety level decreases.

No one knows how a person will cope with stress. An important role in nursing is to help patients decrease stress by anticipating stressful situations and devise a plan that lowers the stress. Fear of the unknown is a trigger for stress. Explaining to the patient events that will be occurring well in advance assists the patient to cope because events are known. Events that cause stress are more than inpatient procedures in a healthcare facility, medical tests, medical procedures and treatments. Events that cause concern also include the patient's lifestyle such as work, caring for family, finances, and how love ones will cope with the patient's illness. The nurse can enlist the services of social workers, case managers, family members, and pastoral care to help address situations before the patient experiences stress.

Behavioral and Mental Health

Behavioral health focuses on the mental well-being of the person. The term behavioral health and mental health are interchangeable. Behavioral health encompasses a broad spectrum of behaviors from how a person feels, thinks, and acts and how a person handles stress throughout their life.

Behavior is the way a person acts, especially toward others in the society. Society determines acceptable behaviors and communicates what is acceptable through attitudes, values, authority, culture, persuasion, and genetics.

Behaviors that deviate from acceptable behavior is considered abnormal, which typically results in society shying away from a person who displays abnormal behavior.

It is fine to be different and strange from others. However, failure to function adequately causes family, friends, and governmental agencies to intervene with or without a person's permission. A person can display abnormal behavior with little or no interference from others until that behavior places the person or places others in risk of harm. It then when government agencies step in to prevent harm by requiring the person to undergo a psychiatric evaluation that might result in treatment for a mental illness.

Mental illness is a disorder that affects a person's behavior, thinking, and mood that can be improved by medical and psychiatric treatments. Mental disorders are described in the Diagnostic and Statistical Manual of Mental Disorders (DSM-5). The DSM-5 organizes mental disorders into classifications and describes diagnostic criteria that must be met for the practitioner to diagnose a person with a mental disorder.

Basis for Abnormal Behavior

The practitioner determines the reason for the abnormal behavior. Abnormal behavior may be attributed to a medical disorder such as diabetes mellitus, dehydration, thyroid disorder, and infection. A person who recently displays abnormal behavior might have an underlying medical disorder that is causing the problematic behavior. The DSM-5 requires that the practitioner rule out a medical disorder as the cause of the behavior before perusing a mental disorder as the cause of the behavior.

Once the patient is medically cleared, the practitioner assesses the patient for a personality disorder and psychotic disorder. A personality disorder is a maladaptive enduring pattern of behavior that is deeply ingrained in a person. The personality disorder causes the patient to experience significant functional impairment in close relationships and functioning in general society. A psychotic disorder is also maladaptive enduring pattern of behavior but the behavioral is caused by an imbalance of neurotransmitters in the brain. A neurotransmitter is a chemical substance released by the end of a nerve to transmit a signal to another nerve.

Personality Disorders

A personality consists of unique characteristics that influence how a person thinks, feels, and behaves. Characteristics may be inherited or result from a person's biology sometimes referred to how a person is "wired up."

Characteristics may result from learning from family, friends, and society in general. Everyone displays a personality but not everyone has a personality disorder. A personality disorder consists of behavior based on a personality that leads to a failure to function. A person diagnosed with a personality disorder typically thinks that his behavior is normal—the person doesn't realize a problem exists. The first step in treating a person who is diagnosed with a personality disorder is to convince the person there is a problem with his behavior. The person then undergoes psychiatric therapy to reduce the abnormal behavior.

Personality disorders are typically organized into clusters. Cluster A is odd or eccentric behaviors. Cluster B is dramatic, emotional, or erratic behaviors. Cluster C is anxious or fearful behaviors.

Cluster A personality disorders:

- Paranoid personality disorder: a person has a pervasive distrust and suspiciousness of others.
- Schizoid personality disorder: a person has a lifelong pattern of being emotionally code and fails to respond to others in a meaningful emotional way.
- Schizotypal personality disorder: a person has disturbances in thought patterns, appearance, and behavior resulting in the person feeling uncomfortable in social situations.

Cluster B personality disorders:

- Antisocial personality disorder: a person has a long-term pattern of manipulating and exploiting the rights of others often associated with criminality.
- Borderline personality disorder: a person has a long-term pattern of being unstable resulting in impulsive actions and having chaotic relations resulting in a fear of being abandoned;
- Histrionic personality disorder: a person is overly emotional and dramatic in order to draw attention to them with a low tolerance of delayed gratification and need to be the center of attention.
- Narcissistic personality disorder: a person has an excessive sense of self-importance and lacks empathy for others—criticism can result in range.

Cluster C personality disorders:

- Avoidant personality disorder: a person has a lifelong feeling of being shy and inadequate for fear of doing something wrong that leads the person to be reluctant to become involved with others.

- Dependent personality disorder: a person depends too much on others to meet the person's emotional and physical needs and overly focused on the fear of being abandoned.

- Obsessive–compulsive personality disorder: a person is preoccupied with orderliness and control and is inflexible with rules and details.

Psychotic Disorders

Psychotic disorders prevent a person to think clearly leading the person to lose touch with reality resulting in psychosis. Psychosis is a symptom of a psychotic disorder that includes delusions (false beliefs) and hallucinations (seeing or hearing things that are not heard or seen by others). Symptoms are categories as positive and negative symptoms. A positive symptom is an obvious abnormal behavior such as having a conversation when no one else is present. A negative symptom is the absence of a normal behavior such as no responding to others when they try to engage in a conversation. A chemical imbalance of neurotransmitters in the brain is believed to be the underlying cause of a psychotic disorder.

Psychotic disorders are treated with medication that helps the body return a balance to neurotransmitters thereby reducing or eliminating symptoms of the psychotic disorder and enables the person to return to normal behaviors. However, the imbalance of neurotransmitters return and so does abnormal behaviors once the patient stops taking medications.

There is a tendency for patients who are diagnosed with a psychotic disorder to become medication noncompliant. Since symptoms subside, the person "feels good" and the person is under the false belief that the medication has cured the disorder. Medication also has adverse side effects such as weight gain and sexual dysfunction. It is for this reason that patients diagnosed with a psychotic disorder return to abnormal behavior to cause readmissions to the healthcare facility to reestablish treatment.

Common Psychotic Disorders are:

- Panic disorder: The sudden feeling of terror in the absence of any sign of terror.

- Obsessive–compulsive disorder: Obsessions are thoughts that continually preoccupy a person even as the person tries to avoid those thoughts. Compulsion is an irresistible urge to behave a way that is opposite of a person's conscious desire.

- Posttraumatic stress disorder: An uncontrollable feeling of stress related to a previous stressful situation that may cause a person to behave as if the stressful situation is current.

- Bipolar Disorder: A person experiences unusual mood changes from very happy (manic) to very sad (depression).
- Depressive Disorder: A person experiences an ongoing loss of interest, loss of energy, feeling worthless that may lead to thoughts of suicide.
- Schizophrenia: Abnormal thinking that causes the person to lose touch with reality and exhibit psychosis.

Conclusion

Human beings are complex beings with physiological and psychosocial needs. Nurses, as members of the healthcare team, play a key role in meeting the healthcare needs of patients, including both their physical and their psychosocial needs. This chapter has spotlighted the psychosocial needs of patients. Key points presented include:

- Identity, body image, and role expectations all contribute to how an individual defines him- or herself and how she or he feels about him- or herself.
- Basic functions of the family may include meeting any of the following needs of the family members: physical, economic, education, socialization, nurturing, and sexual intimacy.
- Values, beliefs, past experiences, health alterations, and life stressors all influence the roles occupied and the relationships that exist within the family structure.
- Human sexuality is defined by multiple factors, including a person's gender, gender role, and sexual orientation.
- A person's physical and psychological status as well as cultural and societal expectations may influence his or her sexuality.
- Spirituality is a highly individualized experience. It is called upon to guide daily living, guide human interaction, and deal with crisis situations.
- Religion may or may not be a component of a person's spiritual dimension.
- Stress occurs when a person encounters a challenging situation. A person is able to adapt to stress if he or she has adequate coping strategies to manage the stressors. Failure to adapt leads to distress.
- Grieving is a normal response to loss (not just death) and is a highly individualized experience. There are several models of grieving, but there is no correct way or time frame for grieving.

- The establishment of a trusting relationship is critical to successful implementation of the nursing process for patients who present with psychosocial stressors.

- Nurses must be in touch with their own values and beliefs to effectively interact with patients who present with needs in the psychosocial realm.

- Behavior is the way a person acts, especially toward others in the society. Behavioral health encompasses a broad spectrum of behaviors from how a person feels, thinks, and acts and how a person handles stress throughout their life. Society determines acceptable behaviors and communicates what is acceptable through attitudes, values, authority, culture, persuasion, and genetics.

- Family, friends, and governmental agencies to intervene with or without a person's permission what a person's abnormal behavior leads to the person's failure to function adequately.

- Mental illness is a disorder that affects a person's behavior, thinking, and mood that can be improved by medical and psychiatric treatments. Mental disorders are described in the DSM-5.

- Abnormal behavior may be caused by a medical disorder, a personality disorder, or a psychotic disorder.

- Personality disorders are typically treated with psychiatric therapy, and psychotic disorders are typically treated with medication.

REVIEW QUESTIONS

1. **A psychiatric nurse is working to develop a rapport with a client in crisis. Attending is one strategy that can be used to achieve this end. Which actions by the nurse demonstrate the use of attending?**

   A. Eye contact
   B. Warm affect
   C. Closed arms
   D. A and B

2. **A client has recently been advised to seek medical treatment in relation to a lump found in her breast. The client has refused to seek the recommended treatment. A nurse assessing the client should recognize that the client's unwillingness to seek treatment may be the utilization of which defense mechanism?**

   A. Compensation
   B. Denial
   C. Displacement
   D. Regression

3. **A nurse is caring for a family that has just lost a loved one. Which is the most important need of the family members at this time?**

    A. To spend time alone with the deceased client

    B. To notify other family members

    C. To talk about their feelings

    D. To arrange for the donation of the client's organs

4. **A psychiatric nurse is counseling a client who has been diagnosed with paranoia. The nurse asks the client about his or her personal identity. Inquiring about a client's personal identity is the first step in assessing the client's overall:**

    A. Body image

    B. Self-concept

    C. Self-interest

    D. All of the above

5. **Social support is defined as a network of people who provide physical, emotional, or spiritual support for a client. Which are potential sources of social support?**

    A. Family members

    B. Church members

    C. Counselors

    D. A and B

    E. All of the above

6. **An obese client with poorly controlled type 2 diabetes says, "Nothing that I do makes a difference. My sugar just stays high." Which is the best response by the nurse?**

    A. "Of course you can make a difference. If you lose weight, your blood glucose will improve."

    B. "You have to make changes in your lifestyle. You will need to exercise more and eat less."

    C. "You sound discouraged. Tell me more about the things you have tried recently."

    D. "It is up to you. If you decide you cannot control your diabetes, you will not be successful."

7. **Which of the following is/are subcomponents of a person's gender role?**

    A. Heterosexuality

    B. Homosexuality

    C. Femininity

    D. Intersex

    E. A and B

8. **Family, friends, and government agencies are likely to intervene in which of the following behaviors?**

    A. The person wears a superhero custom at home after returning from work.

    B. The person looks unkept and dehydrated when a family member visits the person's home after receiving a call from the person's boss saying that the person hasn't showed for work in a week.

C. The person has fallen on the street. A passerby helps the person to her feet. The person refuses further assistance and walks toward the door of her house.

D. The person goes on vacation and emails his boss that he is not returning to work.

E. A person argues with her boss.

9. **You are assigned to a patient who has never been an inpatient until now. What is the best intervention?**

A. Leave the patient alone to give the patient time to adjust to being an inpatient.

B. Introduce yourself then leave patient alone to give the patient time to adjust to being an inpatient.

C. Introduce yourself, acknowledge that you understand this is the patient's first experiencing being a patient in the hospital, and then explain everything that the patient will see, hear, and do.

D. Remind the practitioner that this is the patient's first experience as a patient in a hospital.

E. Make note in the patient's chart that this is the first experience that the patient has as a patient in the hospital.

10. **What is the difference between a personality and a personality disorder?**

A. A personality is a medical disorder, and a personality disorder is a psychiatric disorder.

B. A personality is when a person has failure to function.

C. A personality disorder is a psychiatric disorder that is typically treated with medication.

D. A personality is defined in the DSM-5.

E. A personality consists of unique characteristic that influences how a person thinks, feels, and behaves. A personality disorder consists of behavior based on a personality that leads to a failure to function.

ANSWERS

Routine Checkup 1

1. False.
2. Loss of a family member
   Loss of employment
   Involvement in accidents or disasters
   Illnesses (both acute and chronic)

Routine Checkup 2

1. Physiological, psychological, social.
2. True.
3. False.

Review Questions

1. D
2. B
3. C
4. B
5. E
6. C
7. C
8. B
9. C
10. E

References

Craven RF, Hirnle CJ: *Fundamentals of Nursing: Human Health and Function*, 5th ed. Philadelphia, PA: Lippincott, 2006.

Daniels R: *Nursing Fundamentals: Caring & Clinical Decision Making*. New York, NY: Delmar Thomson Learning, 2004.

O'Brien ME: *Spirituality in Nursing: Standing on Holy Ground*, 3rd ed. Sudbury, MA: Jones and Bartlett, 2008.

Potter PA, Perry AG: *Fundamentals of Nursing*, 6th ed. St. Louis, MO: Mosby Elsevier, 2005.

Additional Resources

American Society for Reproductive Medicine: *Sexual Dysfunction and Infertility*. Available at http://www.asrm.org/uploadedFiles/ASRM_Content/Resources/Patient_Resources/Fact_Sheets_and_Info_Booklets/Sexual_Dysfunction-Fact.pdf.

Cleveland Clinic: *The Importance of Sexual Health*. Available at http://my.clevelandclinic.org/healthy_living/sexual_health/hic_the_importance_of_sexual_health.aspx.

Cleveland Clinic: *Medications that Affect Sexual Function*. Available at http://my.clevelandclinic.org/disorders/Sexual_Dysfunction/hic_Medications_that_Affect_Sexual_Function.aspx.

Mayo Clinic: *Erectile Dysfunction: Treatment and Drugs*. Available at http://www.mayoclinic.com/health/erectile-dysfunction/DS00162/DSECTION=treatments-and-drugs.

Merck: *Sexual Dysfunction in Women*. Available at http://www.merck.com/mmpe/sec18/ch251/ch251a.html.

Sears M: *Using Therapeutic Communication to Connect with Patients.* Available at http://www.stage.dnadialogues.com/wp-content/uploads/2009/10/HC_Using_Therapeutic_Communication_M_Sears.pdf.

Wikibooks: *Sociological Theory/Role Theory.* Available at http://en.wikibooks.org/wiki/Sociological_Theory/Role_Theory.

Wikipedia: *Defence Mechanism.* Available at http://en.wikipedia.org/wiki/Defence_mechanism.

Wikipedia: *Role.* Available at http://en.wikipedia.org/wiki/Role.

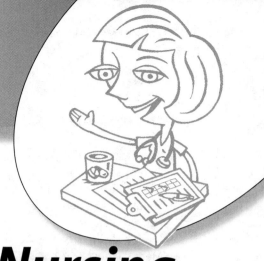

Chapter 18

Mental Health Nursing

KEY WORDS

Active listening	Milieu therapy
Axis	Models of human behavior
Chemical restraint	Nonverbal communication
Defense mechanisms	Process recording
Global assessment of functioning	Psychiatric assessment
Legal commitment	Restraint
Locked seclusion	Seclusion
Mental Health Systems Act of 1980	Therapeutic communication
Mental illness	Therapeutic relationship
Mental Status Examination	

Overview

Mental illness is a psychological or behavioral disorder that alters thinking, mood, and capability of performing activities of daily living and of relating to others. There is no medical test used to diagnose a mental disorder. Instead, practitioners use the Diagnostic and Statistical Manual of Mental Disorders, 5th Edition (DSM-5) published by the American Psychiatric Association to determine if a person is experiencing a mental disorder. The DSM-5 lists categories of mental disorders and clinically significant behaviors that are associated with a diagnosis. The practitioner uses objective and subjective information to assess the person's behavior to determine if the person has a mental disorder and, if so, specifically the disorder. The practitioner differentiates between expected behavioral change such as depression following a death and behavior that is not expected such as depression in the absence of death or other depressive situations.

Models of Human Behavior

The foundation of psychiatric and mental health nursing is based on theoretical models of human behavior. These models provide a basis for understanding a patient and diagnosing and treatment of psychiatric conditions. Models of human behavior are used collectively in caring for a patient rather than basing care on a particular model. The psychiatric nurse can apply the appropriate model to help meet the patient's needs.

- Medical model: Abnormal behavior is caused by an underlying disease that affects neurochemicals in addition to socioenvironmental factors. Treatment of the abnormal behavior focuses on addressing the underlying disease.

- Nursing model: A holistic approach is used to care for the person. The nurse focusing on the person's biopsychosocial needs develops a therapeutic relationship with that person. Nursing interventions are determined by the person's reaction to the therapeutic relationship with the nurse.

- Interpersonal model: A person's behavior is governed by the desire to be satisfied and to avoid anxiety. The nurse's therapeutic relationship with the patient develops trust that is used to satisfy the patient's needs.

- Social model: Abnormal behavior is defined by the patient's sociocultural environment. A behavior may be acceptable in one society and considered abnormal in another society.

- Behavioral model: Behavior is learned through rewards for positive behavior and punishment to prevent negative behaviors. Mental illness is considered a behavior.

- Existential model: A person should be in contact with his or her emotions and needs based on current experience. A person focused on past experiences may become self-alienated and is likely to display abnormal behavior.

- Communication model: The meaning of behavior is dependent on successful communication. Abnormal behavior occurs when communication is clouded. Normal behavior occurs when communication is clear. Degrees of clarity in communication explain degrees of abnormal behavior.

- Psychoanalytic model: Freud proposed five stages of psychosexual childhood development (oral, anal, phallic, latency, and genital). Disruption in psychosexual childhood development results in deviated behavior as an adult.

- Humanistic model: Maslow hierarchy identifies six levels of need. A person needs to meet lower-level needs before striving for higher-level needs.

  - Self-actualization: Acceptance of facts, problem solving, morality, creativity

  - Esteem: Confidence, self-esteem, respects for others and by others, achievement

  - Love/belonging: Sexual intimacy, friendship, family

- Safety: Health, security, morality
- Physiological: Food, sleep, sex, water, excretion

Therapeutic Relationship

A therapeutic relationship is a relationship between a patient and nurse that provides the framework to assist the patient resolve clinical problems, using interpersonal communication techniques. Psychiatric nurse must establish the therapeutic relationship as a clinical relationship and not friendship. At times, there can be a blur in the relationship, especially in an inpatient unit where the patient and the psychiatric nurse may develop a friendlier than clinical rapport. There is a fine but definitive line between a clinical rapport and friendship. It is the psychiatric nurse who must clearly define the difference and maintain the clinical rapport.

A therapeutic relationship also provides the foundation for the psychiatric nurse to assist the patient cope with situations that confront the patients. Processing is thinking logically through a situation to reach an appropriate response to the situation. The psychiatric nurse should not tell the patient what to do. Instead, the psychiatric nurse should ask questions that lead the patient through the process of logical thinking enabling the patient to reach his or her own decision.

The therapeutic relationship framework consists of four phases:

- Preinteraction phase: The nurse assesses unresolved problems presented by the patient with or without the patient's active participation.
- Orientations phase: The nurse is introduced to the patient and defines the nurse's and the patient's roles in the therapeutic relationship. The nurse is working with the patient—not for the patient. The objective is to develop trust and set mutually agreed-upon goals for addressing the patient's unresolved problems based on the results of the preinteraction phase. It is important to tell the patient the rules of confidentiality—what information will be shared and with whom, and what information will not be shared.
- Working phase: The nurse helps the patient examine unresolved problems and achieve goals defined during the orientations phase. A goal is to develop the patient's problem-solving ability to change resistance behaviors and embrace adaptive behaviors.
- Termination phase: The nurse ends the therapeutic relationship by summarizing accomplishments and unachieved goals of the working phase

and explores why any goal was not met. Particular care must be given to recognize that the patient may not want to terminate the therapeutic relationship. The nurse focuses on accomplishments made during the therapeutic relationship and encourages the patient to go forward with follow-up care.

Therapeutic Communication

Therapeutic communication is the primary tool used in a therapeutic relationship and involves both verbal and nonverbal communications. The transactional theory model is a model for therapeutic communication. The transactional model is a communication process where a message is sent using face-to-face communication enabling transmission of verbal and nonverbal messages simultaneously by the psychiatric nurse and the patient. Successful communication occurs when the sender's message is received as intendant by the sender.

Communication is influenced by the following factors:

- Preexisting condition: Preexisting conditions are beliefs, knowledge, developmental level, culture, social status, and religion.
- Environmental conditions: Environmental conditions are distance (the space between the nurse and the patient during the communication process); territoriality (who "owns" the space where the communication takes place; eg, the patient "owns" the space in the patient's room, the nurse "owns" the space at the nurse's station, and a conference room is a neutral territory where no one "owns" the space); and density (the number of participants in the communication).
- Nonverbal communication: Nonverbal communication factors are facial expressions, maintaining eye contact, posture, appearance, and paralanguage that convey emotion (volume, intonation of speech, and pitch that modifies meaning of the verbal message).

Therapeutic Communication Process

Therapeutic communication is effective if the psychiatric nurse follows a communication process that fosters a therapeutic relationship between the psychiatric nurse and the patient. Here are the steps to follow:

- Introduce yourself by name and title to the patient.
- Ask the patient how he or she would like to be addressed.

- Recognize that your nonverbal communication greatly influences your therapeutic relationship with the patient. The patient sees you before he or she listens to you.
- Maintain eye contact with the patient.
- Sit facing the patient using an open, relaxed posture.
- Avoid distractions.
- Provide the patient opportunity to express him- or herself.
- Focus on the patient when he or she is speaking.
- Answer the patient's questions directly and avoid giving immediate advice.
- Assess the patient's nonverbal and verbal messages separately. For example, a patient's verbal message may indicate that he or she is calm and controlled while his or her nonverbal message may indicate anxiety and agitation. Remember that a psychiatric patient's nonverbal communication (ie, behavior) is likely to be considered abnormal, and therefore it can lead to miscommunication with the nurse.
- Assess the patient's preexisting conditions.
- Respect the patient's preexisting conditions (ie, values, beliefs).
- Modify your verbal and nonverbal communications to meet the patient's communication needs.
- Be honest with patient. Explain patient's rights and limitations to confidentiality regarding the patient's treatment team, family, and friends.
- Express empathy for the patient and develop a care plan that leads the patient to self-care within his or her capabilities.

Therapeutic Communication Techniques

Therapeutic communication techniques are methods the psychiatric nurse can use to communicate with the patient so that the communication focuses on addressing the patient's clinical problems. A goal of therapeutic communication is to give the patient an opportunity to express him- or herself freely with the psychiatric nurse. The psychiatric nurse must engage in therapeutic communication using techniques that encourage the patient to speak.

Here are the commonly used techniques to encourage the patient to openly engage in communication:

- Give broad opening: Invite the patient to select the topic for discussion.
  - "I see that you would like to talk about something."

- Recognition: Acknowledge the patient and compliment him or her on the noted changes in his or her progress toward reaching a goal.
  - "You are dressing smartly today."
- Offering: Encourage the patient to continue expressing him- or herself.
  - "Can I sit with you for a few moments?"
- Accepting: Express the feeling that the patient is understood by the nurse.
  - "I understand what you are saying."
- Restating: Express the general meaning of what the patient says to be sure that the nurse correctly understands the patient.
  - "I understand that you said you are having difficulty staying awake."
- Exploring: Ask more about a statement made by the patient.
  - "Tell me more about what you saw."
- Seek clarification: Restate the patient's statement and ask the patient if your understanding is correct.
  - "I'm a little unsure what you said, can you tell me more about the situation?"
- Reflecting: Ask the patient for advice on a problem that the patient faces.
  - "What do you think is appropriate things to do?"
- Silence: The patient is given time to think before responding.
- Sequence event: Explore when events occurred.
  - "What happens next?"
- Making an observation: Verbalize an observable behavior of the patient.
  - "I see that you are picking at your skin, is something bothering you?"
- Describe perceptions: Ask the patient to say what he or she is hearing or seeing. This is useful when a patient experiences hallucinations.
  - "What do you see on the table?"
- Focusing: Return the patient to the topic that is being explored.
  - "Can we go back and talk about your childhood?"
- Reality setting: Clearly state the reality of a situation.
  - "I know you are seeing bugs on the table but there aren't any bugs."
- Translate: De-symbolize a patient's statement into true feelings.
  - "Are you saying that you feel alone?"
- Doubt: Express doubt on what the patient states.
  - "I find that is difficult to believe."

- Offering self: Tell the patient that the nurse is available to assist him or her.
  - "I will stay and talk with you for a while."
- Suggest collaboration: Encourage the patient to work with the nurse to achieve a goal.
  - "Let's come up with a goal together."
- Planning: Help the patient explore options when a problem specified by the patient presents in the future.
  - "The next time that you don't understand what the doctor is saying, ask the doctor or nurse to clarify what was said."
- Summarizing: State your understanding of what the patient stated; then permit the patient to clarify any misstatements.
  - "You and I decided to develop a goal for you the next time we meet."

Barriers to Communication

A barrier to communication is something that impairs transmission of the message or receiving the message for either the psychiatric nurse or the patient. A goal of therapeutic communication is to avoid barriers to communication. Avoiding barriers to communication is challenging since many of them are natural responses most people use in a conversation. Therefore, the psychiatric nurse must make a conscious effort to modify a natural response to a therapeutic communication response.

Here are the common barriers to communication:

- Approval/disapproval: The nurse passes judgment on the patient's statement or action. The nurse should be nonjudgmental about a patient.
  - "You made a good choice."
- Giving advice: The nurse makes a decision for the patient. The nurse should discuss options and let the patient make his or her own decision.
  - "Just say no."
- Defending: The nurse protects a person from verbal attack by a patient. The patient has the right to criticize a person or situation.
  - "Your doctor doesn't make mistakes."
- Denial: The nurse denies that a problem exists with a patient after the patient identifies a problem. This makes it difficult for the nurse to help the patient explore the problem.
  - "Your problems can be solved."

- Trite expressions: The nurse should avoid using meaningless conversations with the patient.
  - "This happens to everyone."
- Minimizing: The nurse's expression leaves the patient feeling that his or her problem is not important. The nurse should empathize with the patient.
  - "That won't hurt you."
- Interpreting: The nurse restates the patient's statement to give the statement meaning. The nurse should encourage the patient to restate his or her remarks to clarify his or her statement.
  - "You really mean to tell me that you don't like taking your medicine."
- Nonverbal negative expression: The nurse disengages from the patient leading to the patient feeling that the nurse is not interested in his or her statement.
- Value judgment: The nurse expresses negative feelings based on the patient's unacceptable behavior. The nurse should focus on acknowledging the behavior and develop a therapeutic rapport enabling the nurse to help the patient correct the behavior.
  - "How come you are eating junk food since you are overweight?"
- Changing the subject: The nurse changes the subject during a conversation with the patient.
  - "Let's talk about your childhood and we'll talk about your medicine another time."
- Reassurance: The nurse should not give the patient any false hopes. The nurse must communicate realistic outcomes.
  - "All your problems will go away in time."
- Probing: The nurse should persistently question a patient about a topic that the patient does not wish to discuss.
  - "Tell me all the times that you were arrested by the police."
- Rejecting: The nurse rejects the patient's ideas. The nurse should use therapeutic communication techniques to enable the patient to discover for him- or herself that idea is unsound.
  - "Enough! Don't tell me that again!"
- Why: The nurse should not ask the patient to provide a reason for their statements or behaviors. This places the patient in a defensive position and breaks down communication with the nurse.
  - "Why do you act that way?"

Active Listening

Active listening requires the psychiatric nurse to be attentive to what the patient is saying and use nonverbal communication to demonstrate that the nurse is listening. Active listening conveys respects for the patient and helps the patient build a trusting relationship with the nurse. Implementing active listening is challenging, especially in an inpatient unit when a psychiatric nurse is multitasking and patients are free to engage the psychiatric nurse at any time. When interacting with a patient, even for a brief moment, give the patient your full attention. If you are unable to do so, then schedule a time (ie, "let talk in 5 minutes") when you can focus fully on the patient.

Techniques for active listening are the following:

- Maintain eye contact with the patient.
- Avoid distraction during a conversation with the patient.
- Listen to the patient. Make sure that you understand what the patient is saying.
- Restate what the patient is saying. Ask the patient validate your understanding of the message.
- Request the patient to clarify any points that are unclear to you.
- Observe the patient's nonverbal communication.
- Provide appropriate feedback to the patient.

Process Recording

A process recording is a document that contains a verbatim record of the conversation between the psychiatric nurse and the patient and is used by the psychiatric nurse to assess if the conversation was therapeutic or not. Information in the processing recording is not part of the patient's chart. Processing recordings are primarily used by student nurses to improve their communication skills.

The psychiatric nurse creates a processing recording following the conversation with the patient and not during the conversation with the patient. There is a risk of distortion in the processing recording because the processing recording is dependent on the psychiatric nurse's memory of the conversation.

Both verbal and nonverbal communications are documented in the processing recording in the order in which they occurred in the conversation as illustrated in Table 18–1.

TABLE 18–1 Here is an Example of a Processing Recording			
Processing Recording			
Nurse's Response	Patient's Response	Therapeutic/Nontherapeutic	Comments
"Good evening Mr. Jones. Can we speak for a few minutes?"		Therapeutic	Giving recognition
Silent		Therapeutic	Encouraging the patient to respond
	"Yes"		Expected response
	Hesitancy and anxious		Increased anxiety noted
"Nothing to be nervous about."		Nontherapeutic	May devalue the patient's nonverbal response

Nonverbal Communication

Nonverbal communications such as facial expressions, eye contact, and tone in the patient's voice express the patient's feelings just as the patient expresses feelings through verbal communication. Nonverbal communication is referred to as a patient's affect. Listen to what the patient says and observe his or her affect. The patient's verbal and nonverbal communications should be congruent. For example, a patient's nonverbal communication should be sad if he or she is talking about his or her current depression.

A patient who is diagnosed with a psychiatric disorder may express one thought while his or her affect displays a contradictory message. The psychiatric nurse must use therapeutic communication to assess which is the true message that the patient is sending.

For example, a patient may be speaking in a calm and controlled tone with a relaxed facial expression while moving quickly toward the psychiatric nurse in a threatening posture. The psychiatric nurse must decide if the patient's intent is to threaten the nurse or to simply engage the psychiatric nurse in conversation. The psychiatric nurse can intervene by engaging the patient in conversation before the patient enters the psychiatric nurse's personal space. The conversation will elicit more information to assess. If the patient continues toward the psychiatric nurse's personal space, the nurse can extend his hand signally to the patient to stop like a police officer stops traffic. This is a nonverbal gesture that the patient should recognize and causes the patient to change his or her behavior. The patient's reaction to the psychiatric nurse's nonverbal gesture implies the patient's intent.

A patient's affect can be bizarre leading to the psychiatric nurse to respond inappropriately to the patient causing the patient to become aggressive. Therefore, the psychiatric nurse should observe and listen to the patient and then assess the patient before reacting to the patient's behavior.

For example, a psychiatric nurse takes vital signs of all patients in the unit's day room where there are jigsaw puzzle pieces spread on a table. A patient who is noted for bizarre behavior sits in a chair then suddenly moves quickly toward the psychiatric nurse. The psychiatric nurse's initial assessment is the patient is going to attack the psychiatric nurse. However, the psychiatric nurse moved to the side and the patient quickly dove under the table to pick up a puzzle piece that had fallen on the floor. The patient was diagnosed with obsessive–compulsive disorder (OCD) among other psychiatric disorders. The patient aggressively takes action to place anything out of order back in order. The situation would have escalated unnecessarily if the psychiatric nurse called for the intervention team. The intervention team, consisting of a psychiatrist, mental health aides, and supervisory staff, is able to take steps to prevent the patient from injuring him- or herself or others.

Special Needs

Normal verbal and nonverbal communication is based on what is normal for the patient based on the patient's culture, native language, education, and medical condition. The psychiatric nurse must assess if miscommunication by the patient is caused by factors other than a psychiatric disorder. Therefore, psychiatric nurses should be trained in cultural sensitivity.

The psychiatric nurse and the healthcare facility are responsible to communicate with patient and to implement processes that remove barrier to communication. For example, a translation service should be used if the patient is unable to communicate because of a language barrier or hearing impairment.

Psychiatric Barriers to Communication

A patient's psychiatric disorder can cause barriers to effective communication with a patient. The psychiatric nurse must employ techniques that overcome those barriers to engage the patient in therapeutic communication.

Here are some tips to help communicate with specific psychiatric disorders.

- Delusion: A patient who has delusions has an irrational belief but believes his or her beliefs are rational and will aggressively defend his or her irrational beliefs. The psychiatric nurse should help the patient focus on reality without agreeing or arguing about the patient's delusion.

- Thought disorders: A patient who has a thought disorder is unable to correctly understand the message sent by the psychiatric nurse. The psychiatric nurse should ask simple concrete questions and permit the patient to express him- or herself. The psychiatric nurse should then clarify the patient's answer by restating the patient's response.

- Dementia: Dementia is irreversible deterioration of the patient's mental capacity affecting memory, language, and logical thinking. The psychiatric nurse must reduce distractions from the environment and ask simple, concrete questions that leave no room for misunderstanding by the patient.

- Paranoid thinking: Paranoid thinking occurs when a patient is mistrusting of the psychiatric nurse and others. The psychiatric nurse should appear nonthreatening and make no movement that could be misinterpreted as a threat.

- Delirium: A patient who is delirious is confused and disoriented and responds inappropriately because the patient misinterprets the psychiatric nurse's statements. The psychiatric nurse should ask simple, direct questions, and reassure the patient that the nurse understands his or her answers.

- Hallucinations: A hallucination occurs when a patient hears or sees something that is not real such as hearing voices or seeing bugs. The psychiatric nurse should acknowledge that the patient is hearing or seeing something but that what he or she is hearing or seeing is not real. The psychiatric nurse should also give concise commands to redirect the patient.

- Inappropriate response: An inappropriate response occurs when the patient changes the topic to avoid answering the nurse's questions. The psychiatric nurse should listen to what the patient is saying without judging the patient. The psychiatric nurse should return to the original topic after the patient completes his or her thought.

Nursing Barriers to Communication

A psychiatric patient may display bizarre behavior during a psychiatric episode. Bizarre behavior can invoke a nontherapeutic response from the psychiatric nurse when the psychiatric nurse reacts intuitively to the patient's bizarre behavior and sends an inappropriate nonverbal message to the patient. It is important that the psychiatric nurse avoid responses that are barriers to effective therapeutic communication.

Here are some traps to avoid:

- Judging or criticizing the patient
- Stereotyping the patient
- Providing false reassurance
- Not focusing on what the patient is saying
- Criticizing other patients and staff in front of the patient
- Becoming angry or argumentative with the patient
- Asking too many questions or not giving the patient time to answer your questions
- Not letting the patient finish talking before you respond

Defense Mechanisms

A patient who experiences increased anxiety will use a defense mechanism as a way to cope with the anxiety. A defense mechanism is an unconscious effort to manipulate reality in order to maintain self-esteem and social acceptance. The psychiatric nurse must be able to identify behavior as a defense mechanism in order to focus on the underlying issue that caused the patient to invoke the defense mechanism.

For example, a patient who denies that he or she has a chronic illness is expressing a defense mechanism as a way of coping with the distressful situation. A patient's denial is likely to interfere with treatment of the illness in that the patient will not take prescribed medication or be compliant with follow-up care. The psychiatric nurse must recognize the defense mechanism and then intervene to address the patient's anxiety related to the diagnosis of a chronic illness. The patient should be able to avoid using the denial defense mechanism once he or she accepts that he or she has a chronic illness. There are many defense mechanisms. Defense mechanisms can be classified as pathological, immature, neurotic, and mature.

Here are the common defense mechanisms:

Pathological

- Conversion: A patient presents with physiological symptoms with no explanation, such as the patient who suddenly limbs for unknown medical reason. Conversion is also known as hysteria.

- Delusional projection: A patient has delusions of being persecuted, such as a patient who states that the staff is picking on him or her.
- Denial: A patient refuses to accept reality such as the patient denies that he or she has a chronic illness.
- Distortion: A patient redefines reality to justify the patient's perception of reality, such as the patient did not abuse prescribe medication. Only a few extra pills make him or her feel better.
- Splitting: A patient views a person or situation as either good or bad, such as the patient telling the nurse that the physician is not a capable medical practitioner.

Immature

- Acting out: A patient expresses destructive behavior to him- or herself or others in an effort to gain attention because of his or her inability to cope with reality, such as a patient who self-inflicts superficial cuts on his or her wrist to gain the attention of the staff.
- Fantasy: A patient enters into unrealistic beliefs when the patient is unable to cope with reality, such as a patient who believes that he or she does not have a mental illness.
- Idealization: A patient perceives that another individual has more positive attributes than that patient has, such as a patient who perceives that a nurse is better than a patient.
- Passive aggression: A patient is an obstructionist demonstrated by procrastination, learned helplessness, stubbornness, and a deliberate attempt to fail, such as a patient who refuses to speak with the physician because the patient dislikes medication that the physician prescribed to him or her.
- Protection: A patient shifts his or her unacceptable feelings to someone else such as prejudice and jealousy, such as a patient saying that a politician was elected because of his or her race.
- Somatization: Negative feelings toward others are transformed in a patient's pain, anxiety, or illness, such as a patient who becomes anxious when seeing a staff member he or she dislikes.

Neurotic

- Dissociation: A patient temporarily postpones feeling to avoid emotional distress, such as a patient who shows no emotions following a motor vehicle accident.

- Intellectualization: A patient distances him- or herself from emotional distress by focusing on the intellectual components of a situation through rituals, magical thinking, and rationalization, such as a patient who procedurally describes a traumatic event.

- Rationalization: A patient makes excuses through faulty reasoning that a wrongful act was either not done or he or she was justified for performing the wrongful act, such as a patient who states that he or she had to take his or her sister's car without permission because he or she had a job interview.

- Isolation: A patient separates feeling from an emotional event while describing the event, such as a patient who describes death of his or her parent in concrete terms.

- Displacement: A patient redirects an emotional response to a less threatening person such as a wife yelling at her husband when she received a traffic ticket rather than to the police officer who issued the ticket.

- Reaction formation: A patient displays a behavior opposite to the behavior that he or she wants to display such as being calm when the patient faces dangerous situation.

- Repression: A patient moves thoughts of a disturbing event to the unconscious, preventing the thoughts from entering consciousness such as lack of awareness or memory lapse, such as a patient who says he or she does not recall if his or her father abused medication when his or her father died of a drug overdose.

- Regression: A patient temporarily reverts to an earlier stage of development rather than coping with a situation in an age-appropriate way such as a patient who throws a tantrum when he or she does not get a room change.

- Undoing: A patient attempts to reverse an unacceptable behavior by doing an acceptable behavior, such as a patient who acts out and then behaves like an ideal patient.

- Withdrawal: A patient removes him- or herself from an interaction fearfully because it will cause the patient to recall painful thoughts, such as an aunt who lost her only son refrains from attending family gatherings.

- Hypochondriasis: A patient is excessively focused on having an illness, such as a patient who frequents a physician asking the physician to authorize unnecessary medical tests.

Mature

- Sublimation: A patient transforms a negative emotion into a positive emotion, such as a patient learns new job skills after losing employment.

- Identification: A patient unconsciously adopts the characteristics and behaviors of another person, such as a patient adopting the perceived characteristics of a celebrity.

- Altruism: A patient experiences personal satisfaction by helping others, such as serving food to residents of a homeless shelter.

- Thought suppression: A patient consciously avoids coping with an unpleasant event by pushing thoughts of the event into the preconscious such as a patient faced with credit card bills.

- Introjection: A patient identifies with an object to the extent that the object becomes part of the person such as a car that brings perceived social status to the patient.

- Anticipation: A patient plans on how to handle a discomfort that will occur in the future such as planning for death of a pet.

- Humor: A patient uses witticism or self-deprecation to express feelings that are too unpleasant to address seriously such as making light of death.

Legal Environment

Psychiatric patients have the same rights as other patients even if the patient's illness leaves them with limited function. The patient has the right to humane treatment and the right to self-determination within the patient's ability to function.

The Mental Health Systems Act of 1980 created a bill of rights for psychiatric patients. The bill of rights states that

- Treatment must be provided by a quality staff in the least restrictive setting based on the patient's treatment plan. The patient has an expectation of privacy and must be provided comfortable accommodations, recreation, and an appropriate diet.

- The psychiatric nurse must ensure to inform the patient of his or her diagnosis and understands and participates in the patient's treatment plan within the patient's ability. It must be clearly documented why the patient is unable to understand or participate in the treatment plan based on objective evidence.

- The patient must be told how to prepare for discharge.

- The patient has the right to consent to treatment, to refuse treatment, and to be discharged from the hospital.

- The patient has the right to marry, have children, choose their own lifestyle, and use contraception.

Legal Commitment

Legal commitment is a process by which a judge requires a patient to undergo treatment. Commitment laws are set by state statue and are therefore unique to each state. Generally, the commitment process is

- The patient demonstrates bizarre behavior that risks injury to him- or herself, others, or property.
- Someone calls the police. Depending on state law, the police may have authority to bring the patient to the hospital's emergency department without the patient's consent. Some states require a crisis psychiatric evaluation to be performed on site by a trained evaluator to assess if the patient should be brought to the hospital without consent. The crisis psychiatric evaluator makes an independent, objective determination if the patient is a danger to him- or herself, others, or property. If so, then the patient is taken to the emergency department.
- Once in the emergency department, two psychiatrists must independently determine if the patient is a danger to him- or herself, others, or property. If so, then the patient is committed to the hospital. The patient becomes an involuntary patient and cannot leave the hospital.
- Within 72 hours of the commitment, the patient has a hearing before a judge. The patient is provided a legal counsel whose job is to guard the patient rights. The patient's healthcare team led by the psychiatrist presents evidence why the patient to remain committed. The judge determines the disposition of the patient.

The judge can also order that the patient receives medication against his or her wishes. The order may describe a three-step process for administering medication.

1. The patient is offered medication as a pill or liquid.
2. If the patient refuses, he or she is offered the medication as an injection.
3. If the patient refuses, then the order states that the medication is administered as an injection.

The psychiatrist can at any time discharge the patient or make the patient a voluntary patient if the psychiatrist determines the patient is no longer a danger to him- or herself, others, or property. For example, a patient diagnosed with schizophrenia may become noncompliant with medication resulting in bizarre behavior. Once the patient becomes medication compliant, then the patient is no longer a danger to him- or herself, others, or property, and therefore must be made voluntary.

A voluntary patient may not have the right to immediate discharge from the hospital. Depending on state law, the patient who wishes to leave the hospital can ask the psychiatrist to discharge him or her. The psychiatrist can refuse to discharge the patient. The patient then signs a document that officially notifies the psychiatrist that the patient wants to be discharged from the hospital. The psychiatrist has 48 hours to respond to the patient's request. During the 48 hours, the psychiatrist assesses the patient to determine if the patient is a danger to him- or herself, others, or property. If so, then the psychiatrist must commit the patient. If not, then the psychiatrist must discharge the patient.

Competency to Give Informed Consent

A patient must be competent to give informed consent for treatment and be of age to give consent based on state law, which is commonly 18 years of age. If the patient is not of age to give consent, then the patient's parents or legal guardian will make the decision for the patient.

For an adult patient, the psychiatric nurse must make sure that the patient is competent to give consent based on assessment of the patient's mental status. The patient must

- Be alert and oriented to time, place, person, and situation
- Be able to be attentive and to concentrate
- Be able to understand
- Be able to reason using abstract concepts
- Be able to reason logically
- Be able to communicate

If the patient is not competent to give consent, then the psychiatrist may commit the patient. If the patient remains incompetent after treatment, then a judge will likely appoint a guardian for the patient until the patient is deemed competent by a psychiatrist.

It is important to understand that a patient can be competent even if the patient has been committed to the hospital by a judge. Commitment means that the patient is a danger to him- or herself, others, or property, and it does not mean that the patient is incompetent.

Patient Rights

The American Hospital Association's Patient's Bill of Rights, the American Nursing Association's Code of Ethics, and Health Insurance Portability and Accountability Act (HIPAA) regulations specify patient's rights. Within these regulations, a hospital has the right to create and enforce policies that limit a patient's right compared to a person who is not hospitalized. For example, smoking might be prohibited and the patient's diet may be restricted to food provided by the hospital.

The patient has the following rights:

- All communications between the patient and healthcare team are confidential.
- The patient's records are confidential.
- The patient can refuse to have his or her photo taken.
- The patient can decide who, if anyone, has access to his or her record. Written consent must be acquired before any information, including if the patient is at the hospital, can be released.
- The patient can rescind consent to share information.

There are three exceptions to the patient privacy rules that allow release of patient information:

1. A patient states he or she will harm another person upon discharge and the patient is being discharged. The healthcare team has a duty to warn the prospective victim.

2. A court order.

3. Education: Patient information contained in the patient's record can be used for educational purpose as long as the patient's identity is expunged from the record.

Seclusion and Restraints

Seclusion is placing the patient in a room that isolates the patient from other patients when the patient becomes agitated and is at risk of injuring him- or herself or others. The seclusion room typically has a bed. There is nothing in the room that can be used by the patient to injure him- or herself.

Open seclusion can be used to give the patient a time-out to compose him- or herself away from the distraction and stimulus of the unit. In this scenario, the seclusion door is open and the patient is free to leave the seclusion room at any time.

Locked seclusion is placing the patient in the seclusion room and locking the door, preventing the patient from leaving the room if he or she becomes violent. The key to the door must always be inserted in the lock so that the door can be opened in an emergency.

Restraint is physically preventing the patient from injuring him- or herself or others through the use of force such as holding a patient or strapping the patient to a bed. Placing a patient in a bed and raising four rails are also considered a restraint because the rails prevent the patient from leaving the bed.

Hospital policy will dictate who can place a patient in seclusion, locked seclusion, and in restraints. For example, a registered nurse can direct the staff to place the patient in seclusion without a follow-up assessment by a practitioner. Likewise in some hospitals, a registered nurse can place the patient in locked seclusion or restraint; however, a practitioner must be notified and assess the patient within an hour and determine if the patient should remain in locked seclusion or restraint.

Special procedures must be followed if the patient is in restraints. Depending on hospital policy,

- The patient must be placed on consent observation.
- The patient must be asked if he or she needs to use the toilet or wants water or food frequently.
- Vital signs are taken at a prescribed frequency.
- The patient's circulation must be assessed every 15 minutes.
- The practitioner must assess the patient and renew the order at a set frequency depending on the age of the patient.
- The patient must be assessed and the restraint must be documented every 15 minutes.
- The practitioner must release the patient from restraints once the patient is no longer a risk of injuring him- or herself or others.

Chemical restraint is restraining the patient through the use of medication, which is illegal. Practitioners commonly prescribe Ativan 2 mg, Haldol 5 mg, and Cogentin 1 mg to the patient for extreme agitation, which is part of the patient's treatment plan. This combination of medication has a clamming effect and reduces the use of locked seclusion and restraints. The patient is offered the medication by mouth or injection. Medication that is part of the patient's treatment plan is not considered a chemical restraint.

Psychiatric Therapies

Psychiatric therapies are treatments that focus on improving a patient psychiatric diagnosis to the point where the patient can be functional in society within the patient's limitations. Psychiatric therapies fall into the following five categories:

- Milieu therapy: Milieu therapy is a therapeutic approach that uses shared responsibilities and rules within a therapeutic community to influence changes in the patient's behavior and attitudes.

- Counseling therapy: Counseling therapy is a therapeutic approach where the therapist helps the patient think through problems by presenting a logical approach to problem solving and encouraging the patient to consider consequences of potential decisions before making the decision.

- Psychotherapy: Psychotherapy is a therapeutic approach that explores the underlying cause of the psychiatric disorder with the goal of changing behavior and attitudes. Common psychotherapies are as follows:

  - Crisis intervention: A crisis is a situation where the patient becomes overwhelmed and lacks the coping skills to address the crisis. Crisis intervention is a therapeutic approach that helps the patient deal with the crisis.

  - Cognitive therapy: Cognitive therapy is a therapeutic approach that identifies and alters the patient's negative feelings about him- or herself.

  - Individual therapy: Individual therapy is a therapeutic approach where a therapist works one-on-one with the patient to identify and resolve the patient's psychiatric problems.

  - Group therapy: Group therapy is a therapeutic approach where a therapist works with a small group of patients who experience the same or similar psychiatric problems to resolve those problems with assistance from other members of the group.

  - Family therapy: Family therapy is a therapeutic approach that focuses on behavior that interferes with a working family relationship. One or more members of the family may have psychiatric problems, which are resolved during family therapy sessions.

- Drug therapy: Drug therapy is a therapeutic approach that uses medications to modify the chemical balance in the brain that results in change in behavior and attitudes.

- Behavior therapy: Behavior therapy is a therapeutic approach that focuses on unlearning unacceptable behaviors and replaces them with acceptable behaviors through training. Here are common behavior therapies:

- Desensitization: Desensitization is used to treat patients who experience phobias by gradually exposing the patient to the situation that causes the patient's anxiety while coaching the patient to relax.

- Flooding: Flooding is used to treat phobias by exposing the patient to the situation that causes the patient's anxiety and allow him or her to experience anxiety. The patient remains in the situation without coaching and is expected to confront the problem. The patient's anxiety will reduce over time and he or she will be able to cope with the situation.

- Positive conditioning: Positive conditioning exposes a patient to positive reinforcement while gradually exposing the patient to the situation that causes the patient's anxiety.

- Aversion therapy: Aversion therapy introduces a painful stimulus whenever the patient has an undesirable behavior with the expectations that the patient will avoid the undesirable behavior to avoid the painful stimulus.

- Response prevention: Response prevention is used to treat patients who experience compulsive behavior by redirecting or distracting the patient when he or she is about to express the compulsive behavior.

- Token economy: A token economy is a behavior therapy technique that rewards a patient with a token each time the patient performs an acceptable behavior. At some point during the day, the patient is able to exchange tokens for a privilege or something that the patient's values.

- Thought stopping: Thought stopping requires the patient to realizing he or she is having unacceptable thoughts and the say "stop" then refocuses on positive thoughts.

- Thought switching: Thought switching requires the patient to substitute positive thoughts with unacceptable thoughts.

- Assertiveness training: Assertiveness training shows the patient how to express feelings and actions without developing guilt over his or her feelings or actions.

Psychiatric Assessment Tests

Psychiatric assessment tests may provide insight into a patient's problem at the moment that the patient is administered the test. A psychiatric test is different than medical tests, it may be used to definitively diagnose a patient, but there is no psychiatric test that definitively diagnoses a psychiatric disorder.

These tests can also be used to estimate the effectiveness of treatment. First, the patient is administered the test and the score is noted in the patient's chart.

This is the patient's baseline score. The test is readministered several weeks after treatment begins. The score is compared to the baseline score to determine if there was any improvement in the patient's condition.

A psychiatric assessment test is no substitution for a thorough psychiatric evaluation. Some practitioners do not administer psychiatric assessment tests to patients who reside in an inpatient facility because a hospitalized patient is contently being observed by psychiatric nurses and seen by a practitioner daily.

It is important to consider the patient's physical and cognitive abilities before administering a psychiatric assessment test. Any impairment or barriers such as language in the patient's ability to comprehend instructions on the test and to take the test may invalidate the results.

Here are commonly administered psychiatric assessment tests:

- Beck depression inventory: The beck depression inventory is a self-administered and self-scored test that asks the patient to identify symptoms of depression that he or she may be experiencing.
- Minnesota multiphasic personality inventory (MMPI): The MMPI is a written test that assesses the patient's personality traits and helps identify if the patient has a potential for being violent and a risk for suicide.
- Thematic apperception test: The thematic apperception test is used to assess the patient's interpersonal relationships and conflicts as well as personality traits. During the test, the patient is presented with pictures of ambiguous situations and asked to tell the examiner what the patient believes is happening in the picture.
- Rorschach test: The Rorschach test is similar to the thematic apperception test except that the patient is shown 10 inkblots and is asked to describe what he or she sees.
- Sentence completion test: The sentence completion test is used to assess the patient's anxieties, aspirations, and other elements of his or her personality. During the test, the test administrator asks the patient to complete a series of sentences such as "When I am angry I…"
- Functional dementia scale: The functional dementia scale measures the patient's ability to perform activities of daily living. During the test, the patient is asked to do things such as putting on clothes and pouring juice to assess how well he or she can care for him- or herself.
- Global deterioration scale: The global deterioration scale assesses primary degenerative dementia. The patient is tested for neurological function such as memory and orientation.

- Cognitive capacity screening examination: The cognitive capacity screening examination assesses the patient's cognitive ability by testing his or her memory, language, and calculation skills.
- Cognitive assessment scale: The cognitive assessment scale measures the patient's cognitive ability by testing his or her psychomotor functions, general knowledge, and mental capability.

American Nurses Association (ANA) Standards of Care

The American Nurses Association (ANA) developed a standard of care that nurses are expected to follow in the care of patients diagnosed with mental illness. The standard provides a framework within which the psychiatric nurse provides clinical actions to care for the patient. The psychiatric nurse is expected to assess the patient, determine one or more nursing diagnoses, and then identify desired outcomes for patient care. Next, the psychiatric nurse develops a care plan and nursing interventions to achieve those outcomes.

Assessment
The psychiatric nurse is expected to collect healthcare information about the patient during the assessment interview to create a database of patient information based on subjective statements made by the patient and objective observation of the patient's behavior. The psychiatric nurse must be aware that the patient's physical speaking capability, culture, and knowledge of the language can limit the patient's responses. Those limitations are not caused by mental illness.

Diagnosis
The psychiatric nurse analyzes the database of patient information to determine if there is a pattern of information that may lead to a psychiatric nursing diagnosis. The nurse psychiatric must be aware that signs and symptoms of a physical illness mimic a mental illness. For example, a patient who has hypothyroidism may experience signs of depression. A patient who has hyperthyroidism may experience signs of anxiety or a hypomanic episode.

Outcome
An outcome is a goal to improve or relieve one or more signs and symptoms of mental illness based on the patient's diagnosis. For example, an outcome for a patient who has anxiety may be to identify two coping skills that reduce the anxiety.

Planning

The psychiatric nurse develops a care plan for the patient to achieve his or her outcome. The care plan defines long-term goals. Each long-term goal is divided into one or more short-term goals. Each short-term goal contains evidence-based interventions that lead to completion of the short-term goal. These are interventions that are known to lead to the desired outcome.

Implementation

The psychiatric nurse implements interventions daily and documents the outcome of the intervention. There are eight categories of interventions in psychiatric nursing:

1. Counseling: The psychiatric nurse provides one-on-one and group counseling that focuses on developing coping skills and behavioral changes that encourage good mental health and reduce the likelihood of relapse.

2. Milieu therapy: A milieu is a therapeutic community structure within which patients reside and interact with staff and other patients. There are community rules, community meetings, and patient assignments to help the community function. The psychiatric nurse is expected to maintain the milieu.

3. Promote self-care activities: The psychiatric nurse develops a care plan with the goal that the patient will perform activities of daily living with minimal support from staff.

4. Psychobiological interventions: The psychiatric nurse will administer medications as prescribed and evaluate the effectiveness of the medication.

5. Health teaching: The psychiatric nurse will teach patients on nutrition and other self-care tasks that result in healthy living.

6. Case management: The psychiatric nurse will coordinate patient care with others on the healthcare team to ensure that patient receives timely, appropriate treatment.

7. Health promotion and health maintenance: The psychiatric nurse implements interventions that encourage the patient to maintain healthy mental health and prevent the patient from experiencing psychiatric illness.

8. Evaluation: The psychiatric nurse is expected to evaluate the patient's goals and intervention ongoing to determine if the care plan is achieving the desired outcome. The care plan is modified if outcomes are not achieved.

Axis

A psychiatric diagnosis is divided into five sections called an axis. Each section provides specific information about a patient's condition. A psychiatric diagnosis is a medical diagnosis made by a practitioner based on a psychiatric evaluation and physical assessment. The psychiatric diagnosis is used to assist the psychiatric nurse to develop the patient's care plan.

Axis I: clinical disorder such as depression, bipolar, anxiety disorders

Axis II: personality disorders and mental retardation

Axis III: general medical condition

Axis IV: psychosocial and environmental problems such as lack of a support system

Axis V: global assessment of functioning (GAF) describes the person's social, psychological, and employment capabilities as a value between 0 and 100.

Global Assessment of Functioning

The GAF is a subjective scale (Table 18–2) assigned to a patient based on his or her social, occupational, and psychological functionality. The value

TABLE 18–2 Global Assessment of Functioning Scale	
91–100	Asymptomatic: The person is able to handle life's problems.
81–90	Minimal symptoms: The person may experience mild anxiety an occasional argument but otherwise can handle life's problems.
71–80	Transient symptoms: Symptoms are expected reactions to stressors. The person experiences slight impairment such as difficulty concentrating after an argument or temporarily falls behind schedule.
61–70	Mild symptoms: The person generally functions well. The person may experience mild insomnia, depressed mood, occasional absence from work without cause, or theft within the family.
51–60	Moderate symptoms: The person has difficulty at work or in social environments. The person presents with occasional panic attacks, flat affect, circumstantial speech, few friends, or conflict with associates.
41–50	Serious symptoms: The person is unable to maintain employment, has no friends, expresses suicidal ideation, antisocial behavior such as stealing, and performs severe obsessional rituals.
31–40	Impaired reality testing: The patient is unable to work, depressed, neglects family, or avoids friends. The person is defiant, assaultive, moody, demonstrates poor judgment, and illogical thinking.
21–30	Behavior influenced by delusions or hallucinations: The person acts grossly inappropriate or unable to function. The patient is incoherent, remains in bed, no friends, unemployed, and preoccupied with suicide.
11–20	Danger of hurting self or others: The patient has attempted suicide no expectation of death, manic, violent, incoherent, or has poor personal hygiene.
1–10	Persistent danger of hurting self or others: The person displays recurrent violence, suicidal attempt with expectation of death or unable to maintain personal hygiene.
0	Unable to assess due to lack of information.

assigned to the patient by a practitioner is associated with his or her ability to perform activities of daily living and the capability of addressing problems associated with living. The practitioner assessment is based on subjective data provided by the patient, family, and friends, and objective data gathered during the practitioner's psychiatric evaluation of the patient. The GAF value is used to evaluate the patient's level of care and treatment outcome. For example, a patient with a GAF value greater than 50 might be treated as an outpatient facility while a patient with a GAF value 50 or lower might be better treated in an inpatient facility. The success of a patient's treatment is measured by an appreciable increase in the patient's GAF value.

Nursing Assessment

The psychiatric nursing assessment follows a process that identifies the patient's psychosocial deficits and strengths that form the foundation for a diagnosis, desired outcome, and care plan that address the patient's deficits. The psychiatric interview is the primary tool used to assess a psychiatric patient. The interview provides the opportunity for the psychiatric nurse to assess the patient's psychological functioning and identify the underlying cause that lead, the patient to seek psychiatric help. The goal of a psychiatric interview is to gather a database of information about the patient that is used to help the psychiatric nurse understand the patient's problems.

Here are the tips for conducting the psychiatric interview:

- Observe the patient's affect and the way the patient answers questions while developing a database of information about him or her. Being fearful that the answer may be embarrassing or expose the patient to undesired consequences such as legal charges, he or she may avoid answering questions that probe sensitive areas of his or her background.

- Do not pressurize the patient for information. If the patient is uncomfortable to answer a question, note the patient's response and move on to the next question.

- Be mindful that the patient may not be a good historian, especially if the patient is experiencing a psychiatric episode. The patient provides subjective data that must be verified by other sources after the interview is completed.

Here are guidelines for conducting the psychiatric interview:

Begin the Interview

- Introduce yourself and ask the patient how the patient would like to be addressed.
- Explain the purpose of the interview and tell the patient that you will be making notes during the interview to help you remember what the patient said.
- Tell the patient how the information will be used in treatment of the patient and who will and who will not have access to this information.
- Explain that information cannot be shared with anyone who is not part of the patient's healthcare team unless the patient grants written consent to share the information with specific individuals such as the patient's spouse.
- Conduct the interview in a private neutral place such as a conference room.
- Position yourself closest to the door and the patient furthest from the door for safety. The patient should not be able to block your egress from the room should the patient become aggressive during the interview.
- Present a calm, nonthreatening, friendly attitude, which encourages the patient to be open and participate in the interview process.

Chief Complaint

- Begin the interview with an open-ended question such as "what brings you here today." The goal is to identify the patient's chief complaint.
- Ask the patient to describe the chief complaint as onset, severity, duration, and impact on his or her life. Some patients may report nothing wrong because they are unaware of their psychiatric problem.
- Write down exactly what the patient says and note the patient's affect.

Biographical and Family Data

- Ask the patient for biographical data such as age, birthplace, marital status, and ethnic origin. The psychiatric nurse must be aware that cultural beliefs can influence the patient's responses to questions.
- Move the interview toward socioeconomic data such as employment, education, financial status, and housing. How does the patient support him- or herself?
- Explore the patient's family. Identify parents, step-parents, foster patients, siblings, and children. Determine if any family member has had a

psychiatric or medical disorder. Assess the relationships between the patient and family members. How frequently does the patient interact with family members? Will family members be involved in the patient's care?

Personality and Psychosocial History

- Inquire about the patient's personality by asking how the patient copes with stress, controls impulses, and judgment. Assess for clues that indicate the patient's capabilities to adapt.
- Explore the patient's lifestyle such as hobbies, spirituality, support network, relationships, marriage, divorce, children, home life, use of drugs and tobacco, diet, and sleeping.

Psychiatric History

- Focus the interview on the patient's psychiatric history. Has the patient ever been seen by a practitioner as outpatient or inpatient for symptoms of psychiatric disorders such as depression or manic episodes? Ask if the patient ever experienced suicidal ideations or attempt to commit suicide. Does the patient have a history of self-mutilation such as cutting his or her arms or legs? Assess if the patient has ever experienced any psychological disturbance?
- Explore any psychiatric episode that the patient mentions during the interview. Gather as much details related to episode including the number of episodes, when they occurred, what preceded the episode, and a complete description of the episode. Focus questioning on treatment and follow-up care. Ask the patient to tell you about the treatment. Find out if the patient was compliant with medication and follow-up care.

Physical and Medical History

- Take a full medical history of the patient. A psychiatric patient's medical condition must also be diagnosed and treated.
- Ask if the patient has any acute or chronic illnesses or has any surgical history.
- Determine if the patient has been diagnosed with a thyroid disorder. Hypothyroidism mimics symptoms of depression. Hyperthyroidism can mimic systems of a hypomanic episode.

- Ask if the patient has been diagnosed with diabetes mellitus. Symptoms of low or high blood sugar may resemble signs of psychiatric conditions.

- Determine medications that the patient takes, including psychiatric and nonpsychiatric medications, over-the-counter medications, and herbal medication. Ask the patient for the dose and frequency of each medication and see if the patient can show you all his or her medication bottles.

- Ask the patient why he or she is taking each medication and if the patient feels the medication is effective.

- Identify allergies.

- The psychiatric nurse or the practitioner should perform a complete physical that includes screening tests to assess body function such as kidney, liver, and metabolic disorders.

- A pregnancy test must be performed on all female patients before any psychiatric medication is administered to the patient. Some psychiatric medications are not safe to take if the patient is pregnant.

Suicide Assessment

The psychiatric nurse must assist and advise a patient against the risk of suicide during each encounter with the patient. A patient may express suicidal ideation with or without a plan. Suicidal ideation is the thought of suicide. Those thoughts may be expressed explicitly by suicidal statements to the psychiatric nurse, staff, other patients, friends, and family. Suicidal ideation may be implied by the patient's actions such as giving away possessions, saying goodbye to family and friends, or preparing to close out their life.

The suicide risk assessment evaluates factors that may lead a patient to suicidal ideation. When performing a suicide risk assessment, evaluate the patient for the following characteristics. The existence of one or more characteristics does not mean the patient may have a tendency to attempt suicide. A thorough psychiatric evaluation must be performed to determine if the patient is a suicide risk.

- Current suicide attempt
- Current suicidal ideation with or without plan
- History of suicide attempt, especially within the last year
- Family history of suicide or suicide attempts
- Depression
- Anxiety
- Impulsivity

- Self-injury behaviors
- Loss of pleasure
- Insomnia
- Hopelessness
- Helplessness
- Poor concentration
- Medical condition
- Psychiatric condition (psychosis, substance abuse, schizophrenia)
- History of physical, emotional, sexual abuse
- Incarcerated

If a patient is a suicide risk based on the suicide risk assessment, ask the patient if he or she has any thoughts of hurting him- or herself. Also, ask the patient to contract for safety. A contract for safety is a verbal agreement between the patient and the staff that states should the patient have feelings to hurt him- or herself, that the patient will tell the staff before taking any actions so the staff can help the patient. If a patient refuses to contract for safety, then he or she should remain on constant observation until a practitioner is able to perform a thorough psychiatric evaluation. Constant observation means that a staff member must be within 5 ft of the patient at all times including when toileting.

Patients who are high risk for suicide must be placed in a safe environment that includes

- No strings, shoe laces, belts, electrical cord.
- No sharp objects such as scissors, knives, pens, pencils, and nail clippers.
- Controlled access to the outside such as locked doors to the unit and windows that have limited openings.
- All glass in the unit must be safety glass.
- Only safety razors and supervised shaving.
- Telephone cords must be shortened.
- All items on the unit that can be used as a weapon including furniture, pipes, and fixtures that can be broken by the patient must be removed.

A patient who contracts for safety may still have suicidal ideation and may attempt suicide on the unit. A patient may have a secret plan to commit suicide; therefore, the staff must be on constant alert for activities that may indicate the patient's intentions. For example, the patient may be pretending to take medication but instead saving medication to be taken all at one time in an attempt to overdose on medication.

Likewise, a patient may carefully monitor the unit's routine to discover a time when staff is distracted and not watching the patient such as meal time and shift change. This gives the patient time to attempt suicide. It takes less than 15 minutes to tie a sheet over the bathroom door and around the patient's neck, stand on the toilet, and jump, breaking the patient's neck.

Always assess for change in behavior when a patient is deemed a suicide risk. A patient who is hopeless, helpless, depressed, and remains in bed all day probably lacks the energy to attempt suicide. However, be on high alert when that same patient is happy, socializing, and engaging with staff because the patient has the energy to commit suicide. The practitioner must evaluate the patient to assess if the change in behavior is related to successful treatment or a façade presented by the patient to conceal his or her suicidal ideation.

Mental Status Examination

A mental status examination is used to assess the patient's psychological function and dysfunction that might have led the patient to ask for help. The mental status examination focuses on the patient's cognitive functions such as judgment, reasoning, problem solving, thought pattern, and other factors that can provide insight into the patient's mental function.

Here are questions to ask when conducting the mental status examination. Figure 18–1 illustrates where the examination results are documented in an electronic medical record (EMR).

Appearance

- Is the patient appropriately groomed and dressed?
  - Abnormal: Disheveled, inappropriately applied cosmetics.
- Does the patient dress appropriately for his or her age?
  - Abnormal: Dresses older or younger for his or her age.
- Does the patient maintain proper hygiene?
  - Abnormal: Odor, poorly maintained teeth, nail, and hair.
- Does the patient hold an erect posture?
  - Abnormal: Slouch, stiff posture, head lowered.
- Is the patient's weight appropriate to his or her height and have good nutritional status?
  - Abnormal: Overweight, underweight

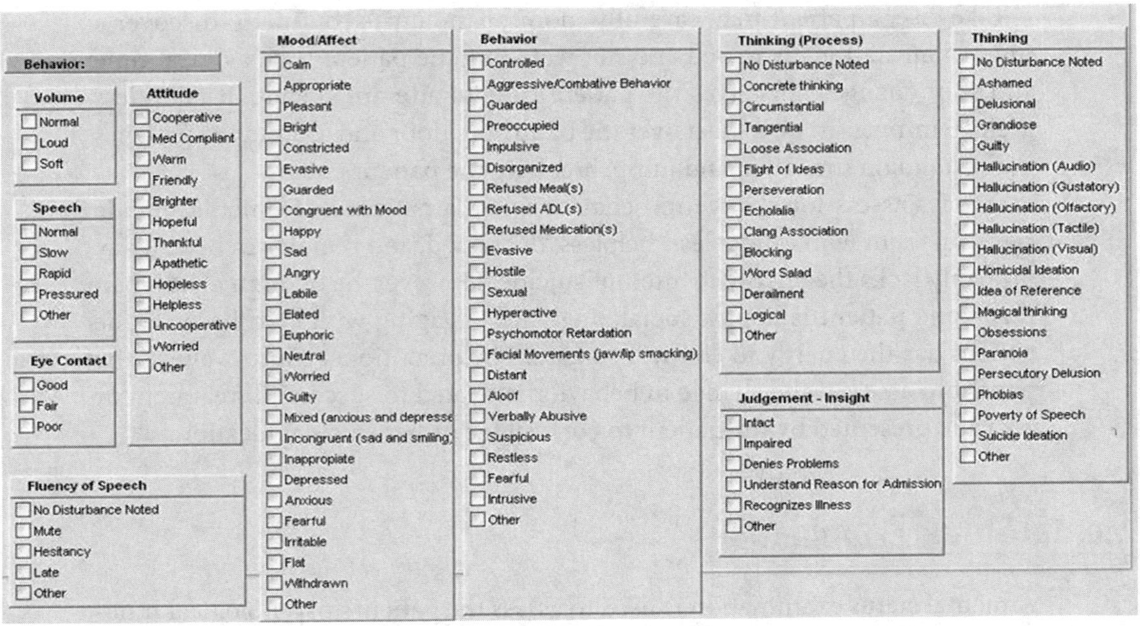

Behavior:

Volume
- Normal
- Loud
- Soft

Attitude
- Cooperative
- Med Compliant
- Warm
- Friendly
- Brighter
- Hopeful
- Thankful
- Apathetic
- Hopeless
- Helpless
- Uncooperative
- Worried
- Other

Speech
- Normal
- Slow
- Rapid
- Pressured
- Other

Eye Contact
- Good
- Fair
- Poor

Fluency of Speech
- No Disturbance Noted
- Mute
- Hesitancy
- Late
- Other

Mood/Affect
- Calm
- Appropriate
- Pleasant
- Bright
- Constricted
- Evasive
- Guarded
- Congruent with Mood
- Happy
- Sad
- Angry
- Labile
- Elated
- Euphoric
- Neutral
- Worried
- Guilty
- Mixed (anxious and depresse
- Incongruent (sad and smiling)
- Inappropriate
- Depressed
- Anxious
- Fearful
- Irritable
- Flat
- Withdrawn
- Other

Behavior
- Controlled
- Aggressive/Combative Behavior
- Guarded
- Preoccupied
- Impulsive
- Disorganized
- Refused Meal(s)
- Refused ADL(s)
- Refused Medication(s)
- Evasive
- Hostile
- Sexual
- Hyperactive
- Psychomotor Retardation
- Facial Movements (jaw/lip smacking)
- Distant
- Aloof
- Verbally Abusive
- Suspicious
- Restless
- Fearful
- Intrusive
- Other

Thinking (Process)
- No Disturbance Noted
- Concrete thinking
- Circumstantial
- Tangential
- Loose Association
- Flight of Ideas
- Perseveration
- Echolalia
- Clang Association
- Blocking
- Word Salad
- Derailment
- Logical
- Other

Judgement - Insight
- Intact
- Impaired
- Denies Problems
- Understand Reason for Admission
- Recognizes Illness
- Other

Thinking
- No Disturbance Noted
- Ashamed
- Delusional
- Grandiose
- Guilty
- Hallucination (Audio)
- Hallucination (Gustatory)
- Hallucination (Olfactory)
- Hallucination (Tactile)
- Hallucination (Visual)
- Homicidal Ideation
- Idea of Reference
- Magical thinking
- Obsessions
- Paranoia
- Persecutory Delusion
- Phobias
- Poverty of Speech
- Suicide Ideation
- Other

FIGURE 18–1 • After examining the patients, results of the mental status examination are recorded by checking appropriate boxes in the electronic medical record.

- Does the patient have a normal gait?
  - Abnormal: Slow, fast, unsteady gait.
- Does the patient appear alert and have normal facial expressions?
  - Abnormal: Sleepy, flat expression.
- Does the patient make and maintain proper eye contact?
  - Abnormal: Poor eye contact, blank stare, stares at you, breaks eye contact, looks at the floor, or around the room.
- Is the patient's affect congruent with what the patient is saying?
  - Abnormal: Sadness, overly happy.
- Is the patient's behavior appropriate during the examination?
  - Abnormal: hostile, uncooperative, indifferent, distance, tense, overly responsive, nonresponsive.
- Are mannerisms appropriate?
  - Abnormal: Restlessness, nail biting, appears to listening to someone who is not there or seeing things that are not there.

- Is the patient's speech appropriate?
  - Abnormal: Fast or slow place, illogical responses, over productive (uses too many words), under productive (uses too few words), loud or soft, defects in speech, delays responding to questions, or flight of ideas.

Affect and Mood

- Does the patient experience a full range of emotions?
  - Abnormal: Depressed, manic, no emotion, mood swings, or patient is unable to discuss his or her emotions.
- Is the patient's affect congruent with his or her mood?
  - Abnormal: Neutral, flat, depressed, hypomanic, manic, liable (rapid change in a range of emotions), or mood is inconsistent with body language.
- Is the patient calm and in control?
  - Abnormal: Overly excited, depressed, trembling, angry, provoking, sweating, or crying.

Orientation

- What is your name? Where are you? What is today's date?
  - Abnormal: Unable to respond with the correct answers.

Memory

- Ask the patient to repeat the words apple, house, and umbrella immediately to test immediate recall.
  - Abnormal: Patient is unable to repeat all the words.
- Continue with the assessment. After 5 minutes, ask the patient to recall the three words to test delayed recall.
  - Abnormal: Patient is unable to repeat all the words.
- Ask the patient about something that happened to the patient in the past day to test the patient's recent memory.
  - Abnormal: Patient is unable to recall the event.
- Ask the patient about the neighborhood where he or she grew up to test the patient's remote memory.
  - Abnormal: Patient is unable to recall the neighborhood.
- Ask the patient to count backward from 100 by subtracting 7 to test the patient's attention status. Stop after five or six irritations.

- Abnormal: Patient is unable to perform the subtraction.
- Ask the patient to read and explain a news story to test the patient's comprehension ability.
  - Abnormal: Patient is unable to explain the news story.
- Ask the patient what is meant by the expression "no man is an island" to assess the patient's ability to think abstractly.
  - Abnormal: Patient is unable to explain the expression or explains the expression in concrete terms.

Judgment, Perception, and Insight

Explore the patient's ability to make rational judgments and have a realistic sense of reality. Also, assess the patient's insight into the patient's clinical problem.

- Ask the patient what he or she would do if he or she was unable to keep an outpatient appointment.
  - Abnormal: Any response that implies the patient would not reschedule the appointment.
- Ask the patient what is the role of the practitioner?
  - Abnormal: Any response that implies the patient does not perceive that the practitioner is there to help the patient.
- Ask the patient what might be causing his or her symptoms?
  - Abnormal: The patient's response shows no insight into his or her disorder.

Thought, Delusions, and Sensory Perception

Thought processing explores how the patient thinks and what the patient says and whether what the patient says is based on reality. The patient should be focused on answering the nurse's questions and not be easily distracted or seems to be responding to internal stimuli.

Abnormal thought processing occurs when the patient experiences one of the followings:

- Circumstantial thinking: The conversation drifts off the point of discussion and then eventually returns and addresses the point.
- Flight of ideas: The conversation changes quickly to a series of unrelated topics.
- Loose associations: The conversation moves to a different but related topic.
- Tangential thinking: The patient's response is without reference to the question.

- Thought blocking: The patient's speech is interrupted before the patient completes the thought.

- Preservation: The patient uses few words to respond to questions.

- Word salad: The patient responds using real words when sentences are incoherent.

- Thought broadcasting: The patient believes his or her thoughts are being transmitted into the environment.

- Thought insertion: The patient believes someone is inserting thoughts into his or her mind.

- Magical thinking: The patient has an irrational belief that causes an event such as placing a spell on a person will cause the person to experience an adverse event.

- Ideas of reference: The patient believes that an event has occurred although the patient has no involvement in the event such as the patient feels this is the cause of an air crash.

- Depersonalization: The patient loses all sense of identity and expresses feelings that are different from his or her normal feelings. For example, the patient may feel as if he or she is outside his or her body.

- Delusion: The patient has false belief even when presented with evidence to the contrary.

- Phobias: The patient has an irrational fear of a situation such as fear that an elevator will fall when he or she rides an elevator.

- Obsession: The patient is unable to stop thinking about an idea such as becoming a billionaire.

- Sensory perception: The patient experience misperceptions referred to as an illusion or hallucination. An illusion is caused by the presence of an external stimulus such as reflection of the sun on the desert giving the illusion of water. A hallucination occurs in the absence of an external stimulus such as hearing voices when no one is speaking (auditory), seeing things that are not there (visual), touching things that are not there (tactile), tasting things that are not present (gustatory), and smelling things that are not there (olfactory).

Cognitive Ability

Cognitive ability is the patient's capacity to remember, understand, reason, and problem solve. Be aware of factors that may influence the patient's response. For example, a patient who has been inpatient for several days may not recall the month and date because he or she is disoriented related to disruption in his or her normal schedule. Likewise, the patient's culture and primary language may provide misleading results. A patient whose primary language is other than English may have difficulty responding to questions. The patient may not have completed formal education.

Level of Consciousness

- Ask the patient his or her name, where he or she is, and the date and month.
  - Abnormal: Confused, slow to respond or sedated.

Memory

- Immediate memory is assessed by telling the patient a series of numbers. Wait 10 seconds and ask the patient to repeat those numbers forward and backward.
  - Abnormal: The patient is unable to repeat the series of numbers forward and backward.
- Recent memory is assessed by asking the patient about an event that he or she was involved in yesterday. Be sure that you can verify the event.
  - Abnormal: The patient is unable to recall any portion of the event.
- Remote memory is assessed by asking the patient where he or she was born or about schools he or she attended.
  - Abnormal: The patient is unable to recall those events.

Concentration

- Ask the patient to start with 100 and continue to subtract 7 the remainder for five iterations.
- Ask the patient to say the months of the year backward.
  - Abnormal: The patient is unable to answer these questions within a reasonable time period.

Abstract Thinking

- Ask the patient to interpret the meaning of common proverbs such as
  - A stitch in time saves nine
  - A bird in the hand is worth two in the bush
- Ask the patient to identify similarities between

- A bicycle and bus
- Orange and apple
- Abnormal: The patient is unable to interpret proverbs or compare similarities between pairs of objects.

Judgment

- Ask the patient questions whose answers give you insight into the ability to make rational judgment.
  - Abnormal: The patient describes situations where demonstrated poor judgment such as blaming others for his or her poor behavior.

Psychosocial Assessment

The psychosocial assessment collects objective data about the patient's responsibilities, education, employment, family, spirituality, resources, and culture. Each element of the psychosocial assessment can introduce stressors into the patient's life that could be an underlying cause of his or her mental status.

Summarize the data and ask the patient to verify that the information you recorded is accurate based on the patient's knowledge. Remember that the information is based on the patient's ability and willingness to share the information with you. The patient may not be a good historian. The information you collected may not be accurate. You must be aware of the patient's culture and cultural healthcare practices because the patient's culture may influence the patient's responses.

Validate the information provided by the patient with a secondary source after the patient gives you written consent. Secondary sources are family, friends, social services agencies, and healthcare providers, who were treating the patient prior to admission.

Ask the patient the following questions:

- What is your primary language?
- How do you support yourself (ie, employed, disability benefits, unemployment insurance, state subsidy)?
- Where do you live (ie, house, apartment, homeless)?
- Who do you live with (ie, significant other, alone)?
- Tell me about your family.
- Do you have children? If so, then ask for detailed information about each child.
- What is a typical day like for you?

- Do you practice or belong to any religion or spiritual group?
- What role does religion or spirituality play in your life?
- Describe your cultural background.
- What do you do when you are upset?
- What relieves your stress?
- Does the patient have a positive attitude?
- Is the patient able to meet basic needs?
- Can the patient live independently?
- Is the patient able to make rational decisions?
- Does the patient have insight into his or her illness?
- Does the patient want to participate in treatment?
- Does the patient have a support system of family and friends?

Medication and Medical Assessment

The medication assessment collects objective data about the patient's medication. The assessment must explore the patient's use of prescribed, over-the-counter, and herbal/supplements medication, and street drugs. Keep in mind that the patient may not be a good historian, and therefore the psychiatric nurse should verify all reported medication with the patient's prescriber and pharmacy, if possible. Always ask the patient or the patient's family to bring the patient's medication to the facility to enable you to properly identify medication prescribed to the patient.

The medial assessment collects information about the patient's general health. These include allergies, diet, acute or chronic medical conditions, pregnancy, and recent labs and medical tests result. Enter the results into the patient's EMR (Figure 18–2).

Here are the following questions to answer:

- What is the name of medication?
- What is the dosage?

Home Meds	Dose	Route	Frequency
SEROQUEL	300MG	BY MOUTH	BEDTIME
NEURONTIN	300 MG	BY MOUTH	3 XDAY
BACLOFEN	10 MG	BY MOUTH	3 X DAY
LISINOPRIL	10 MG	BY MOUTH	DAILY
VENLAFAXINE	75 MG	BY MOUTH	3 X DAY
NALTREXONE	50 MG	BY MOUTH	DAILY
CARISOPRODOL	350 MG	BY MOUTH	2 X DAY

FIGURE 18–2 · It is important that all medications taken by the patient are documented in the electronic medical record.

- How do you take the medication (route)?
- How frequently do you take the medication?
- What is the prescriber's name and contact information?
- How long have you been taking the medication?
- Why the medication is prescribed.
- Has the patient experienced side effects?
- Has the patient experience good results taking the medication?
- Is the patient compliant taking the medication? If not then, why?

If the patient uses street drugs, then ask the following questions

- What street drugs do you use?
- How much do you use?
- How frequently do you use?
- What is your behavior when you are under the influence of street drugs?
- When was the drug last used? Be alert that the patient may experience withdrawal symptoms if the patient uses street drugs regularly but has not used in the past several hours. Withdrawal symptoms can be severe and lead to seizures and delirium, depending on the drug.
- Have you ever overdosed? If so, was it intentional or accidental?
- Have you ever attended a drug rehabilitation program? If so, ask for details.

Summarize the Nursing Assessment

The psychiatric nursing assessment summary is a document that describes the psychiatric nurse's findings and becomes a database of information used by the healthcare team to treat the patient. The psychiatric nursing summary contains the following sections:

Identifying Data
This section identifies the patient to the reader.

- "The patient is a 45-year-old-single Caucasian man."

Chief Complaint
This section is the patient's description of why the patient came to the hospital.

"I want to get off street drugs."

History of Present Illness

The psychiatric nurse describes background of the patient's chief complaint based on the psychiatric nursing assessment of the patient.

- "The patient presented with symptoms of alcohol and opioid withdrawal and is seeking detox. The patient has a history of dependence on alcohol, opioid, and cocaine that has led to severe impairment in his functioning. The patient denies any suicidal or homicidal ideations."

Present Medications

This section contains a listing of all medications prescribed to the patient along with any herbal or over-the-counter medications and supplements.

- Trazodone 100 mg PO at bedtime for insomnia.
- Metoprolol-XL 50 mg PO daily for hypertension.
- Lisinopril 20 mg PO twice a day for hypertension.
- Vistaril 50 mg PO every six hours as needed for anxiety.
- Spironolactone 25 mg PO twice daily for fluid retention.

Past Psychiatric History

In this section, the psychiatric nurse describes the patient's psychiatric history based on interviews with the patients and review of the patient's medical records.

- "The patient has a history of polysubstance dependency for more than 20 years. The patient uses alcohol, opioid, cocaine, and benzodiazepine daily. The patient has had five inpatient admissions in the Mentally Ill Chemically Addicted (MICA) unit and six inpatient admissions in the detox unit. The patient is currently being seen in the outpatient clinic."

Past Medical History

This second describes the patient's medical problems.

- "Hypertension, edema"

Social and Family History

This section describes the patient's psychosocial assessment.

- "The patient is a single unemployed construction worker living alone in an apartment. The patient last worked 9 months ago. The patient's parents are deceased from natural causes. The patient has one sibling, a brother who has a history of polysubstance dependence (alcohol, opioid, cocaine) and has been in recovery for 5 years. The patient has no other living relative."

Mental Status Examination

This section describes the nurse's assessment of the patient's mental status.

- "Alert and orient X3. Appearance appropriate. Speech normal. Though processes coherent. Thought associations intact. Mood and affect anxious. Denies auditory and visual hallucinations. Denies suicidal and homicidal ideations. Memory, attention span, and concentration are intact. Insight, judgment, and impulse control adequate."

Assessment of Risk or Violence to Self or Others

This section describes if the patient's behavior could put the patient or others in danger.

- "The patient denies any suicidal or homicidal ideations. Imminent risk is minimal."

Strengths

This section describes positive features displayed by the patient.

- "The patient is seeking help and willing to participate in treatment."

Weaknesses

This section describes negative features displayed by the patient.

- "History of substance abuse."

Initial Formulation

This section summarizes the nurse's assessment of the patient.

- "This is a 45-year-old man who is seeking inpatient treatment for polysubstance dependence that leads to severe impairment of his functioning."

Problem List

This section itemizes problems that must be addressed during the patient's admission:

- Polysubstance dependence
- Withdrawal
- Anxiety
- Hypertension

Developing a Nursing Diagnosis

A nursing diagnosis provides the basis for a nursing short- and long-term outcomes and nursing interventions that will achieve those outcomes.

The North American Nursing Diagnosis Association (NANDA) defines acceptable nursing diagnosis.

There are three elements of a nursing diagnosis:

1. Problem: The problem describes the deficiencies that are presented by the patient during the nursing assessment.

Example: Substance dependency.

2. Etiology: The etiology is the probable cause that contributes to nursing diagnosis.

Example: Substance dependency related to ineffective coping skills.

3. Supporting data: Supporting data are the objective evidence that support the nursing diagnosis.

Example: Substance dependency related to ineffective coping skills as evidenced by multiple relapses.

Two categories of goals are established for each nursing diagnosis: one long-term goal that specifies the long-term treatment objective and one or more short-term goals each creating short-term treatment objectives. The long-term goal is achieved when all short-term goals are achieved.

1. Long-term goal

Example: The patient will achieve and/or maintain sobriety.

2. Short-term goal

Example: Identify 2 or 3 stressors in their lives and identify 2–3 coping skills or strategies to handle the stressors.

The final step in developing a nursing diagnosis is to identify nursing interventions for each short-term goal. A nursing intervention is an activity performed by a nurse whose outcome helps to achieve the related short-term goal. Goals and interventions should be entered in the patient's care plan (Figure 18–3).

Example: The nurse will speak with the patient for 15 minutes each shift to help the patient identify a stressor and help the patient identify coping skills to handle the stressor.

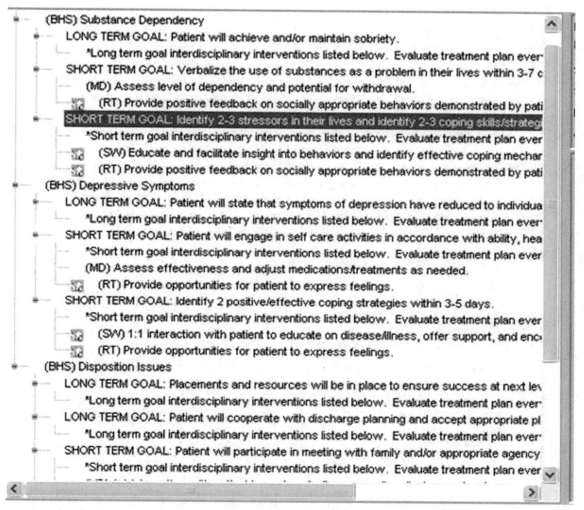

(BHS) Substance Dependency
    LONG TERM GOAL: Patient will achieve and/or maintain sobriety.
        *Long term goal interdisciplinary interventions listed below. Evaluate treatment plan ever·
    SHORT TERM GOAL: Verbalize the use of substances as a problem in their lives within 3-7 c
        (MD) Assess level of dependency and potential for withdrawal.
        (RT) Provide positive feedback on socially appropriate behaviors demonstrated by pati
    SHORT TERM GOAL: Identify 2-3 stressors in their lives and identify 2-3 coping skills/strateg·
        *Short term goal interdisciplinary interventions listed below. Evaluate treatment plan ever
        (SW) Educate and facilitate insight into behaviors and identify effective coping mechar
        (RT) Provide positive feedback on socially appropriate behaviors demonstrated by pati
(BHS) Depressive Symptoms
    LONG TERM GOAL: Patient will state that symptoms of depression have reduced to individua
        *Long term goal interdisciplinary interventions listed below. Evaluate treatment plan ever·
    SHORT TERM GOAL: Patient will engage in self care activities in accordance with ability, hea
        *Short term goal interdisciplinary interventions listed below. Evaluate treatment plan ever
        (MD) Assess effectiveness and adjust medications/treatments as needed.
        (RT) Provide opportunities for patient to express feelings.
    SHORT TERM GOAL: Identify 2 positive/effective coping strategies within 3-5 days.
        *Short term goal interdisciplinary interventions listed below. Evaluate treatment plan ever
        (SW) 1:1 interaction with patient to educate on disease/illness, offer support, and enc·
        (RT) Provide opportunities for patient to express feelings.
(BHS) Disposition Issues
    LONG TERM GOAL: Placements and resources will be in place to ensure success at next lev
        *Long term goal interdisciplinary interventions listed below. Evaluate treatment plan ever·
    LONG TERM GOAL: Patient will cooperate with discharge planning and accept appropriate pl
        *Long term goal interdisciplinary interventions listed below. Evaluate treatment plan ever·
    SHORT TERM GOAL: Patient will participate in meeting with family and/or appropriate agency
        *Short term goal interdisciplinary interventions listed below. Evaluate treatment plan ever

FIGURE 18–3 · Long-term and short-term goals along with corresponding interventions are entered into the patient's care plan in the electronic medical record.

CASE STUDY

CASE 1

A 23-year-old female patient diagnosed with depressive disorder and personality disorder has hospitalized in an inpatient acute psychiatric unit for 3 days. Hospital policy states that patients are permitted to use the telephone at the nurse's desk for 10 minutes each shift. The patient made a 10-minute phone call at the beginning of the shift and asks the charge nurse for permission to make another telephone call. The charge nurse says no. The patient tells the charge nurse that the staff on the previous shift let her make three phone calls because they were important phone calls. A few minutes later after noticing that the charge nurse is in the chart office, the patient asks the (Certified Nursing Assistant) CNA to make another telephone call. The CNA says no and the patient responds with the same statement.

QUESTION 1. What is the patient doing?

ANSWER The patient is splitting staff by asking each staff member for permission to use the phone knowing that the patient has exhausted her phone privileges for the shift.

QUESTION 2. How would you respond to this situation?

ANSWER The best response is to set boundaries for the patient such as enforcing the policy on when a patient is permitted to use the telephone at the nurse's station. Each staff member must enforce the policy. The patient will realize that she will not be rewarded by receiving additional telephone privileges by rewarding staff.

REVIEW QUESTIONS

1. **The psychiatric nurse on an inpatient acute unit notices a patient pacing the floor looking side-to-side quickly. What should the psychiatric nurse first?**
   A. Call the practitioners
   B. Medicate the patient
   C. Use therapeutic communication
   D. Place the patient in the seclusion room

2. **A 53-year-old woman is nearing discharge from an inpatient acute unit. The patient was admitted 15 days ago for chronic depression following 2 months of noncompliant with medication. The patient lives alone in an apartment that is subsided by social services. The social worker wants the patient to move to a group home where she can have assisted living and socialize with her peers. The**

patient approaches the psychiatric nurse and asks what should she do? How should the psychiatric nurse respond?

A. Tell the patient that she will enjoy living in the group home because others will be there to help her.

B. Tell the patient that she should live independently but need to take her medication as prescribed by the practitioner.

C. Tell the patient to speak with the social worker.

D. Help the patient process her options letting the patient make the final decision.

3. A 73-year-old man is wandering the hallway in the dementia unit during dinner time. The hallway is lined with many doors some opening to patient rooms and others to closets. All doors are clearly marked. What should the psychiatric nurse do first?

A. Take the patient to the dining room.

B. Ask the patient if he needs to use the bathroom.

C. Ask the patient if he is a little confused.

D. Medicate the patient.

4. A 34-year-old man is admitted to the acute inpatient unit with a diagnosis of schizophrenia paranoid type. He arrives in a wheelchair then stands at the nurse's station staring in all directions. The psychiatric nurse introduces herself and the patient stares silently in her direction. What should the psychiatric nurse do first?

A. Medicate the patient.

B. Call the practitioner.

C. Calmly walk the patient into the seclusion room.

D. Maintain a friendly tone and calmly explain the admission process and explain any activity that the patient may be seeing around the nurse's station.

5. A 63-year-old divorced woman, mother of four adult children, is admitted voluntarily to an acute inpatient unit for detoxing from Xanax. The patient says, "I get a little anxious since all my kids moved out of the house 4 years ago. My doctor prescribed me Xanax to help me." According to the report from the emergency department, the patient was prescribed a 30 day supply of Xanax and used the entire supply in 3 days. The patient has six practitioners each prescribing Xanax unbeknown to the others. The patient is careful to have prescriptions filled in different pharmacies throughout the county to prevent pharmacists from discovering her plan. The patient tells the psychiatric nurse, "I don't know why they put me here with all these drug addicts. I'm not one of them. My doctor prescribes me my medication." What is the best explanation for the patient's statement?

A. The patient is displaying the distorted defense mechanism.

B. The high dose of Xanax has made the patient delusional.

C. The patient is displaying dissociation defense mechanism.

D. The patient is displaying the undoing defense mechanism.

6. A 20-year-old man is brought to the acute inpatient unit and diagnosed with major depressive disorder. Two days before admission to the unit, the patient told his mother that he did not want to live anymore since his girlfriend broke up with him over the weekend. The patient's mother called the police who convinced the patient to go to the emergency department for medication. The patient calmly told the ER psychiatrist that he had no suicide plan and really had no intention to kill himself. With some arm twisting, the patient agreed to be admitted for overnight observation. Early the next morning, the patient tells the psychiatric nurse that he is ready to go home. What is the best response?

   A. I'll get your paperwork ready now. You'll be discharged in a couple of hours.
   B. Talk to the psychiatrist.
   C. You cannot be discharged for 48 hours.
   D. Speak with the psychiatrist. The psychiatrist can discharge you or ask you to stay for further observation or treatment. If you disagree with the psychiatrist, you can sign a 48-hour notice that informs the psychiatrist that you want to be discharged within the next 48 hours. According to our state law, the psychiatrist must discharge you at the end of the 48 hours if the psychiatrist does not feel you are a danger to yourself or others.

7. A 43-year-old female patient is brought to the hospital for bizarre behavior. The patient had been noncompliant with medication for 2 months. The patient was committed to the acute involuntary unit of the hospital. Four weeks after being medicated the patient showed normal behavior but remained involuntary. The charge psychiatric nurse asked a new psychiatric nurse to have the patient sign consent forms. What is the best response?

   A. The new psychiatric nurse should explain the consent form to the patient and ask the patient to sign the form.
   B. The new psychiatric nurse should tell the charge psychiatric nurse that the patient is not competent to sign the form because she is an involuntary patient.
   C. The new psychiatric nurse should assess the patient to determine if the patient is competent. If so, then explain the consent form to the patient and ask the patient to sign the form.
   D. The new psychiatric nurse should tell the charge psychiatric nurse that she is not comfortable asking the patient to sign the document.

8. A 33-year-old male patient is admitted to an acute inpatient unit for anxiety disorder enters a verbal altercation with another patient over selection of a television program for evening viewing. The psychiatric nurse separated the patients. The 33-year-old male walked the hallway shouting flaring his arms. What is the psychiatric nurse's first response?

   A. Medicate the patient.
   B. Place the patient in the seclusion room in four point restraints.
   C. Place the patient in the seclusion room.
   D. Use active listening and therapeutic communication to de-escalate the patient.

9. A new psychiatric nurse is conducting the admission assessment with a 24-year-old female patient diagnosed with bipolar I disorder and borderline personality.

The patient is calm and cooperative. On the report the new psychiatric nurse learns that the patient stopped taking medication 1 month ago and voluntarily took herself to the hospital to have her medication adjusted. The only interviewing area available was in a vacant social worker's office down the hallway from the nurse's station. The new psychiatric nurse sat at the desk located in the center of the room and the patient sat in a chair near the door. The door was open during the interview. All the other patients were in group therapy while the interview was being conducted. Upon learning of the assessment, the charge psychiatric nurse reprimanded the new psychiatric nurse. Why was it necessary to reprimand the new psychiatric nurse?

A. The psychiatric new nurse was using the social worker's office for the assessment.

B. The new psychiatric nurse placed herself at risk.

C. The new psychiatric nurse violated HIPAA law.

D. The charge psychiatric nurse had no cause to reprimand the new psychiatric nurse.

10. **A 42-year-old woman, single, living alone, is brought to the emergency department by her sister. Her sister received a call from the patient's employer saying that the patient had missed work for the past week and he was concerned about her safety. Her sister found the patient lying in bed, the apartment was in disarray, dishes unwashed in the sink, and the patient had poor hygiene. The patient told her sister that she had lost interest in everything over the past several months. All she wanted to do is sleep. What should the psychiatric nurse in the emergency do first?**

A. Place the patient on constant observation knowing that a patient with depression may attempt suicide.

B. Ask the practitioner if she wants to order a thyroid test panel.

C. Ask the practitioner if she wants to order a CT scan of the brain.

D. Prepare the paperwork so the practitioner can commit the patient.

ANSWERS

Review Questions

1. C. Use therapeutic communication. Rationale: The patient is displaying anxiety that can easily escalate to agitation. Therapeutic communication helps to explore and addresses the underlying cause of anxiety.

2. D. Help the patient process her options letting the patient make the final decision. Rationale: Do not give advice or make a decision for the patient. Help the patient reach a decision.

3. B. Ask the patient if he needs to use the bathroom. Rationale: Ask simple, concrete questions that leave no room from misunderstanding by the patient.

4. D. Maintain a friendly tone and calmly explain the admission process and explain any activity that the patient may be seeing around the nurse's station. Rationale: The psychiatric nurse should appear nonthreatening and make no movement that

could be misinterpreted as a threat. Explaining what the patient is seeing helps the patient to recognize that those activities are nonthreatening. The patient will become less paranoid and more functional in due course.

5. A. The patient is displaying the distorted defense mechanism. Rationale: The patient redefines reality to the justify the patient's perception of reality.

6. D. Speak with the psychiatrist. The psychiatrist can discharge you or ask you to stay for further observation or treatment. If you disagree with the psychiatrist, you can sign a 48-hour notice that informs the psychiatrist that you want to be discharged within the next 48 hours. According to our state law, the psychiatrist must discharge you at the end of the 48 hours if the psychiatrist does not feel you are a danger to yourself or others. Rationale: The psychiatric nurse explained the discharge process to the patient.

7. C. The new psychiatric nurse should assess the patient to determine if the patient is competent. If so, then explain the consent form to the patient and ask the patient to sign the form. Rationale: An involuntary status does not make a patient incompetent. The psychiatric nurse assesses if the patient is:
   • Alert and oriented to time, place, person, and situation
   • Able to be attentive and to concentrate
   • Able to understand
   • Able to reason using abstract concepts
   • Able to reason logically
   • Able to communicate

8. D. Use active listening and therapeutic communication to de-escalate the patient. Rationale: The psychiatric nurse must use the least restrictive technique to control the situations such therapeutic communication, medication by mouth, open seclusion (give the patient time out away from distractions), intramuscular medication, four-point restraints.

9. B. The new psychiatric nurse placed herself at risk. Rationale: Position yourself closest to the door and the patient furthest from the door for safety. The patient should not be able to block your egress from the room should the patient become aggressive during the interview.

10. B. Ask the practitioner if she wants to order a thyroid test panel. Rationale: Determine if the patient has a thyroid disorder. Hypothyroidism mimics symptoms of depression.

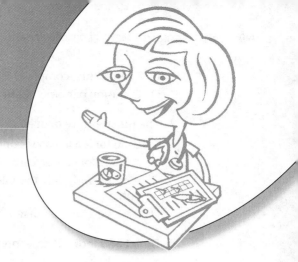

Final Exam

1. **Nurses can best avoid or defend negligence or lawsuits by following which principles?**
   A. Providing proper care and documenting such care accurately
   B. Knowing the standard of care, delivering the care that meets the standard, and documenting care accurately and concisely
   C. Knowing the standard of care, delivering the care that meets the standard, and taking responsibility for such care
   D. Knowing the standard of care, knowing state laws, and gaining the client's confidence

2. **The Registered Nurse derives diagnoses based on:**
   A. Assessment data
   B. Medical diagnoses
   C. Expected outcomes
   D. Strategies and alternatives for expected outcomes

3. **Planning nursing care requires which of the following?**
   A. Critical thinking
   B. Complete knowledge of the client's condition

C. Client's chief complaint

D. Exclusion of home treatment measures

4. **The nursing care plan is:**

A. Used for legal reasons only

B. A guide for clinical care

C. A guide with only the interventions necessary to meet the client's expected outcomes

D. Reserved for the nurse who writes the plan

5. **Direct and indirect care interventions include those that are:**

A. Specified in protocols

B. Specified in standing orders

C. Performed through interaction with the client

D. Nurse initiated, physician initiated, and collaborative

6. **During evaluation, the nurse determines the effectiveness of a specific nursing action by:**

A. Speaking with the client

B. Speaking with the family

C. Comparing the client's response with expected outcomes

D. Comparing the client's response with other clients who have received such care

7. **Empathy is:**

A. A nontherapeutic technique

B. Expressing approval or disapproval

C. The ability to understand and accept another person's reality, accurately perceive feelings, and communicate this understanding

D. The ability to express concern, sorrow, or pity for the client generated by the nurse's personal identification with the client's needs

8. **The nurse demonstrates active listening to the client by:**

A. Facing the client, assuming a relaxed posture, and making intermittent eye contact

B. Facing the client, assuming a relaxed posture, and making constant eye contact

C. Facing the client and nodding to show agreement

D. Smiling, making eye contact, and crossing arms and legs to appear relaxed

9. **Who conceptualized the five stages of grief?**

A. Dorothea Lynde Dix

B. John Bowlby

C. Elisabeth Kubler-Ross

D. L.H. Levy

10. **The five stages of grief are:**
    A. Disbelief, anger, questioning, spirituality, and acceptance
    B. Shock, anger, guilt, disbelief, and anger
    C. Denial, guilt, bargaining, shock, and depression
    D. Denial, anger, bargaining, depression, and acceptance

11. **The point at which a stimulus is perceived as painful is:**
    A. Breakthrough pain
    B. Pain
    C. Pain tolerance
    D. The pain threshold

12. **Which of the following contribute to development of pressure ulcers?**
    A. Immobility, friction and shear forces, increased moisture, impaired sensory perception, disease process, and age-related skin changes
    B. Immobility, decreased tissue perfusion, decreased nutrition, friction and shear forces, increased moisture, impaired sensory perception, and age-related skin changes
    C. Immobility, decreased tissue perfusion, friction and shear forces, bone fractures, and age-related skin changes
    D. Immobility, decreased tissue perfusion, decreased nutrition, increased moisture, bone fractures, use of anticoagulants, and age-related skin changes

13. **A client has pneumonia with thick, tenacious secretions. Which of the following initial actions would help liquefy the secretions?**
    A. Immediately obtain a prescription for an expectorant.
    B. Keep the room temperature cool.
    C. Keep the room temperature warm.
    D. Encourage the client to increase oral fluid intake.

14. **Pain is categorized according to its duration, location, and etiology. Three basic categories of pain are:**
    A. Acute, breakthrough, and chronic
    B. Acute, chronic (nonmalignant), and cancer related
    C. Acute, chronic, and stable
    D. Dull, aching, and throbbing

15. **Which of the following is an example of an opioid antagonist commonly used to reverse respiratory depression?**
    A. Naloxone (Narcan)
    B. Naltrexone (Depade, RiVia)

    C. Morphine sulfate

    D. Acetaminophen (Tylenol)

16. When assessing a child's pain level, one pain scale that is especially suited is the:

    A. Faces Pain Scale

    B. Verbal Pain Scale

    C. The 10-cm Baseline Scale

    D. Written Pain Scale

17. Approximately what percent of a typical adult male's weight consists of fluid (water and electrolytes)?

    A. 40%

    B. 50%

    C. 60%

    D. 80%

18. Body fluid is located in two fluid compartments. Approximately two-thirds of body fluid is in which compartment?

    A. The extracellular compartment

    B. The intracellular compartment

    C. The intravascular compartment

    D. The interstitial compartment

19. Major electrolytes in body fluids that carry positive charges are:

    A. Chloride, bicarbonate, phosphate, sulfate, and organic acids

    B. Chloride, bicarbonate, sodium, calcium, and sulfate

    C. Sodium, potassium, chloride, phosphate, and hydrogen ions

    D. Sodium, potassium, calcium, magnesium, and hydrogen ions

20. Fluid volume deficit can develop rapidly. Important characteristics that the nurse should watch for are:

    A. Thirst, decreased skin turgor, and increased blood urea nitrogen (BUN) level

    B. Thirst, nausea, orthostatic hypotension, and decreased skin turgor

    C. Thirst, nausea, decreased BUN level, and orthostatic hypotension

    D. Thirst, edema, distended neck veins, and increased BUN level

21. A high arterial pH with increased bicarbonate concentrations is:

    A. Metabolic acidosis

    B. Metabolic alkalosis

    C. Respiratory alkalosis

    D. Respiratory acidosis

22. **A low arterial pH with reduced bicarbonate concentrations is:**
    A. Metabolic acidosis
    B. Metabolic alkalosis
    C. Respiratory alkalosis
    D. Respiratory acidosis

23. **When assessing a client for circulatory overload, what are some of the signs and symptoms the nurse should look for before giving additional fluids?**
    A. Dyspnea, weight gain in 24 hours, clammy skin, and edema
    B. Dyspnea, distended neck veins, edema, and elevated blood pressure
    C. Puffy eyelids, flattened neck veins, edema, and cough
    D. Nausea, lassitude, muscle weakness, and edema

24. **What is the significance of a profuse amount of mucus that is yellow or green or has changed in color?**
    A. Indicates a bacterial infection
    B. Indicates a viral infection
    C. Little significance unless the client has other complaints
    D. No significance

25. **Relief of dyspnea is sometimes achieved by placing the client in what position?**
    A. Knee–chest position
    B. Trendelenburg position
    C. High Fowler position
    D. Semi-Fowler position

26. **A behavioral theory that involves giving persons information about physiological responses and ways to exercise voluntary control over those responses to obtain nonpharmacologic pain relief is:**
    A. Contralateral stimulation
    B. Biofeedback
    C. Guided imagery
    D. Massage

27. **When a normotensive person develops symptoms of low blood pressure on rising to an upright position, this is known as:**
    A. Hypotension
    B. Orthostatic hypotension
    C. Fainting
    D. Syncope

28. Cyanosis, a bluish discoloration of the skin, is:

    A. An indicator of 10 g/dL of unoxygenated hemoglobin
    B. A true indicator of polycythemia
    C. An early indicator of hypoxia
    D. A very late indicator of hypoxia

29. Respirations characterized by cycles in which respirations gradually increase in rate and depth, peak, and then decrease followed by a period of apnea are:

    A. Biot's respirations
    B. Cheyne-Stokes respirations
    C. Bradypnea
    D. Bradypnea and tachypnea

30. A normal range for plasma pH is which of the following?

    A. 7.35–7.45
    B. 7.35–7.9
    C. 6.35–7.8
    D. 6.8 –7.45

31. The process of digestion of food begins in the

    A. Esophagus
    B. Mouth
    C. Small intestine
    D. Gallbladder

32. If a nurse notices a reddened area on a client at a pressure site, the nurse should perform which of the following interventions?

    A. Remove pressure sources, such as wrinkles in the sheets, and massage the site.
    B. Reposition the client and exercise the part as appropriate.
    C. Massage the site.
    D. Apply an ice pack to the site.

33. A nurse is administering an injection to a client. Which actions should be taken by the nurse to prevent a needlestick injury?

    A. Recap the needle after use to prevent injury.
    B. Ask the client to recap the needle.
    C. Place the needle into a puncture-resistant sharps container.
    D. Place the recapped needle into a pocket for disposal at a later time.

34. **A nurse in a clinic is observing all personnel to ensure that correct handwashing technique is demonstrated. Which step does the nurse expect to see first?**

    A. Apply soap to the hands.
    B. Clean under the fingernails.
    C. Rub the hands vigorously for at least 15–30 seconds.
    D. Wet the hands thoroughly.

35. **Which is the most accurate description of a family?**

    A. A group of people related by birth, adoption, or marriage
    B. A group of people living together in the same household
    C. A social group whose members share common values
    D. A woman and a man and their offspring

36. **A community health nurse is engaged in health program planning. The nurse's goal is to provide wellness information to people in rural settings where healthcare services are limited. Which is the best way for the nurse to get wellness information to rural clients?**

    A. Apply for a grant to get additional healthcare providers into the area.
    B. Display posters in the local community center.
    C. Conduct door-to-door visits.
    D. Use videotapes, health fairs, and church social events to promote healthful practices.

37. **A client with chronic back pain and a history of addiction has an order for morphine 2–4 mg every 2 hours as needed for pain. At shift report, a nurse states that this client is "drug seeking" and use of the morphine "needs to be limited." Which response by the nurse receiving the report is most appropriate?**

    A. "Giving the morphine means fewer call lights, so I would rather give it."
    B. "I agree with you. Giving morphine will just make the addiction worse."
    C. "It is ethically wrong to withhold medication. I am reporting this to the manager."
    D. "The physicians really should stop giving in to people like this!"

38. **A client has recently been advised to seek medical treatment in relation to a lump found in her breast. The client has refused to seek the recommended treatment. A nurse assessing the client should recognize that the client's unwillingness to seek treatment may be the utilization of which defense mechanism?**

    A. Displacement
    B. Regression
    C. Denial
    D. Compensation

39. **A psychiatric nurse is working to develop a rapport with a client in crisis. The nurse understands that he or she must use attending behavior to make the client feel more comfortable. All of the following actions by the nurse demonstrate the use of attending behavior EXCEPT:**

    A. Eye contact

    B. Warm affect

    C. Closed arms

    D. Relaxed posture

40. **A nurse is caring for a client to whom immediate and extended family is extremely important. Which action should be taken by the nurse to determine the structure of the client's family?**

    A. Identify the age of each family member.

    B. Identify the gender of each family member.

    C. Identify the head of the household.

    D. Identify the relationships among the individual family members.

41. **Self-concept is the mental image or picture a client has of him-or herself. All of the following factors are used to assess self-concept EXCEPT:**

    A. Body image

    B. Self-esteem

    C. Self-awareness

    D. Role performance

    E. Personal identity

42. **When a nurse works with older clients, many clients experience diminished self-concept associated with the process of aging. Which intervention should a nurse use to enhance and maintain a client's self-esteem?**

    A. A nurse should treat an elderly client no different than a child.

    B. A nurse should encourage an elderly client to maintain the same level of activity as a younger client.

    C. A nurse should talk to an elderly client's family and advise them not to treat the client any differently throughout the aging process.

    D. A nurse should provide a safe environment for an elderly client to communicate concerns about potential losses.

43. **A nurse is preparing to obtain a health history from a newly admitted client. Which is the best way for the nurse to obtain the medical history?**

    A. Enter the room and ask the client his or her name.

    B. Enter the room, maintain eye contact, and introduce oneself.

    C. Enter the room and take the client's vital signs.

    D. Enter the room and ask the client if he or she is ready to begin.

44. **A nurse is preparing to administer a unit of packed red blood cells to a client. All of the following actions should be taken by the nurse before administering the blood EXCEPT:**

    A. Ask another nurse to check the blood before administration.
    B. Obtain baseline vital signs before administering the blood.
    C. Ask a nursing assistant to check the blood before administration.
    D. Verify the client's blood type before administering the blood.

45. **A client receiving a blood transfusion requests medication for pain in the lower back. Which action should be taken by the nurse first?**

    A. Assess the patient's vital signs.
    B. Determine the pain level.
    C. Notify the physician.
    D. Stop the transfusion.

46. **Contents of a client's health history include:**

    A. Biographical data, chief complaint, and past history
    B. Chief complaint, family history, and cultural concerns
    C. Chief complaint, past history, and home assessment
    D. Biographical data, chief complaint, and ethical concerns

47. **When palpating pulses, the nurse may mistake his or her own pulse for that of the client. To prevent this, the nurse should**

    A. Use the back of the hand.
    B. Use firm touch with the first two or three fingers but not the thumb.
    C. Use light touch with all five fingers.
    D. Press hard to ensure that the pulses felt are those of the client.

48. **Water-soluble vitamins are**

    A. Vitamin A, vitamin B_1, and vitamin B_6
    B. Vitamin C, vitamin D, and vitamin K
    C. Vitamin B_{12} and vitamin E
    D. Vitamin B complex and vitamin C

49. **Which of these vitamins is most likely to accumulate in the body, causing vitamin toxicity?**

    A. Vitamin C
    B. Vitamin D
    C. Vitamin B_1
    D. Vitamin B_6

50. **Physical examination of a client's abdomen is done in which order?**
    A. Inspection, auscultation, percussion, and palpation
    B. Auscultation, percussion, inspection, and palpation
    C. Auscultation, percussion, palpation, and inspection
    D. Percussion, palpation, auscultation, and inspection

51. **Which model of human behavior suggests that abnormal behavior is caused by an underlying disease that affects neurochemical in addition to socio-environment factors?**
    A. Medical model
    B. Nursing model
    C. Interpersonal model
    D. Behavioral model

52. **What phase of the therapeutic relationship framework is where the nurse helps the patient examine unresolved problems and helps the patient achieve goals?**
    A. Preinteraction phase
    B. Orientations phase
    C. Working phase
    D. Termination phase

53. **What model of therapeutic communication is used when a message is sent using face-to-face communication enabling transmission of verbal and non-verbal messages simultaneously by the psychiatric nurse and the patient?**
    A. Environmental model
    B. Transactional model
    C. Cultural model
    D. Orientation model

54. **What type of communication occurs through facial expressions, maintaining eye contact, posture, appearance, and paralanguage that convey emotion?**
    A. Transactional communication
    B. Verbal communication
    C. Nontherapeutic communication
    D. Nonverbal communication

55. **What type of therapeutic communication technique is illustrated by "I'm a little unsure what you said, call you tell me more about the situation?"**
    A. Restating
    B. Seek clarification

    C. Recognition

    D. Reflecting

56. **What type of therapeutic communication technique is illustrated by "Can we go back and talk about your childhood?"**

    A. Making an observation

    B. Describe perceptions

    C. Focusing

    D. Exploring

57. **What type of therapeutic communication technique is illustrated by "Let's come up with a goal together."**

    A. Offering self

    B. Suggest collaboration

    C. Focusing

    D. Reality setting

58. **What type of therapeutic communication technique is illustrated by "Tell me more about what you saw."**

    A. Exploring

    B. Restating

    C. Accepting

    D. Making an observation

59. **What type of therapeutic communication technique is illustrated by "I see that you would like to talk about something."**

    A. Give broad opening

    B. Recognition

    C. Offering

    D. Exploring

60. **What type of therapeutic communication technique is illustrated by "You are dressing smartly today."**

    A. Offering

    B. Recognition

    C. Accepting

    D. Making an observation

ANSWERS

1.	B	21.	B	41.	C
2.	A	22.	A	42.	D
3.	A	23.	B	43.	B
4.	B	24.	A	44.	C
5.	D	25.	C	45.	D
6.	C	26.	B	46.	A
7.	C	27.	B	47.	B
8.	A	28.	D	48.	D
9.	C	29.	B	49.	B
10.	D	30.	A	50.	A
11.	D	31.	B	51.	A
12.	B	32.	B	52.	C
13.	D	33.	C	53.	B
14.	B	34.	D	54.	D
15.	A	35.	C	55.	B
16.	A	36.	D	56.	C
17.	C	37.	C	57.	B
18.	B	38.	C	58.	A
19.	D	39.	C	59.	A
20.	B	40.	D	60.	B

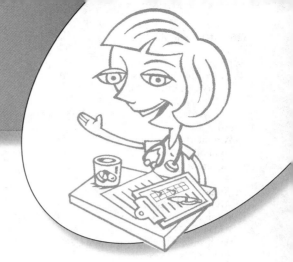

Index

Page numbers followed by "f" denote figures; those followed by "t" denote tables; those followed by "b" denote boxes